ESASO Course Series

Vol. 2

Series Editors

F. Bandello Milan
B. Corcóstegui Barcelona

Selected contributions from ESASO modules 2009 and 2010

Surgical Retina

Volume Editors

Francesco Bandello Milan

Maurizio Battaglia Parodi Milan

89 figures, 56 in color, and 23 tables, 2012

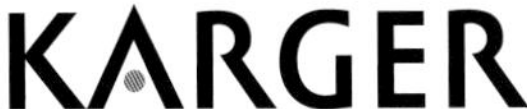

Basel · Freiburg · Paris · London · New York · New Delhi · Bangkok ·
Beijing · Tokyo · Kuala Lumpur · Singapore · Sydney

Francesco Bandello
Department of Ophthalmology
University Vita-Salute
Scientific Institute San Raffaele
IT–20132 Milan (Italy)

Maurizio Battaglia Parodi
Department of Ophthalmology
University Vita-Salute
Scientific Institute San Raffaele
IT–20132 Milan (Italy)

Library of Congress Cataloging-in-Publication Data

Surgical retina / volume editors, Francesco Bandello, Maurizio Battaglia Parodi.
    p. ; cm. -- (ESASO course series, ISSN 1664-882X ; v. 2)
  At head of title: Selected contributions from ESASO modules 2009 and 2010
  Includes bibliographical references and index.
  ISBN 978-3-318-02158-5 (soft cover : alk. paper) -- ISBN 978-3-318-02159-2 (e-ISBN)
  I. Bandello, F. (Francesco) II. Battaglia Parodi, M. (Maurizio) III. European School for Advanced
Studies in Ophthalmology. IV. Title: Selected contributions from ESASO modules 2009 and 2010. V.
Series: ESASO course series ; v. 2. 1664-882X
  [DNLM: 1. Retinal Diseases--surgery--Practice Guideline. 2. Retina--surgery--Practice Guideline.
WW 270]

  617.7'35068--dc23

                                                                                      2012026424

Bibliographic Indices. This publication is listed in bibliographic services, including Current Contents®.

© Copyright 2012 by S. Karger AG, P.O. Box, CH–4009 Basel (Switzerland)
www.karger.com
Printed in Germany on acid-free and non-aging paper (ISO 9706) by Kraft Druck GmbH, Ettlingen
ISSN 1664–882X
e-ISSN 1664–8838
ISBN 978–3–318–02158–5
e-ISBN 978–3–318–02159–2

Contents

List of Contributors

George William Aylward, MD
Consultant Vitreoretinal Surgery
Moorfields Eye Hospital
City Road
London EC1V 2PD (UK)
E-Mail bill.aylward@moorfields.nhs.uk

Carme Macia Badia, MD
Hospital Vall Hebrón, 119–129
Passeig de la Vall d'Hebron
ES–08035 Barcelona (Spain)
E-Mail cmaciabadia@gmail.com

Prof. Francesco Bandello
Department of Ophthalmology
University Vita-Salute
Scientific Institute San Raffaele
Via Olgettina 60
IT–20132 Milano (Italy)
E-Mail bandello.francesco@hsr.it

Maurizio Battaglia Parodi, MD
Department of Ophthalmology
University Vita-Salute
Scientific Institute San Raffaele
Via Olgettina 60
IT–20132 Milan (Italy)
E-Mail battagliaparodi.maurizio@hsr.it

Naomi Fischer, MD
Department of Ophthalmology
Tel-Aviv Medical Center
6 Weizman Street
Tel Aviv 64239 (Israel)
E-Mail naomi797@hotmail.com

Jose Garcia-Arumi, MD
Instituto de Microcirugía Ocular
c/ Josep Maria Lladó no 3
ES–08022 Barcelona (Spain)
E-Mail jgarcia.arumi@gmail.com

Prof. Alain Gaudric
Service d'Ophtalmologie
Hôpital Lariboisière AP-HP
Université Paris 7 Diderot
2 rue Ambroise Paré
FR–75010 Paris (France)
E-Mail alain.gaudric@lrb.aphp.fr

Prof. Dr. Anselm Kampik FEBO
Augenklinik der LMU, Klinikum der Universität München
Campus Innenstadt
Mathildenstrasse 8
DE–80336 München (Germany)
E-Mail akampik@med.uni-muenchen.de

Ainat Klein, MD
Department of Ophthalmology
Tel-Aviv Sourasky Medical Center
6 Weizman Street
Tel Aviv 64239 (Israel)
E-Mail euriya@gmail.com

Elad Moisseiev, MD
Department of Ophthalmology
Tel Aviv Sourasky Medical Center
Weitzman 6 St.
Tel Aviv 64239 (Israel)
E-Mail elad_moi@netvision.net.il

Constantin J. Pournaras, MD
Department of Ophthalmology
Vitreo-Retinal Unit
Geneva University Hospitals
22 rue Alcide-Jentzer
CH-12 11 Geneva 14 (Switzerland)
E-Mail constantin.pournaras@hcuge.ch

Stanislao Rizzo, MD
Ospedale Cisanello
Via Paradisa
Edificio 30A
Azienda Ospedaliera Universitaria Pisana
IT–56100 Pisa (Italy)
E-Mail stanislao.rizzo@gmail.com

Marco A. Zarbin, MD, PhD
Institute of Ophthalmology and
Visual Science-New Jersey Medical School
Room 6156, Doctors Office Center
90 Bergen Street
Newark, NJ 07103 (USA)
E-Mail zarbin@earthlink.net

Preface

We are delighted to have the opportunity to offer this book to the ophthalmological community. ESASO has progressively grown into a definite project with the objective to spread of the knowledge and innovation among young ophthalmologists.

This book is specifically intended for those who have attended the ESASO modules and want to refresh their memory with all the teachings, but it can also be directed at all the young ophthalmologists who are looking for simple and clear indications regarding the surgical management of vitreoretinal disorders. Many renowned international experts have striven to bring their experience to common practice, gradually describing principles and surgical phases of the most common procedures. We hope that their efforts can be of help to everyone.

Francesco Bandello, Milan
Maurizio Battaglia Parodi, Milan

Bandello F, Battaglia Parodi M (eds): Surgical Retina.
ESASO Course Series. Basel, Karger, 2012, vol 2, pp 1–34

Diabetic Retinopathy Management

Marco A. Zarbin[a] · William E. Smiddy[b]

[a]Institute of Ophthalmology and Visual Science-New Jersey Medical School, Newark, N.J., and
[b]Bascom Palmer Eye Institute, Miami, Fla., USA

Abstract

Strict control of blood glucose and blood pressure is critical for reduction of the incidence and progression of diabetic retinopathy (DR). Follow-up of patients with diabetes mellitus is protocol based and not based solely on the presence of symptoms. Staging of the level of DR (mild, moderate, or severe nonproliferative DR vs. proliferative DR, PDR) drives the follow-up interval. The most common cause of visual loss in diabetic patients is diabetic macular edema (DME). The results of multicenter, randomized studies suggest that the best visual results for DME currently are achieved with intravitreal ranibizumab injections ± focal laser photocoagulation. Results using bevacizumab seem quite comparable to those with ranibizumab. In addition to treating DME, this approach also seems to reduce the likelihood of progression of DR. Selected patients also may benefit from intravitreal steroid treatment + focal laser therapy, but there is a relatively higher rate of glaucoma and cataract formation. Panretinal photocoagulation is currently the most effective treatment for high-risk PDR. Panretinal photocoagulation also should be considered for patients with severe nonproliferative DR and early PDR, particularly if follow-up cannot be assured and/or if the patient has type 2 diabetes mellitus. Pars plana vitrectomy is used to manage severe complications of DR such as nonclearing vitreous hemorrhage, severe fibrovascular proliferation, and retinal detachment. Adjunctive anti-vascular endothelial growth factor agents might enhance those results in selected subsets of patients.

A substantial body of scientific data, much of it in the form of randomized, controlled clinical trials, underlies current treatment recommendations for patients with diabetic retinopathy (DR) [1–36]. These data define recommendations for patient follow-up, indications for focal and scatter laser photocoagulation, indications for pharmacological intervention (intraocular), and indications for vitrectomy. The main purpose of this chapter is to review these data in the context of contemporary treatment options. In addition, the pathophysiology of DR and associated clinical findings will be mentioned in the context of clinical management paradigms.

Pathological Processes

A detailed review of the pathophysiology of DR is beyond the scope of this chapter but has been published elsewhere (fig. 1, 2) [34, 37, 38].

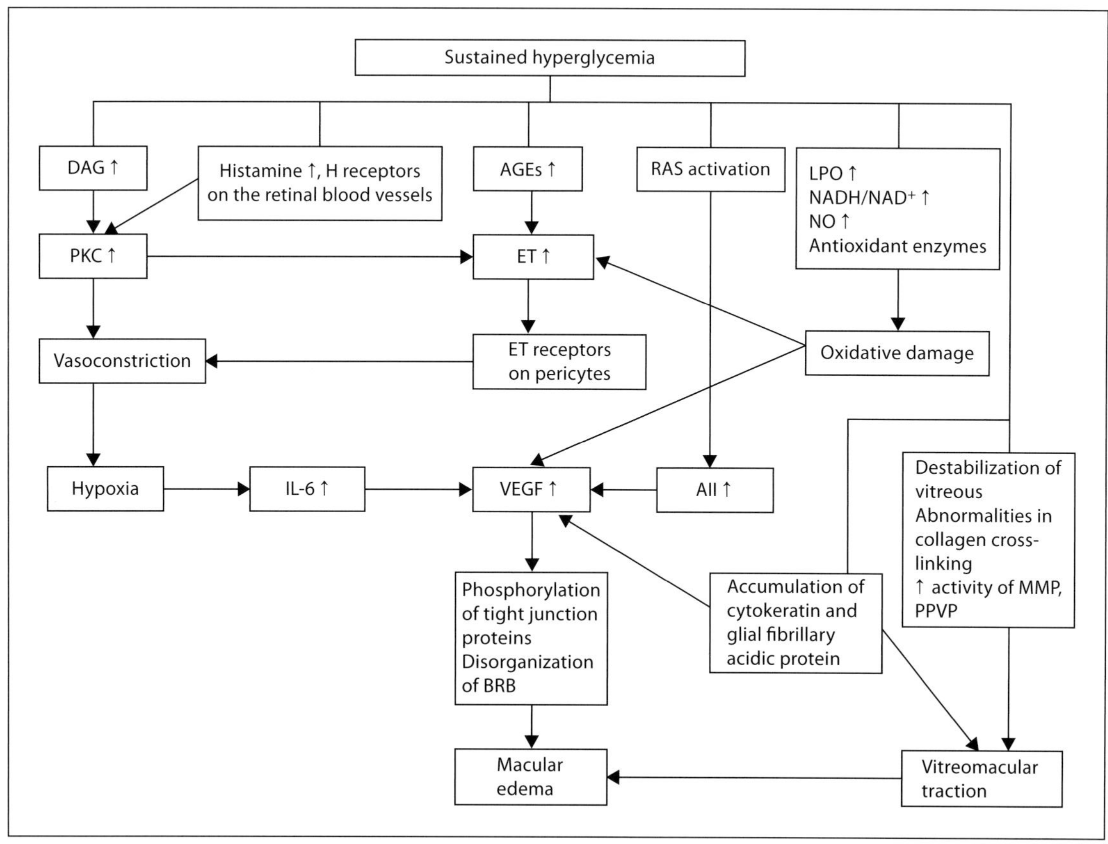

Fig. 1. Pathogenesis of DME. AII = Angiotensin II; DAG = diacylglycerol; ET = endothelin; LPO = lipo-oxygenase; NO = nitric oxide; PKC = protein kinase C; RAS = renin-angiotensin system. Reproduced with permission from Bhagat et al. [34].

Briefly, hyperglycemia leads inter alia to high intracellular levels of glucose, free radical formation (oxidative stress), and protein kinase C activation [39]. Chronic hyperglycemia generates advanced glycation end products (AGEs), which may incite processes leading to DR and maculopathy. Hypoxia, altered blood flow, retinal ischemia, and inflammation also are associated with DR. Increased vascular endothelial growth factor (VEGF) levels, decreased pigment epithelium-derived factor levels, increased protein kinase C production, endothelial dysfunction, and leukocyte adhesion are associated with breakdown of the blood-retinal barrier and, thus, increased diabetic retinal vascular permeability. In preclinical models, AGEs seem to be involved in of all these processes [40–42]. There is evidence that neuronal dysfunction precedes the retinal vascular abnormalities in DR [43]. For example, abnormalities of the ERG and multifocal ERG as well as apoptosis of retinal neurons have been demonstrated early in patients with diabetes mellitus, before the appearance of retinopathy [44–46]. Accordingly, early DR may be a neurovascular disease of the retina [47]. Eventually, ischemia may result in retinal neovascularization (mediated in part by the 121 and 165 amino acid isoforms of VEGF), vitreous hemorrhage (VH),

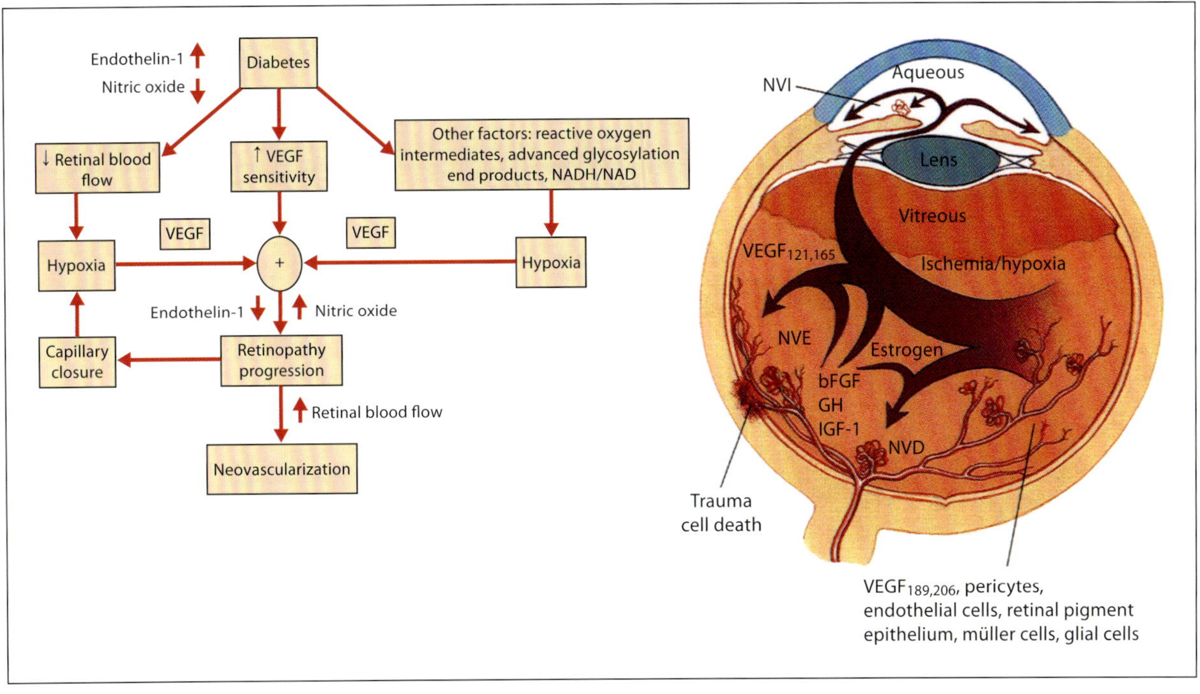

Fig. 2. Pathogenesis of retinal neovascularization in DR. VEGF and its isoforms, basic fibroblast growth factor (bFGF), growth hormone (GH), insulin-like growth factor-1 (IGF-1), inflammation, and ischemia all play important roles in disease progression. Reproduced with permission [114–116].

retinal detachment, rubeosis iridis, and neovascular glaucoma.

Clinical Findings

Microaneurysms (MAs) are foci of retinal capillary endothelial proliferation and are the earliest clinical sign of DR (fig. 3). Vascular damage resulting in ischemia and increased vascular permeability include *cotton wool spots* (signs of nerve fiber layer ischemia), *intraretinal microvascular abnormalities* (IRMA, areas of retinal vascular remodeling that occur within the plane of the retina), *venous loops* (areas of endothelial cell proliferation associated with partition of the venous lumen) [48], and *venous beading*, as well as in the development of capillary non-perfusion (fig. 3). Macular capillary non-perfusion can be associated with visual loss (particularly if the foveal avascular zone (FAZ) is enlarged to more than 875 μm in diameter) [49]. More severe degrees of ischemia induce proliferation of *abnormal blood vessels* arising from the retinal vasculature or, in severe cases, on the iris. These vessels may bleed, giving rise to *preretinal or vitreous hemorrhage* or *hyphema*, depending on their location (fig. 4). With time, fibrous tissue proliferation (cicatrization) results from the abnormal blood vessels (fig. 4). These cells have myofibroblastic properties and can contract to the point of causing *traction and combined traction-rhegmatogenous retinal detachment* (compounding the ischemia), causing severe visual loss. Cellular proliferation within the premacular vitreous cortex can cause *opacification of the posterior hyaloid face* (recognizable clinically

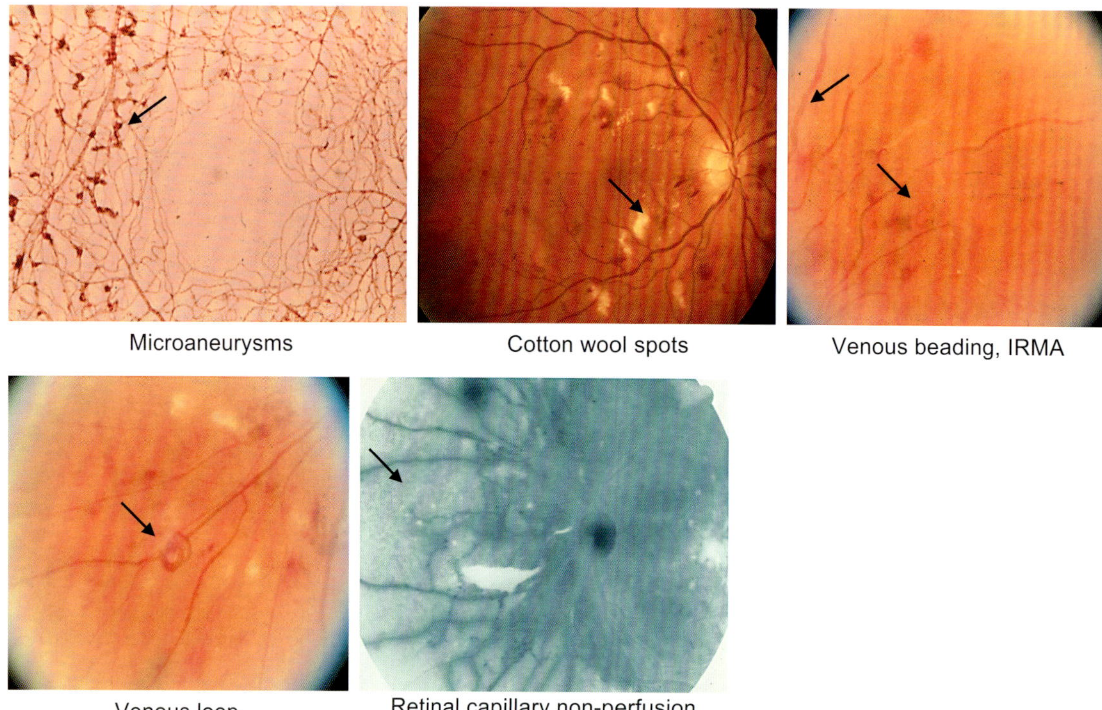

Fig. 3. Signs of DR. Arrows point out MAs (shown here in an India ink histopathology preparation), cotton wool spots (areas of superficial retinal whitening), venous beading, IRMA, venous loops, and retinal non-perfusion (shown on fluorescein angiography).

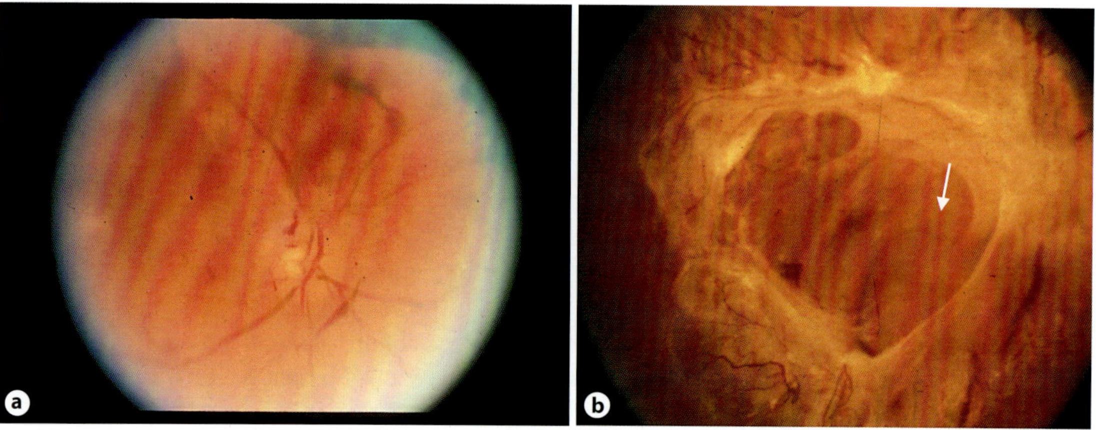

Fig. 4. a VH arising from retinal neovascularization. **b** Untreated retinal neovascularization has undergone cicatrization and contracture resulting in traction retinal detachment.

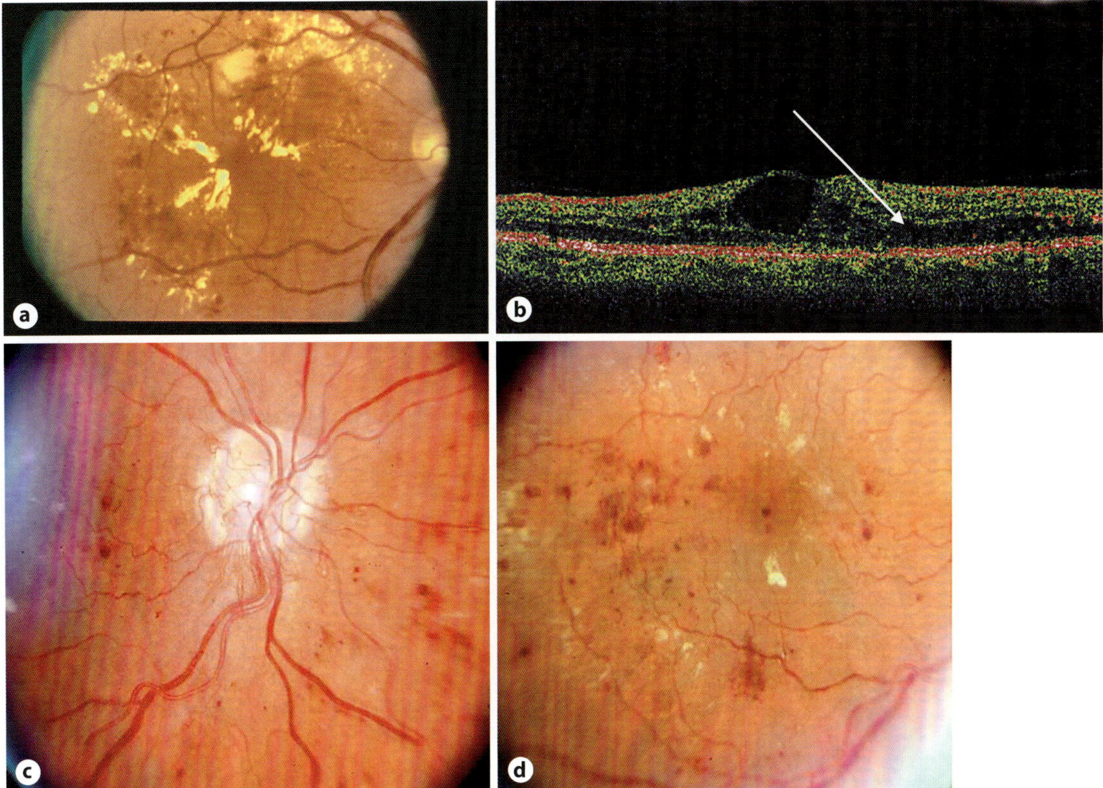

Fig. 5. a Hard exudates in a case of NPDR. **b** OCT of a case with macular edema showing fluid accumulation in the outer plexiform layer (arrow). **c** Neovascularization at the optic nerve head. **d** Same eye as **c** showing macular edema with loss of the foveal light reflex and cystic change in fovea.

and with optical coherence tomography, OCT) and macular edema. Growth of abnormal vessels in the anterior chamber angle is associated with *neovascular glaucoma*.

Increased vascular permeability is evidenced by *lipoprotein exudates*; *hemorrhages* and *edema* develop in the early stages of DR and may occur to remarkable degrees in later stages, especially when systemic hypertension coexists (fig. 5). Breakdown of the inner blood-retinal barrier results in retinal edema (most prominent in the outer plexiform layer, nerve fiber layer of Henle) as well as intraretinal hemorrhage. Severe lipoprotein deposits (hard exudates) can be a manifestation of hyperlipidemia as well as vascular

incompetence [50]. Hard exudates normally are cleared by phagocytosis, and edema is corrected by dehydration of the retina via RPE active transport and, in some cases (e.g. after pharmacological therapy), by reestablishment of the blood-ocular barrier.

Classification of Diabetic Retinopathy

An empirically defined and validated classification of the different stages of DR is based on specific clinical findings (detailed below) identified with a variety of examination techniques (table 1).

Table 1. Examination techniques to identify clinically significant findings of DR

Technique	Indication
Fundus contact lens	Macular examination; generally gives higher resolution and better stereopsis than non-contact indirect exam with 78- or 90-dpt lenses
Three-mirror or panfundus contact lens	Midperipheral fundus examination; generally gives better resolution than indirect ophthalmoscopy to detect early retinal NV
Gonioscopy	To detect rubeosis iridis, particularly in the anterior chamber angle
Color fundus photography	To document the fundus appearance before surgery To document severe changing disease To establish a baseline exam in the setting of significant disease (e.g. CSME) for subsequent comparison To document fundus appearance immediately after laser treatment (uncommonly)
Fluorescein angiography	To assess macular capillary perfusion in the setting of unexplained visual loss To guide laser treatment for CSME To identify occult NV To distinguish IRMA from NV (occasionally)
OCT	To document degree of macular thickening (e.g. during treatment of CSME) To detect potential vitreomacular traction induced by an opacified posterior hyaloid face To assess unexplained visual loss (i.e. integrity of outer limiting membrane)

Nonproliferative versus Proliferative Diabetic Retinopathy

Previously, DR was classified into background, pre-proliferative, and proliferative DR (PDR). The current classification is based on the location/extent/degree of various clinically significant features (MAs, hemorrhage, venous beading, IRMA, neovascularization) as defined by standard photographs (7 stereo fields; grade: absent, questionable, definite, moderate, severe, very severe). This classification scheme is complex and is used for clinical research but may be simplified by recognizing the threshold clinical features of severe nonproliferative DR (NPDR), clinically significant macular edema (CSME), and high-risk PDR (HR-PDR).

A simplified grading scheme for NPDR is: 'less severe' versus 'more severe'. Less severe refers to severity ≤moderately severe NPDR. More severe refers to severity ≥severe NPDR and is defined by the '4-2-1 rule' (fig. 6):

- 4 quadrants of hemorrhages/MAs ≥standard photograph 2A
- 2 quadrants of venous beading ≥standard photograph 6B
- 1 quadrant of IRMA ≥standard photograph 8A

'Very severe NPDR' is present if two or more of the findings establishing 'severe NPDR' are present (e.g. 4 quadrants of hemorrhages/MAs ≥standard photograph 2A + 2 quadrants of venous beading ≥standard photograph 6B).

Macular edema refers to retinal swelling in the macular region. Macular edema is the most common cause of moderate visual loss in diabetic patients and is clinically diagnosed with biomicroscopy (either high-magnification indirect ophthalmoscopy, e.g. with a 90- or 78-diopter

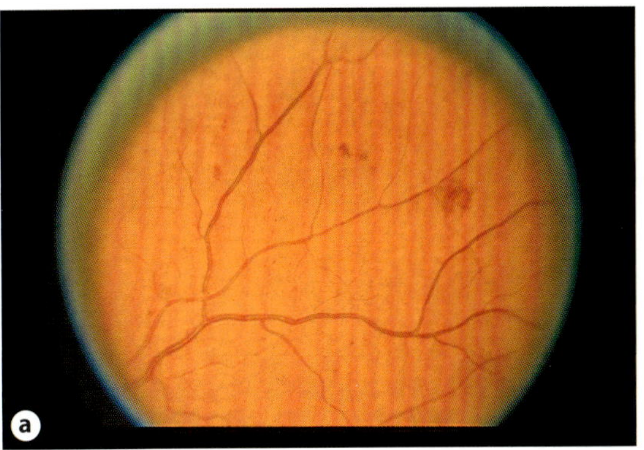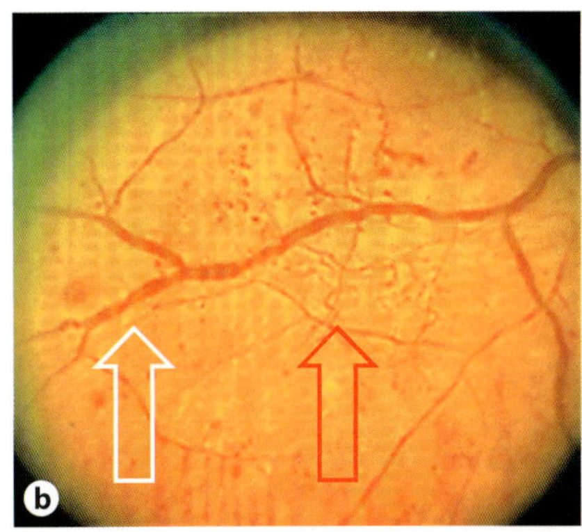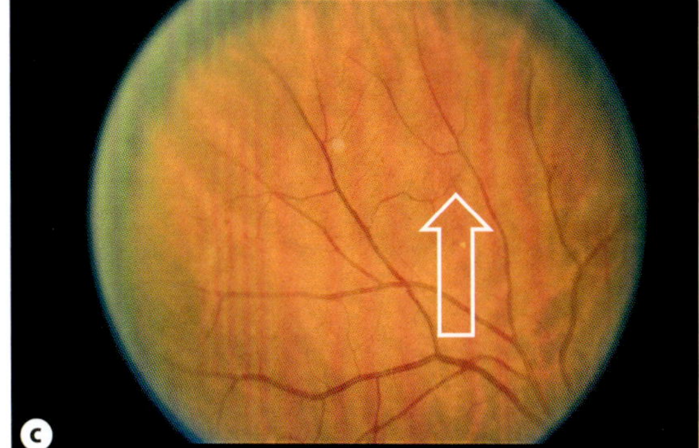

Fig. 6. **a** ETDRS standard photograph 2A showing hemorrhage severity consistent with severe NPDR if present in four quadrants. **b** ETDRS standard photograph 6B showing venous beading (white arrow) consistent with severe NPDR if present in two quadrants and a severe level of IRMA (red arrow). **c** ETDRS standard photograph 8A showing IRMA (arrow) consistent with severe NPDR if present in one quadrant.

lens, or contact lens exam). OCT provides a very sensitive way to document macular edema and follow the response to treatment, but OCT was not available during seminal studies assessing the potential benefits of laser treatment for diabetic macular edema (DME). In contrast to OCT, clinical exam, including 78-dpt lens or contact lens, is not reliable for detecting macular thickening less than 300 μm [51, 52]. *Fluorescein leakage does not correlate strictly with retinal thickening.* Leakage reflects breakdown of the blood-retinal barrier, which increases fluid flow into the retinal interstitial space. RPE active transport moves water from the interstitial space into the choroid. Edema results when the bulk flow of intravascular fluid into the interstices exceeds the bulk flow into the choroid. In diabetic eyes, macular thickness does not correlate directly with visual acuity, but there is a correlation between the integrity of the photoreceptor inner segment-outer segment junction and visual acuity [53]. There is also a correlation between photoreceptor outer segment length and visual acuity [54]. Stereo fundus photographs, stereo fluorescein angiography and OCT are reasonably well correlated for assessment of macular edema (as distinct from visual acuity) [55, 56].

Macular edema can be present in the setting of NPDR and/or PDR. Macular edema occurs in various patterns: focal, multifocal, and diffuse (fig. 7). Focal or multifocal leakage is characterized by the presence of circinate lipid rings that typically have leaking MAs in the center of the ring. (The ring probably arises from the precipitation of lipoproteins in areas where the lipoprotein concentration in the interstitial space exceeds the solubility

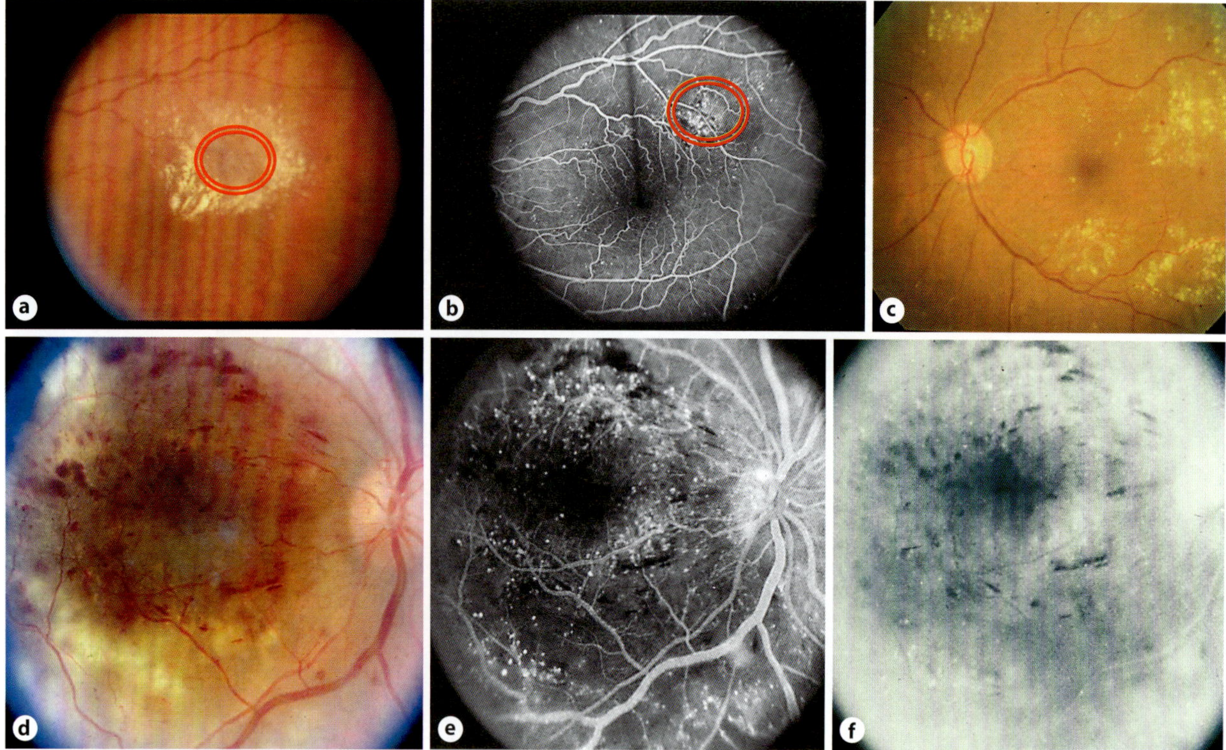

Fig. 7. Patterns of macular edema. **a** Focal leakage. Red circle surrounds MAs in the center of a lipid ring. **b** Fluorescein angiography demonstrates that the leaking lesions are in the center of the lipid ring (red circle, left). **c** Color fundus photograph of an eye with multifocal leaks and multiple circinate lipid rings. **d** Color fundus photograph of a patient with diabetes mellitus, renal failure, and diffuse macular edema. **e** Early frame of the fluorescein angiogram demonstrates numerous MAs. **f** Late frame of the fluorescein angiogram demonstrates leakage from virtually all the vessels in the area centralis with diffuse dye leakage into the retina.

coefficient.) These cases have the best prognosis with focal laser treatment. Diffuse leakage is characterized by leakage from a variety of vessels (e.g. capillaries, arterioles, venules) throughout the area centralis. These cases tend to have a poorer prognosis, even with laser treatment. Subfoveal lipid and edema associated with macular ischemia (most readily identified with fluorescein angiography) usually are associated with a poor visual prognosis (fig. 8). CSME is edema that threatens or involves the macular center and is defined by the following findings:

- Retinal thickening at or within 500 µm of the macular center

- Retinal thickening more than 500 µm from the macular center if associated with lipid at or within 500 µm of macular center
- Retinal thickening within 1 disc diameter of the macular center if the area of thickening is ≥1 disc area in size
- Notably, the definition does NOT depend on visual acuity (even 20/20 vision is compatible with CSME), fluorescein leakage, or OCT findings. Clinicians generally cannot reliably recognize macular edema clinically unless retinal thickness is 300 µm or more [51, 52]. On the other hand, retinal thickening <300 µm may not be important prognostically.

Zarbin · Smiddy

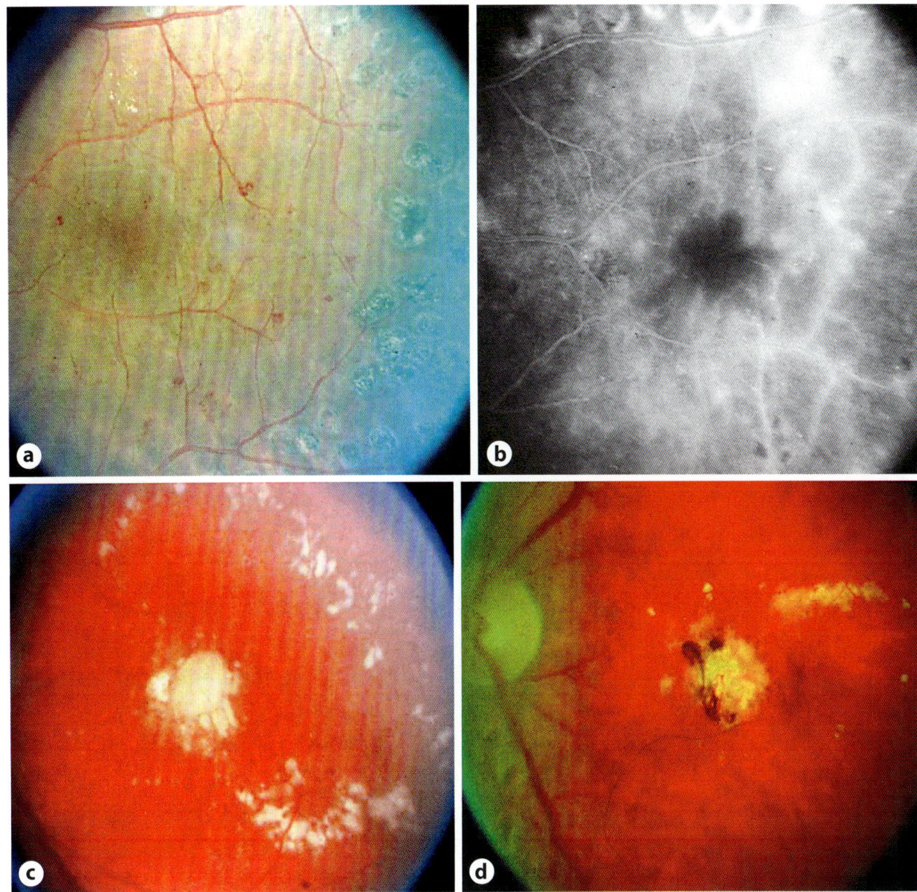

Fig. 8. Macular edema associated with poor visual prognosis. **a**, **b** Macular edema associated with ischemia. **c**, **d** Macular edema associated with subfoveal lipid.

PDR refers to new blood vessel (NV) growth arising from the retinal vasculature or on the iris. Generally, NV grow at the border zone of perfused and non-perfused retina, which sometimes can be recognized clinically by the bland appearance of ischemic retina and the ghost vessels that can be seen occasionally in non-perfused retina. Retinal NV tends to grow just inside the posterior vitreous cortex adjacent to the retinal surface. These vessels are permeable, and the leakage of plasma contents probably causes a structural change in the adjacent vitreous that can lead to local liquefaction and separation of the hyaloid from the internal limiting membrane of the retina. As a result, suspended retinal NV may be subjected to vitreo-retinal traction that can cause bleeding (vitreous and/or subhyaloid hemorrhage) and traction or traction-rhegmatogenous retinal detachment. This anatomic relation also can be exploited surgically by developing a cleavage plane between the hyaloid face and underlying retina to dissect NV off of the retinal surface in an en bloc fashion. Neovascularization arising from the optic disc can grow directly into the vitreous cavity (possibly along Cloquet's canal) or onto the adjacent retina.

Retinal NV is identified best using high magnification contact lens biomicroscopy at the slit lamp. Indirect ophthalmoscopy is a notoriously poor detection method, even by experienced examiners, particularly in the case of fine, early NV. Fluorescein angiography is even more sensitive because retinal NV leak dye early and profusely in the early phases of the angiogram. In contrast, IRMA leak dye relatively later in the transit phase of the angiogram, and also is confined between the paired artery and vein, in contrast to NV, which often cross these borders.

Neovascularization of the iris (NVI) usually is recognizable at the slit lamp, but in early stages, the vessels are subtle and tend to appear first at the pupillary margin or in the anterior chamber angle. As a result, NVI are seen most easily on an undilated iris. Occasionally, NVI is present in the anterior chamber angle first, and these NV can be identified only by gonioscopy. Without treatment, NVI gradually causes the formation of peripheral anterior synechiae and secondary angle closure glaucoma. Many patients with DR have dilated normal iris vessels that can resemble NVI. Normal iris vessels leak fluorescein dye weakly (if at all), in contrast to NVI, which leaks profusely.

Protocols for Patient Follow-Up

First Exam
The Wisconsin Eye Survey of Diabetic Retinopathy (WESDR) study showed that among patients with age at onset 0–29 years (generally type 1), the prevalence of any DR at less than 5 years was 17% and of PDR was close to 0% [2]. Thus, the first dilated eye exam is an effective screening procedure 5 years after diagnosis with annual follow-up exams thereafter until retinopathy appears. By year 20, the prevalence of DR, PDR, and DME was ~99, ~50, and ~30%, respectively [2, 4]. A reasonable estimate is that annually 2% will develop DME, and 3% will develop PDR, with a higher incidence

if the baseline level of disease severity is worse or if the hemoglobin A1c is elevated [7].

Among patients with age at onset ≥30 years (generally type 2), the prevalence of any DR at 5 years was ~30% and of PDR was ~2% [3]. By year 15, the prevalence of DR and PDR was ~80 and ~15%, respectively. Thus, an effective time to conduct the first dilated eye exam is at the time of diagnosis and annually thereafter until retinopathy appears.

Additional studies show higher rates of DR in non-Hispanic blacks and Mexican Americans (33%) than among non-Hispanic whites [57, 58]. The risk of DR in rural Asian populations is comparable [59].

Pregnancy
Pregnancy increases the risk of DR progression [60]. Ideally, diabetic patients contemplating pregnancy should be examined before conception, and all treatable retinopathy should be treated. Some physicians recommend that pregnant patients have a dilated fundus exam each trimester and 6 weeks after delivery or at any time if visual loss develops. Some experts feel that this recommendation can be safely relaxed for patients with little or no retinopathy by the end of the first trimester. If CSME develops, it can be observed (fluid overload associated with pregnancy might reverse after pregnancy with resolution of DME) or treated with focal laser. Concern about possible risk to the fetus with anti-VEGF agents has limited its use in this setting, although one case report indicates it may be safe [61]. Patients with HR-PDR (see below) should undergo prompt panretinal photocoagulation (PRP).

Puberty
Routine screening is not recommended until patients are 12 years old. In one study, for example, the 10-year incidence of PDR and DME was 0% in a cohort whose age was <10 years old at baseline. Furthermore, the 14-year incidence of PDR (6%)

and DME (10%) was low in patients <10 years old at baseline [6, 7].

Follow-Up Exam: Less Severe Diabetic Retinopathy
Their low rate of progression in population-based studies suggests that patients with no or minimal DR can be followed with dilated fundus exams every 6–12 months. If DME that is not clinically significant is present, follow-up every 3–4 months is advised (to identify and treat CSME promptly). If CSME is present, generally one will treat the patient, but occasionally one will observe to give time for correction of fluid overload (renal failure, congestive heart failure) or blood pressure control or due to patient preference for observation. In these cases, follow-up every 1–3 months is advised.

Follow-Up Exam: More Severe Diabetic Retinopathy with or without Diabetic Macular Edema
In contrast, epidemiological data suggest that patients with more severe DR should be followed more frequently, every 2–4 months, particularly if very severe NPDR is present, in which case there is a 45% 1-year incidence of HR-PDR, i.e. neovascularization at the optic disc greater than standard photograph 10A or neovascularization elsewhere greater than 1/2 disc diameter in size combined with vitreous or preretinal hemorrhage (see below for detailed description of HR-PDR) [12]. One option for these patients is immediate PRP, particularly if follow-up is not assured or if the other eye has severe DR with or without visual loss.

Follow-Up Exam: Early Proliferative Diabetic Retinopathy with or without Diabetic Macular Edema
The Diabetic Retinopathy Study (DRS) and Early Treatment Diabetic Retinopathy Study (ETDRS) did not mandate treatment for early PDR, but immediate PRP is a feasible option, particularly if follow-up is not assured or if the fellow eye has severe DR with or without visual loss. Another option is follow-up every 2–4 months with a plan to treat with PRP once high-risk characteristics develop.

Follow-Up Exam: Treated Proliferative Diabetic Retinopathy
After patients with PDR have been treated successfully, they usually are followed every 3–4 months to monitor for complications such as retinal detachment and CSME. Some experts feel that once PDR has regressed and has not led to hemorrhaging or NV regrowth for a year or so, the follow-up intervals can be correspondingly lengthened. The incidence of progressive traction retinal detachment involving the macula is fairly low and was reported as 14%/year in one study [62].

Treatment

General Health
Control of blood glucose, blood pressure, and serum lipids reduces the incidence and severity of DR. The Diabetes Control and Complications Trial (DCCT) showed that among type I diabetic patients, strict control of blood glucose (typically ~4 insulin injections/day) was associated with a 76% reduction in the development of DR vs. the conventional management cohort (typically 2 insulin injections/day; fig. 9) [8]. In addition, there was a 54% reduction in retinopathy progression vs. the conventional management cohort. Patients in the strict control cohort experienced an initial worsening of retinopathy that was visually insignificant and that resolved after one year. In addition, they experienced an increased risk of life-threatening hypoglycemia (fig. 9). At 8 years' follow-up, the incidence of retinal NV was ~10% in the strict control cohort versus ~20% in the conventional management cohort. Of note, strict control did not produce clinical benefit until year 4 of the study. (In fact, many patients in the strict

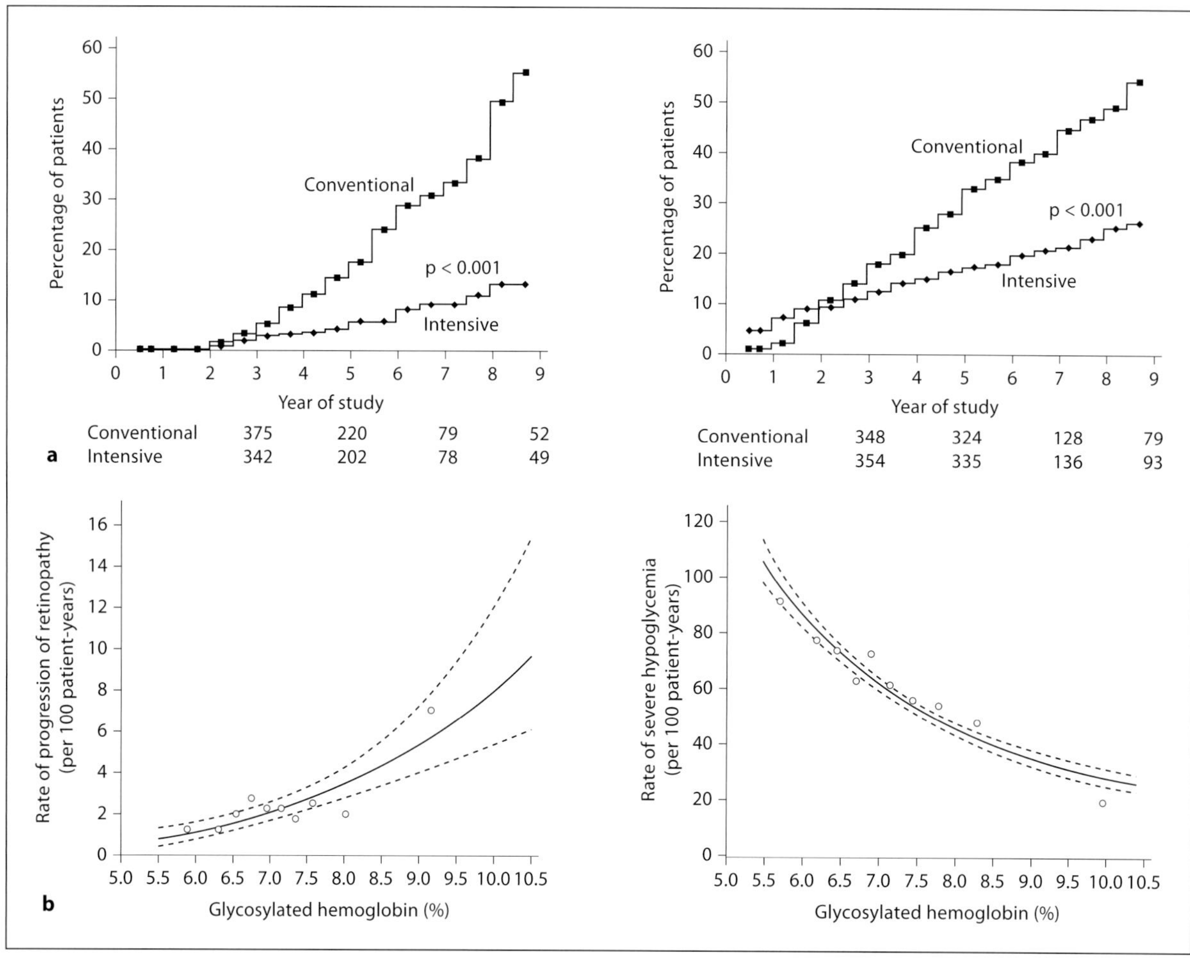

Fig. 9. Results of the DCCT [8]. **a** Percentage of patients developing (left) or experiencing (right) progression of DR under conventional vs. intensive blood glucose management. **b** Rate of progression of DR (left) and rate of severe hypoglycemia (right) as a function of hemoglobin A1c. Reproduced with permission.

control group initially experienced a paradoxical worsening during the first year; some of this effect has been attributed to gaining strict control too rapidly and might be mitigated by a slower phase-in.) This outcome may reflect the fact that the extracellular matrix proteins damaged by hyperglycemia have a relatively long half-life [63]. Similarly, loss of strict control may require several years for the beneficial effects of strict control to be lost. In the DCCT, a 10% reduction in the hemoglobin A1c during the study was associated with a 43% lower risk of progressive retinopathy in the strict control cohort and a 45% lower risk in the conventional management cohort [64]. This result was observed across all ranges of hemoglobin A1c and was unaffected by covariates.

The United Kingdom Prospective Diabetes Study (UKPDS) found that among type 2 diabetic patients, tighter blood glucose control and blood pressure control were associated with a lower rate

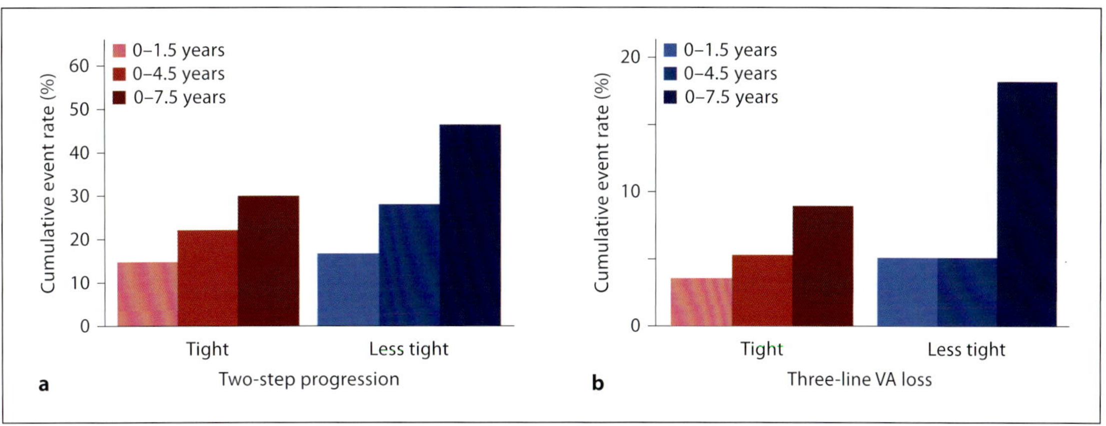

Fig. 10. UK Prospective Diabetes Study [9, 10]. **a** Rate of progression of DR. **b** Rate of visual loss. Reproduced with permission from Skyler [117].

of DR progression, a lower rate of laser surgery for DR, and a lower rate of moderate visual loss (fig. 10), although the event rates were somewhat less than in ETDRS reports, probably in large part because the UKPDS studied type 2 diabetics exclusively [9, 10, 65, 66].

A number of studies have examined the effect of various interventions on DR, e.g. fenofibrate to lower cholesterol, aspirin, ticlopidine (antiplatelet), sorbinil (aldose reductase inhibitor), ruboxistaurin (PKC inhibitor), octreotide (somatostatin analogue), atorvastatin, and rosiglitazone (activates intracellular peroxisome proliferator-activated receptor to uptake insulin better), but the results have not demonstrated great impact, or the studies have been limited in their design, thus calling into question the ability to generalize the results.

Diabetic Macular Edema: Focal Laser Photocoagulation

The ETDRS was a randomized, multicenter clinical trial that asked three questions:
- Does focal laser treatment of DME prevent visual loss? Answer: Yes
- Does early PRP prevent visual loss? Answer: Yes, for DR ≥severe NPDR
- Does aspirin treatment influence visual loss? Answer: No

The ETDRS enrolled a wide variety of patients, ranging from those with no retinal thickening (but with hard exudates in the macula) and visual acuity ≥20/40 to those with retinal thickening and vision ≥20/200 [11–13]. The primary end point was moderate visual loss (3-line loss on a Bailey-Lovie eye chart) or gain (3-line improvement; fig. 11). Among patients with CSME, the 3-year risk of moderate visual loss with treatment was 13% vs. 22% among controls. The benefit was evident for *all* levels of initial visual acuity (including Snellen acuity of 20/20) [28] but only for patients with CSME. If CSME involved the macular center, the 3-year risk of moderate visual loss was higher (33% in controls and 14% in the treatment group), and the magnitude of the treatment benefit was greater (table 2). Although only ~10% of treated patients overall had improved visual acuity, among those with vision ≤20/40 at entry into the study, 40% gained ≥6 letters at 3-year follow-up [11, 12, 67]. A randomized clinical study showed that approximately 1/3 of eyes with vision ≤20/40 gain ≥2 lines at 2 years follow-up and approximately 20% worsen by ≥2 lines [22].

Although the results of randomized, multicenter studies can provide the highest level of

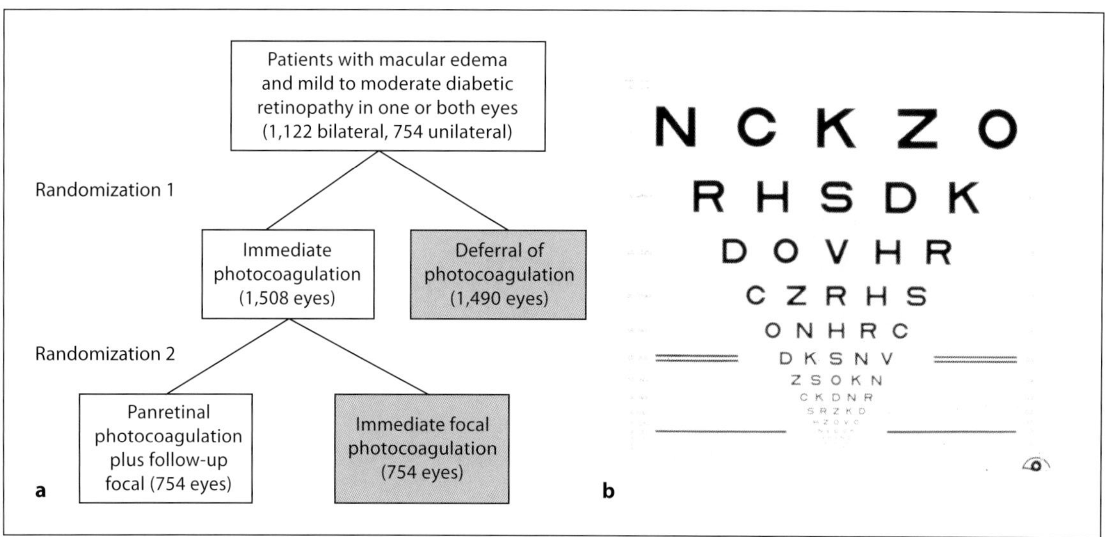

Fig. 11. a Structure of the ETDRS study. **b** Bailey-Lovie eye chart. Gain of 15 letters equals halving of the visual angle (e.g. improving from 20/80 to 20/40). Loss of 15 letters equals doubling of the visual angle (e.g. declining from 20/20 to 20/40).

Table 2. Risk of moderate visual loss (doubling of the visual angle) in the ETDRS

Retinopathy	Follow-up, years	Control patients, %	Treated patients, %
CSME-macular center *not* involved	1	7.5	1.0
	2	15.8	6.1
	3	22.1	13.2
CSME-macular center involved	1	13.3	7.5
	2	23.6	9.4
	3	33.0	13.8

scientific evidence on which to base treatment paradigms, it is important to remember that many patients in a typical practice do not fit the enrollment criteria of these studies. Thus, clinicians often must extrapolate the results to daily clinical practice. For example, patients with DME causing vision ≤20/400, with DME associated with HR-PDR, and patients with DME in pregnancy were not studied systematically in the ETDRS. In addition, the timing of cataract extraction in the setting of DME was not studied.

Focal laser photocoagulation can be applied using different treatment patterns: *direct* and *grid* (table 3; fig. 12). In practice, *combination treatment* is applied in most patients, which involves direct treatment of leakage points (identified on pretreatment fluorescein angiography) and grid treatment in areas of diffuse leakage and in areas of capillary non-perfusion. In general, one treats all lesions in thickened retina located between 0.5–3 mm from the macular center. One generally does not treat lesions located 300–500 μm from

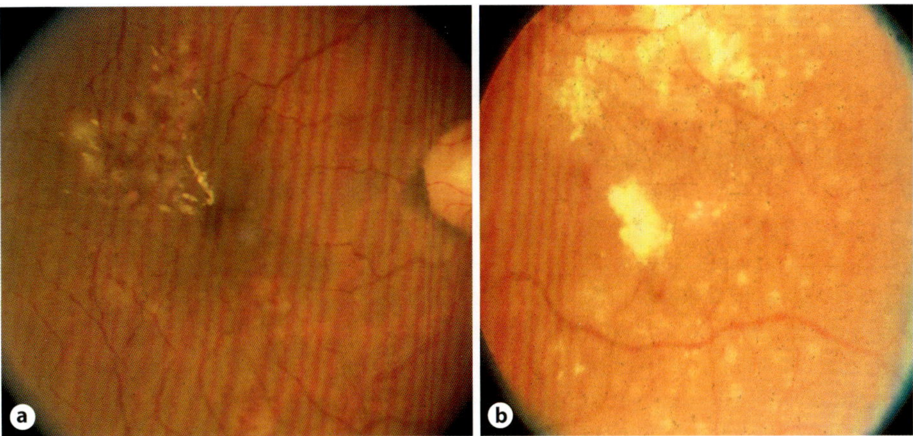

Fig. 12. a Appearance of focal laser treatment. **b** Appearance of grid laser treatment. In practice, one applies laser treatment opportunistically so that most treatments have features of both the focal and grid paradigms.

Table 3. Focal laser treatment paradigms: direct versus grid pattern

Parameter	Direct	Grid pattern
Spot size	50–100 µm (use 50 µm when working near FAZ)	50–100 µm
Duration	0.05–0.10 s	0.05–0.10 s
Topography of laser application	Apply burns to leaking lesions in thickened retina	Space burns at least one burn width apart in grid pattern
Clinical end point	Mild whitening of underlying RPE	Mild whitening of underlying RPE

the FAZ center initially, but if the visual acuity is ≤20/40 and CSME persists after initial treatment, one may treat leaking lesions in this zone in a further follow-up session. It is not necessary to treat all leaking lesions for the edema to resolve. Thus, one can add more treatment if needed, but one cannot reverse the scotoma that a laser spot induces. Laser spot size can range from 50 to 200 µm. One generally uses a 50 µm spot size when treating near the FAZ to avoid creating a symptomatic paracentral scotoma. Treatment duration ranges from 0.05 to 0.10 s (unless micropulse laser is used, see below). When treating near the FAZ, 0.05 s duration may be preferred to minimize the chance of inadvertent foveal treatment

arising from an unanticipated saccadic eye movement. The laser power should be reduced if the laser duration is increased or if the spot size is decreased to avoid creating an undesirably intense laser burn. Argon blue-green laser is commonly avoided to decrease the lifetime risk of induced problems in the surgeon's blue color sensitivity. Argon green (514 nm) or dye yellow (577 nm, the authors' preference) laser (good uptake by MAs) are the most commonly used wavelengths, but krypton red (647 nm) and diode (810 nm) laser also work well (see below). Typically, patients are reevaluated for retreatment at 4-month intervals. The mean number of treatments required to induce resolution of retinal edema in the ETDRS was 3–4. At each retreatment, many surgeons repeat the fluorescein angiogram to identify sites of persistent dye leakage and, perhaps more importantly, to reconfirm the location of the FAZ so that inadvertent treatment at the edge or into the FAZ does not occur. If a patient has focal leakage with a circinate lipid ring, it may not be necessary to perform fluorescein angiography preoperatively since the leaking lesions are in the center of the lipid ring. In one randomized clinical trial, a modified macular grid treatment (mild grid treatment without direct treatment, very mild burns applied throughout the macula whether or not edema is present) was not superior to ETDRS style treatment [20].

One study indicates that control of blood glucose may be important for the success of focal laser treatment for DME [25].

Alternative laser modalities have been used to treat DME successfully. Krypton red laser and diode laser, for example, have been shown to be effective in treating CSME [68–70]. Micropulse laser also is effective in the treatment of DME [71–77]. Micropulse laser consists of brief energy delivery such that the pulse duration is shorter than the thermal relaxation time of RPE cells. Thus, heat is more selectively confined to the RPE, sparing surrounding tissues (e.g. overlying retina, subjacent choriocapillaries) but only to the RPE. A pulse of 0.1 ms duration corresponds to a thermal diffusion distance of 10 μm, which is the typical diameter of an RPE cell. Brief laser pulses alternate with periods of no laser treatment that allow heat to dissipate before the next laser pulse is delivered (fig. 13). This approach to delivery of laser energy might minimize retinal and choroidal damage, even with repeat treatments, thus permitting greater preservation of visual function [74].

Diabetic Macular Edema: Pathway-Based Therapy

DME is associated with a number of processes (e.g. oxidative stress, inflammation, increased intravascular hydrostatic pressure, tight junction

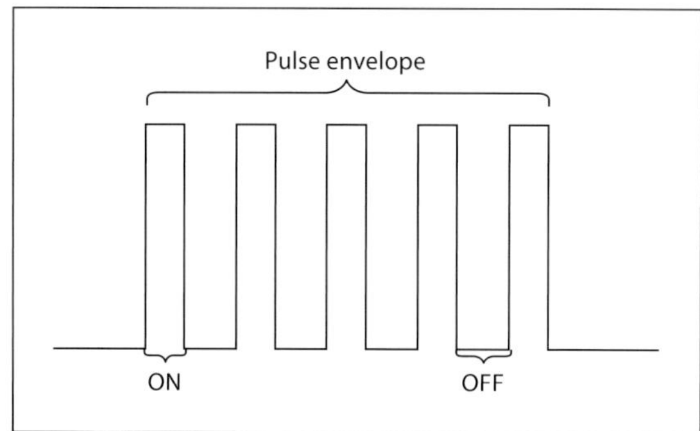

Fig. 13. Schematic of laser delivery using micropulse laser. See text for details. Reproduced with permission from Bhagat et al. [34].

breakdown; fig. 1, 2) [78–81]. Therapeutic targets include VEGF-A, PKC, oxidative reactions, aldose reductase, VEGF-A receptors, growth hormone, tight junction proteins, and the renin-angiotesin-aldosterone system.

VEGF inhibitors (e.g. pegaptanib, ranibizumab, bevacizumab, aflibercept) have been explored as a treatment for macular edema and for PDR with good reason. VEGF is upregulated by hypoxia, and VEGF induces vasopermeability by: (1) inducing phosphorylation of tight junction proteins (occludin, ZO-1), (2) induction of Fas-mediated endothelial cell apoptosis, and (3) promotion of production of other inflammatory factors. VEGF levels are increased in ocular tissues from diabetic patients and in preclinical models, and blockade of VEGF is therapeutic [41, 82–86]. Use of VEGF inhibitors for DME has been reviewed in detail by Nicholson and Schachat [87].

A randomized, multicenter clinical study has demonstrated that intravitreal ranibizumab with prompt or deferred modified ETDRS laser treatment is more effective (at 1-year follow-up) than laser treatment alone (fig. 14) [88]. On average, both ranibizumab treatment cohorts gained +9 ETDRS letters by the end of the first year of treatment (vs. +4 in the triamcinolone + prompt laser, and +3 in the sham injection + prompt laser cohorts); 50% of the ranibizumab cohorts gained ≥10 letters, and 30% gained ≥15 letters (vs. 28 and 15% for 10- and 15-letter gain in the sham injection + laser treatment cohort; fig. 15, 16). OCT results generally paralleled the visual acuity results for the ranibizumab cohorts but not for the laser-only cohort, which showed continued decline in retinal thickness that was not matched by visual acuity improvement (fig. 17). Treatment benefits were independent of whether the edema was focal or diffuse. There was a greater risk of 10- and 15-letter vision loss in the laser-only cohort (13%, 8%, respectively) versus the ranibizumab cohorts (4%, 2%, respectively). Eyes assigned to ranibizumab treatment were less likely to show progression of retinopathy (e.g. development of PDR, VH, need for PRP) than the laser only cohort. The mean number of injections in both ranibizumab groups was 8–9 during the first year and 2–3 in the 2nd year, but only 1/5 (ranibizumab + deferred laser)–1/3 (ranibizumab + prompt laser) of patients required no injections in the 2nd year. On average, two additional laser treatments were given to theranibizumab + prompt laser cohort during the first year of treatment. These results mean that patients with DME require ongoing follow-up, and probably will need additional treatment (often including focal laser photocoagulation), during the first 2 years after initiating anti-VEGF treatment for DME.

Very similar results have been reported in a randomized trial of ranibizumab versus sham treatment (with laser rescue) in patients with DME [89]. Similar beneficial effects also have been reported in a randomized trial comparing intravitreal bevacizumab with modified ETDRS macular laser therapy [90].

Although there are reports that anti-VEGF therapy might increase macular ischemia [91, 92], a number of reports indicate that if this effect occurs, it is outweighed in the majority of patients by the benefits of anti-VEGF treatment [88, 90, 93]. Results of a small randomized study indicate that administration of bevacizumab (1.25 mg/0.05 ml) may improve visual outcome after cataract surgery [35]. (Of note, all patients had undergone macular laser photocoagulation 3–4 months before surgery.)

In pseudophakic eyes, intravitreal triamcinolone plus prompt laser are more effective than laser alone, but there is a significant chance for increased intraocular pressure (fig. 18) [88]. Intravitreal triamcinolone plus prompt laser seems to reduce the likelihood of progression of DR, including the development of PDR and/or VH [88]. However, intravitreal triamcinolone injection is more likely to be associated with cataract progression (fig. 19) and intraocular pressure elevation (IOP; 50% had IOP ≥30 mm Hg and/or needed antiglaucoma medication and 1% needed glaucoma surgery versus 11 and <1%, respectively, in the laser only cohort) [88]. Randomized clinical trials have shown that sustained intravitreal delivery of 700 µg dexamethasone (Ozurdex, Allergan, Irvine, Calif., USA) at day 90 is associated with a 33% chance of ≥10 ETDRS letters visual improvement (vs. 12% in the observation group) [94]. Approximately 15% gained ≥15 letters (vs. ~7% in the observation group). The benefits seemed to persist for at least 6 months. Increased IOP of ≥10 mm Hg occurred in 15% of the 700 µg cohort versus 1% of the observation group. No eye required glaucoma surgery. There was no increased risk of cataract formation.

An important consideration is that the foregoing clinical trials only studied eyes with visual acuities of 20/32–20/40 or worse, whereas the ETDRS did not exclude eyes with macular edema and visual acuity of 20/20.

In view of the above results, while the first-line treatment for focal patterns of DME, especially with visual acuity better than 20/32 remains focal laser photocoagulation, the authors currently favor consideration of the use of combined intravitreal ranibizumab (0.5 mg/0.05 ml to 1.0 mg/0.1 ml) or bevacizumab (1.25 mg/0.05 ml) and prompt laser therapy for eyes with CSME and vision <20/32. Intravitreal triamcinolone, particularly in pseudophakic eyes with no history or increased risk of

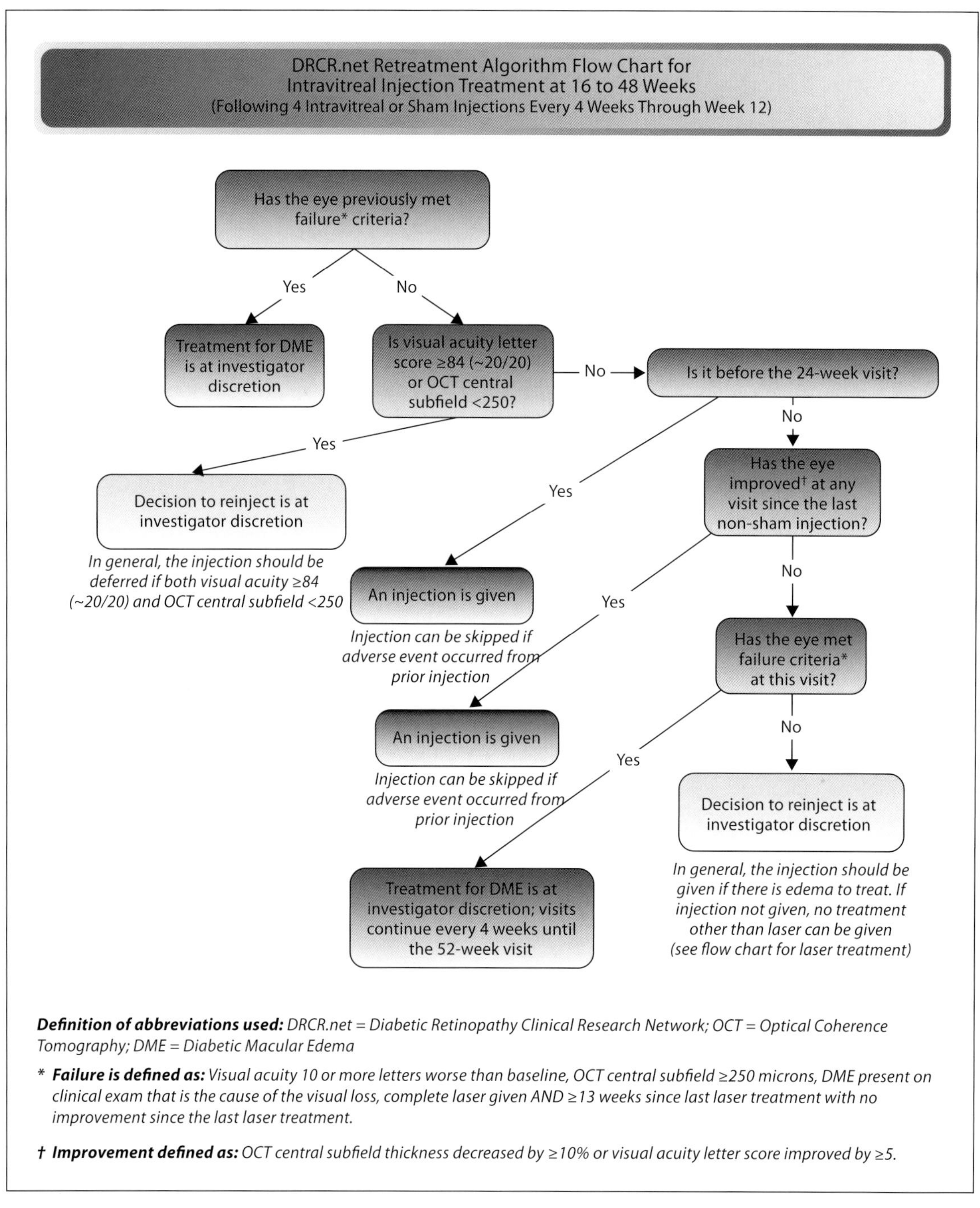

Fig. 14. Treatment algorithms for intravitreal injection and laser treatment in the DRCR.net trial of ranibizumab, triamcinolone, and macular laser treatment for DME [88]. Reproduced with permission.

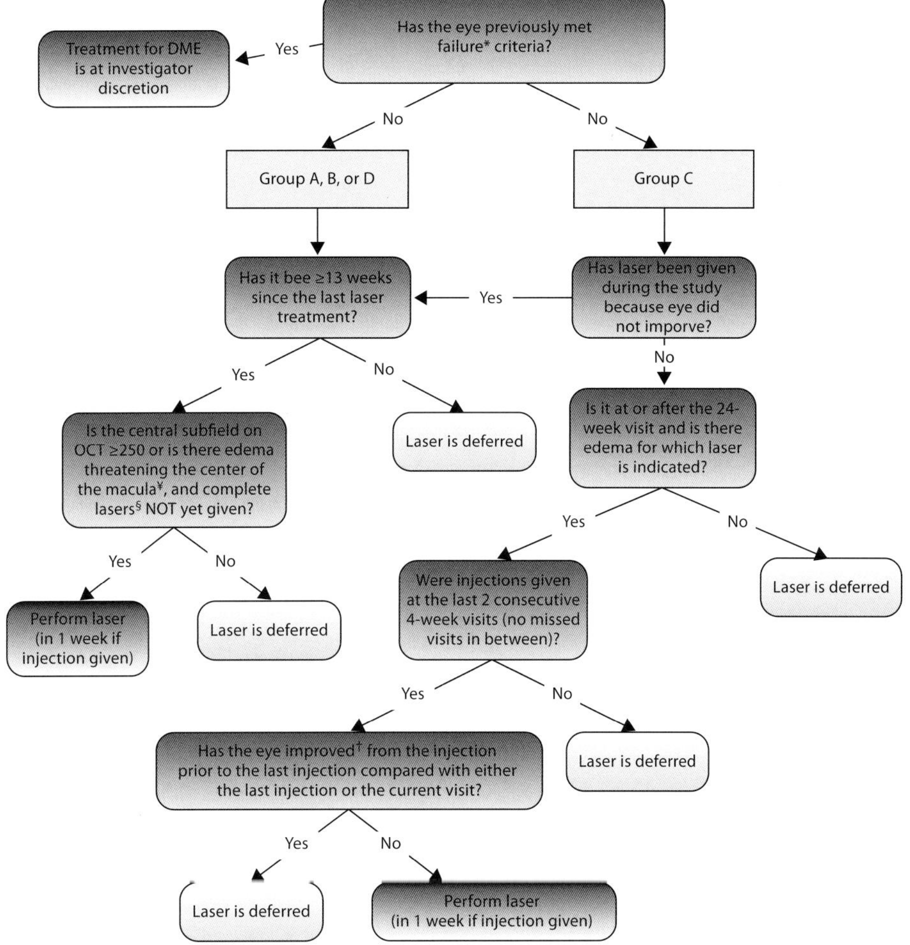

Definition of abbreviations used: *DRCR.net = Diabetic Retinopathy Clinical Research Network; OCT = Optical Coherence Tomography; DME = Diabetic Macular Edema*

* **Failure is defined as:** *Visual acuity 10 or more letters worse than baseline, OCT central subfield ≥250 microns, DME present on clinical exam that is the cause of the visual loss, complete laser given AND ≥13 weeks since last laser treatment with no improvement since the last laser treatment.*

† **Improvement defined as:** *OCT central subfield thickness decreased by ≥10% or visual acuity letter score improved by ≥5.*

§ **Complete laser:** *Direct treatment to all microaneurysms within areas of macular edema and grid treatment to all other areas of macular edema.*

¥ **Edema threatening the center of the macula:** *Edema on clinical exam within 500 microns of the foveal center or edema associated with lipid with 500 microns of the foveal center of 1 disc area of edema within 1 disc area of the foveal center.*

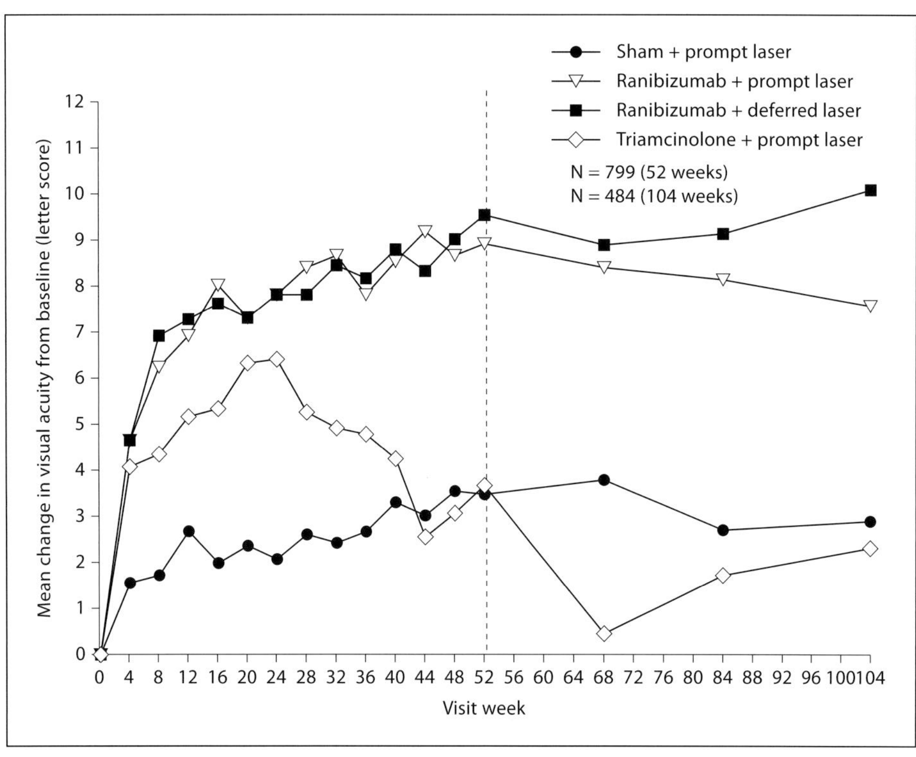

Fig. 15. Mean change in visual acuity at follow-up visits after treatment for DME. Values that were ±30 letters were assigned a value of 30. p values for difference in mean change in visual acuity from sham + prompt laser at 52 weeks: ranibizumab + prompt laser <0.001, ranibizumab + deferred laser <0.001, and triamcinolone + prompt laser groups <0.31. Each visit week includes visits that are ±14 days, except the 52-week visit, which includes visits that occur between 308 and 420 days (between 44 and 60 weeks) from randomization, and the 104-week visit, which includes visits that occur between 616 and 840 days (between 88 and 120 weeks) from randomization. Reproduced with permission from Elman et al. [88].

glaucoma, is viable second-line choice. Sustained release corticosteroid delivery systems have the advantage of a lower incidence of cataract than intravitreal triamcinolone, but the degree of visual improvement may not be as great as with triamcinolone and may not be substantially longer in duration compared with single bolus intravitreal triamcinolone injections. For patients with DME that will undergo combined focal laser and intravitreal injection therapy, one possible treatment protocol is described in table 4. Intravitreal injection of anti-VEGF agents has a low risk of complications that include endophthalmitis (0.1%),

retinal detachment, and cataract. To minimize complications, a standard approach to sterile injection is followed for patients who are not iodine allergic (fig. 20).

In addition to VEGF, hypoxia-inducible factor-1, erythropoietin, placental growth factor, angiopoietin-2, and platelet-derived growth factor may play a role in hypoxia-induced retinal vascular changes associated with the development of DME. Insulin-like growth factor, basic fibroblast growth factor, hepatocyte growth factor, integrins, and components of the mitogen-activated protein kinase signaling cascade (e.g. c-Raf kinase) also may play a role in the pathogenesis of DR. These molecular targets may become the focus of different therapeutic modalities in the future through, for example, the use of therapeutic oligonucleotide, including antisense oligonucleotide (e.g. short interfering RNA) and oligonucleotide aptamers [95]. Pegaptanib is an aptamer directed against the 165-amino acid isoform of VEGF-A, and has been shown to be beneficial in the treatment of DME [96].

Diabetic Macular Edema: Vitrectomy
Although some initial studies indicated clinical benefit for vitrectomy with posterior hyaloid face peeling [32, 97], evidence from subsequent larger series does not strongly support this approach as first-line therapy for DME [98, 99]. In a prospective, multicenter study of 241 eyes [98], 6 months after surgery, mean visual acuity was unchanged (20/80). More than half (55%) of the eyes had PDR, and 72% had received previous treatment for DME. Corticosteroids in some form were administered to 68%. Visual acuity improved by ≥10 letters in 26% and worsened by ≥10 letters in 22%. Only two factors were associated with greater mean visual acuity improvement from baseline to month 6: worse baseline visual acuity and epiretinal removal at surgery. Pseudophakic eyes fared similar to phakic eyes. Retinal thickness (OCT) did decrease after surgery despite the limited visual benefit for most patients. In view of these data, one might offer pars plana vitrectomy (PPV) to patients with DME unresponsive to combined anti-VEGF-laser and/or triamcinolone-laser provided that they accept the 1/5 risk of visual loss and the expected need for cataract surgery (in phakic eyes), with the primary goal of visual stabilization. (For patients with vision in the range 20/20–20/80, the ETDRS study showed that chronic edema is likely to reduce vision, albeit slowly.) Patients without demonstrable vitreoretinal attachment clinically or by OCT are probably even less likely to experience visual improvement with surgery. It may be of interest to note that a small randomized trial of intravitreal plasmin without vitrectomy showed significantly reduced central macular thickness (241 μm from 541 μm before injection and vs. 530 μm in fellow control eye) and improved vision (from 0.62 to 0.45) at month 1 follow-up, which was sustained at the month 6 follow-up [100].

Proliferative Diabetic Retinopathy: Panretinal Photocoagulation
The DRS demonstrated that PRP reduces the risk of severe visual loss (defined as best-corrected visual acuity <5/200 on 2 consecutive visits separated by 4 months) by 50% during a 5-year period of follow-up [15, 16]. Four risk factors were identified: (1) any neovascularization; (2) location of neovascularization at or within 1-disc diameter of the optic disc; (3) severity of neovascularization [at the optic disc >standard photograph 10a (1/4–1/3 disc area, fig. 21), elsewhere ≥1/2 disc diameter]; (4) vitreous or subhyaloid hemorrhage. Eyes with 3 or 4 risk factors are said to have HR-PDR, since the risk of severe visual loss without treatment in this cohort is 50% at the 5-year follow-up. Xenon photocoagulation was associated with severe visual loss in this study, but this modality is no longer in use due to the unwieldy delivery system and the visual field defects that the large laser spots induce. PRP is generally administered in 2–3 sessions, each separated by 1–2 weeks. One treatment technique is outlined in table 5 and figure 22. Regression of NV typically occurs within 3 weeks of treatment (fig. 23). PRP can be associated with visual field constriction, nyctalopia, serous retinal and choroidal detachment, and cycloplegia. In one study [101], ~8% of patients had decreased central vision >2 lines due to persistent macular edema. Biweekly treatment may reduce this risk [102, 103]. In cases where full PRP treatment must be administered quickly (e.g. 1–2 sessions), one can administer topical corticosteroid and cycloplegia therapy (e.g. prednisolone acetate 1% q.i.d. and atropine 1% b.i.d.) to prevent the development of choroidal

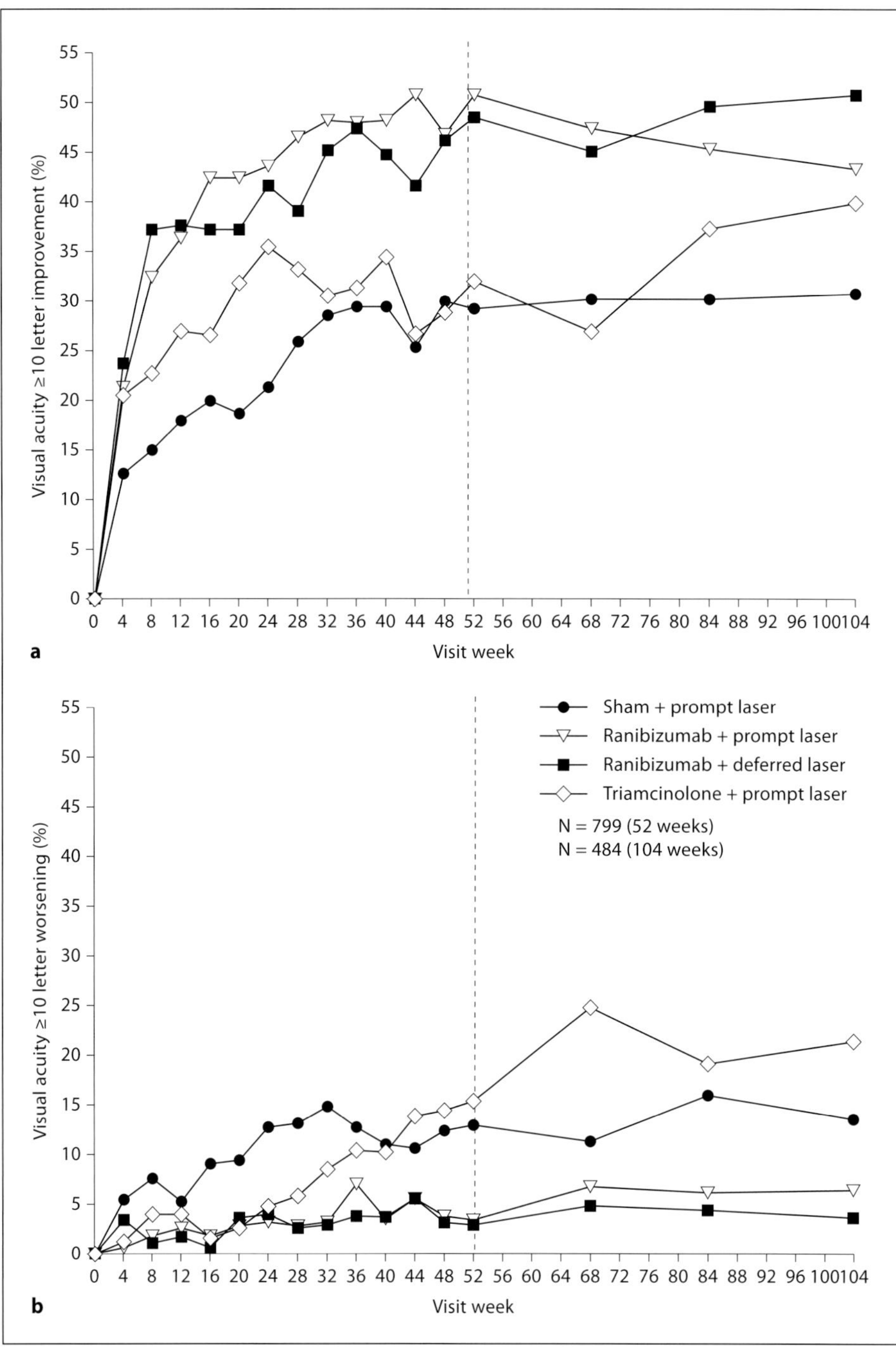

Visual acuity ≥10 letter improvement (%)
Visit week
a
Visual acuity ≥10 letter worsening (%)
Visit week
b
Sham + prompt laser
Ranibizumab + prompt laser
Ranibizumab + deferred laser
Triamcinolone + prompt laser
N = 799 (52 weeks)
N = 484 (104 weeks)

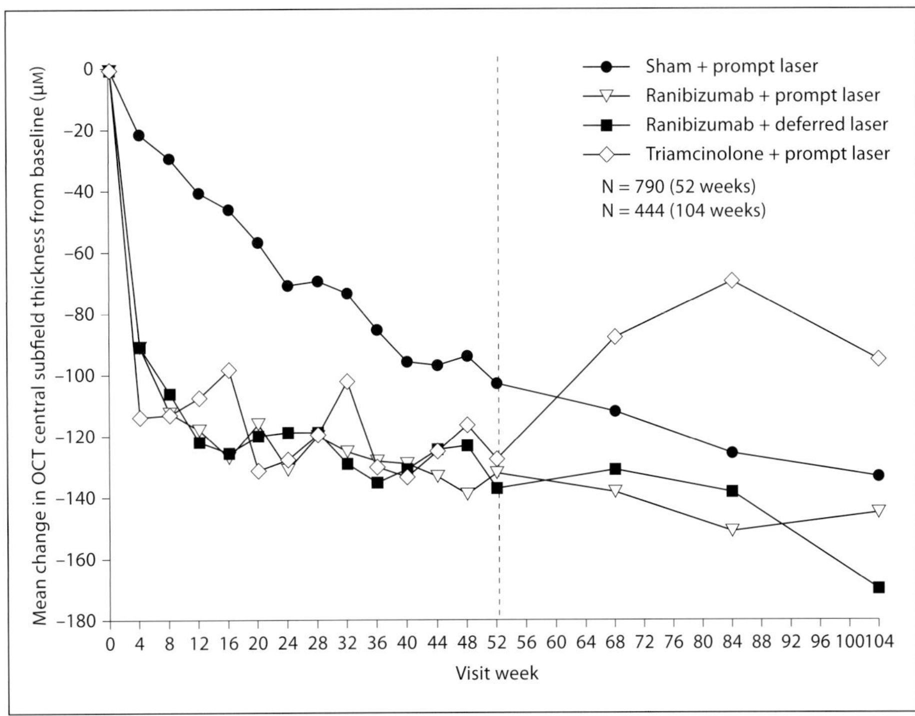

Fig. 17. Mean change in OCT central subfield retinal thickening at follow-up visits. p values for difference in mean change in OCT central subfield retinal thickness from sham + prompt laser at the 52-week visit: ranibizumab + prompt laser <0.001, ranibizumab + deferred laser <0.001, and triamcinolone + prompt laser <0.001. Each visit week includes visits that are ±14 days, except the 52-week visit, which includes visits that occur between 308 and 420 days (between 44 and 60 weeks) from randomization, and the 104-week visit, which includes visits that occur between 616 and 840 days (between 88 and 120 weeks) from randomization. Reproduced with permission of Elman et al. [88].

Fig. 16. a Ten letter or greater improvement in visual acuity at follow-up visits. p values for difference in proportion of ≥10 letter improvement in visual acuity from sham + prompt laser at the 52-week visit: ranibizumab + prompt laser <0.001, ranibizumab + deferred laser <0.001, and triamcinolone + prompt laser <0.16. Each visit week includes visits that are ±14 days, except the 52-week visit, which includes visits that occur between 308 and 420 days (between 44 and 60 weeks) from randomization, and the 104-week visit, which includes visits that occur between 616 and 840 days (between 88 and120 weeks) from randomization. **b** Ten-letter or greater loss in visual acuity at follow-up visits. p values for difference in proportion of 10 letter loss in visual acuity from sham + prompt laser at the 52-week visit: ranibizumab + prompt laser <0.001, ranibizumab + deferred laser <0.001, and triamcinolone + prompt laser <0.75. Each visit week includes visits that are ±14 days, except the 52-week visit, which includes visits that occur between 308 and 420 days (between 44 and 60 weeks) from randomization, and the 104-week visit, which includes visits that occur between 616 and 840 days (between 88 and120 weeks) from randomization. Reproduced with permission from Elman et al. [88].

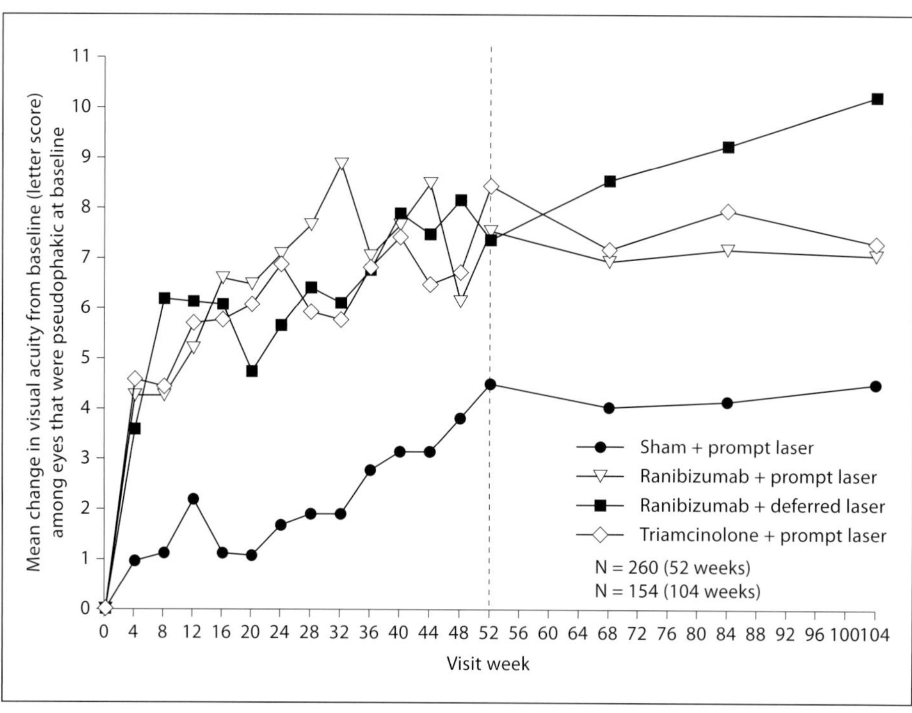

Fig. 18. Mean change in visual acuity at follow-up visits among eyes that were pseudophakic at baseline. Values of ±30 or more letters were assigned a value of 30. Each visit week includes visits that are ±14 days, except the 52-week visit, which includes visits that occur between 308 and 420 days (between 44 and 60 weeks) from randomization, and the 104-week visit, which includes visits that occur between 616 and 840 days (between 88 and 120 weeks) from randomization. Reproduced with permission of Elman et al. [88].

detachment and secondary angle closure glaucoma. In the setting of combined CSME and HR-PDR, one can use prophylaxis against the exacerbation of DME by providing sub-Tenon triamcinolone injection prior to PRP [104] or by administering intravitreal ranibizumab or bevacizumab just before or shortly after PRP is applied. These agents can help promote prompt regression of retinal neovascularization (and rubeosis iridis), which gives time for the full, presumably more long-lasting effect of PRP to become evident [105]. If significant retinal neovascularization is present, however, intravitreal anti-VEGF agent injection might precipitate development of or progression of retinal detachment [106, 107]. The DRS showed that PRP, in contrast, does not

exacerbate or precipitate traction retinal detachment in PDR.

Both the DRS and the ETDRS showed that PRP reduces the risk of severe visual loss in the setting of severe NPDR (table 6). One should consider PRP in patients with severe NPDR or non-HR-PDR, especially for type 2 diabetes mellitus patients without macular edema [108]. This recommendation is particularly worthy of consideration in patients who have significant visual loss due to PDR in the fellow eye or who cannot be followed reliably. PRP before HR-PDR characteristics develop is associated with an increased risk of moderate visual loss during the first year after PRP, but it is associated with a decreased risk by years 2–5 after treatment.

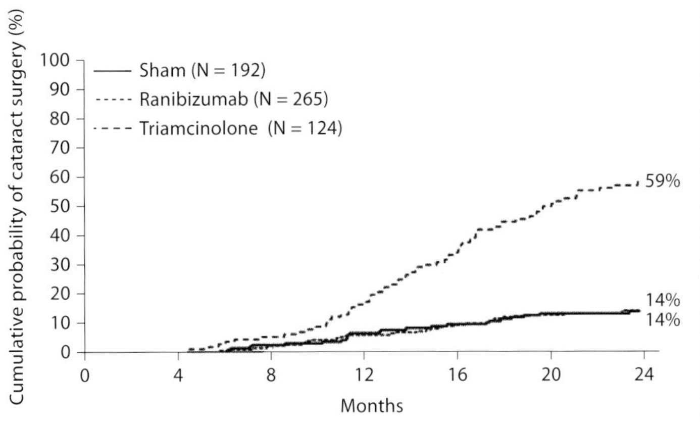

Sham						
• Eyes at risk*	192	183	174	163	148	140
• Cataract surgeries**	0	4	7	5	6	1
Ranibizumab						
• Eyes at risk*	265	252	242	231	213	201
• Cataract surgeries**	0	5	9	8	8	3
Triamcinolone						
• Eyes at risk*	124	120	112	98	77	57
• Cataract surgeries**	0	6	13	20	19	10

Fig. 19. Cumulative probability of cataract surgery through 2 years of follow-up for all eyes phakic at baseline. Eyes pending a 2-year visit or that were lost to follow-up were censored at their last visit. The number of eyes phakic at baseline is shown in parentheses. The number of eyes at the start of the interval without previous cataract surgery is indicated by asterisk. Double asterisk indicates the number of eyes with cataract surgery during the subsequent 4-month period. Reproduced with permission of Elman et al. [88].

Proliferative Diabetic Retinopathy: Pars Plana Vitrectomy

Full review of the techniques and use of vitrectomy in DR is beyond the scope of this chapter but has been described elsewhere [110]. Indications for PPV include media opacity, traction-related complications of fibrovascular proliferation, glaucoma, and fibrinoid syndrome (table 7) [111].

The objectives of PPV include: (1) removal of media opacities; (2) release of traction (anteroposterior and tangential) through excision of the posterior hyaloid face, core vitreous, and epiretinal membranes; (3) hemostasis; (4) identification and treatment of all retinal breaks; (5) application of full PRP from outside the temporal arcades to anterior to the equator (usually to the ora serrata) if PDR is present or if there is severe retinal ischemia in the absence of PDR (to reduce the likelihood of developing rubeosis iridis and/or anterior hyaloid fibrovascular proliferation after surgery).

The Diabetic Retinopathy Vitrectomy Study (DRVS) was a randomized multicenter study that addressed the following questions: (1) Does early vitrectomy for severe (causing vision ≤5/200 for at least 1 month) nonclearing VH improve visual outcome? (2) Does early (before macular detachment) vitrectomy for severe, active fibrovascular proliferation improve visual outcome? The DRVS showed that at 2-year follow-up, early vitrectomy for nonclearing VH primarily increased the chance for retaining vision ≥20/40 [25% (surgery 1–6 months after VH onset) versus 15% in the conventional management cohort (surgery 1 year or more after VH)]. This difference was most pronounced for type 1 diabetic patients (36 vs. 12% in the conventional management cohort) versus type 2 diabetic patients (16 vs. 18% in the conventional management cohort) [112]. In practice, most type 2 patients with nonclearing VH are offered vitrectomy within 1–3

Table 4. Potential treatment protocols for eyes with CSME, vision 20/40 or worse, and selected for combination therapy involving intravitreal ranibizumab/bevacizumab or triamcinolone with modified ETDRS focal laser photocoagulation

---

Ranibizumab/bevacizumab plus focal laser photocoagulation
1. Inject ranibizumab/bevacizumab: at week 0, week 4, week 8, and week 12.
2. Perform complete focal laser: at week 1 follow-up visit.
3. At and after week 16, if visual acuity is worse than 20/20 or central subfield OCT is ≥250 μm and retinal edema is present and is a cause of visual loss:
    a. ollow patient every month and provide injection every month unless patient deemed unresponsive (<10% change in central subfield OCT thickness or <5 letter gain in vision).
    b. Repeat laser every 4 months if previous treatment deemed incomplete unless patient deemed unresponsive.
4. If patient achieves VA 20/20 and OCT central subfield <250 μm, one can gradually increase follow-up intervals to every 4 months with return to treatment protocol (steps 1–3 above) if macular edema causing visual loss occurs.
5. If, after steps 1–3, there is >10 letter loss of vision, OCT central subfield is ≥250 μm, CSME that is a cause of visual loss is present, and complete laser treatment was given at least 4 months earlier, then the patient is deemed a treatment failure and intravitreal triamcinolone (IVTA) or other therapy is considered.
    a. IVTA injection (4 mg/0.1 ml) every 4 months until patient is deemed a success or unresponsive or develops unacceptable IOP or other complications.
    b. PPV in selected cases (e.g. taut posterior hyaloid face).
6. In any case, follow-up continues at 4-month intervals to monitor for progression of DR and complications such as cataract and increased IOP.

Triamcinolone plus focal laser photocoagulation
1. Consider this option particularly if patient is pseudophakic and has no history or increased risk of glaucoma.
2. IVTA injection (4 mg/0.1 ml) at week 0.
3. Perform complete focal laser: at week 1 follow-up visit.
4. Follow patient every 4 months:
    a. At and after week 16, if visual acuity is worse than 20/20 or central subfield OCT is ≥250 μm and retinal edema is present and is a cause of visual loss and IOP is not unacceptably elevated, provide repeat IVTA injection unless patient deemed unresponsive (<10% change in central subfield OCT thickness or <5 letter gain in vision).
    b. Repeat laser every 4 months if previous treatment deemed incomplete unless patient deemed unresponsive.
5. If, after steps 1–3, there is >10-letter loss of vision, OCT central subfield is ≥250 μm, CSME that is cause of visual loss is present, and complete laser treatment was given at least 4 months earlier, then the patient is deemed a treatment failure, and other therapy is considered (e.g. PPV).
6. In any case, follow-up continues at 4-month intervals to monitor for progression of DR and complications such as cataract and increased IOP.

---

months after VH onset unless medical problems preclude it. Approximately 80% of diabetic eyes undergoing vitrectomy for nonclearing VH achieve visual improvement of 2 Snellen lines or more after surgery, although nearly all patients over age 50 years develop progressive nuclear sclerotic cataract. Patients who present with severe subhyaloid hemorrhage are given full PRP (if not done already) and are observed for 1–2 months. If substantial clearing of the hemorrhage is not evident by ~2 months, vitrectomy usually is offered to avoid the development of severe epiretinal fibrosis in the area of subhyaloid hemorrhage (fig. 24). Patients with severe, active PDR and vision ≥20/400 also have a greater chance to retain/recover vision ≥20/40 with

- Sterile lid speculum

- Topical anesthesia (lidocaine gel)

- 5–10% povidone-iodine prep (× 2 or 3) of lid margin, lashes, and conjunctiva

- Inject with a ½ inch 30-gauge needle attached to TB syringe (10 s)

- Tamponade injection site with sterile Q-tip

- Topical antibiotic (e.g. gatifloxacin, 5 ml bottle) every hour while awake

- Follow-up exam (or phone interview) within one week of injection to monitor for complications

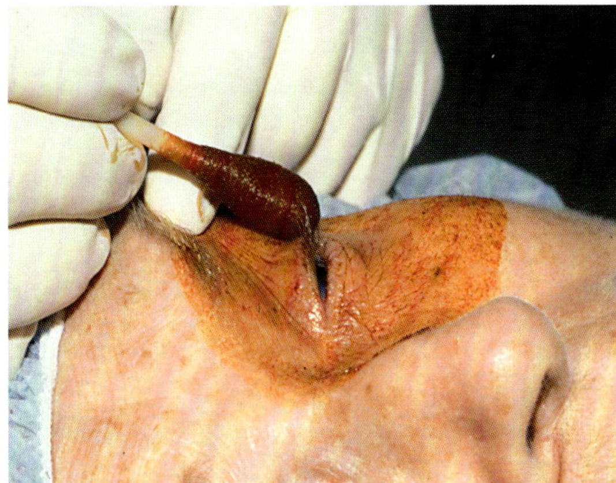

Fig. 20. Intravitreal injection technique. After medication is injected, the needle is left in the eye for 10 s before withdrawal to permit diffusion of medication throughout the vitreous cavity. Patients are instructed to report to the physician immediately if they develop decreasing vision, increasing pain, or increasing floaters after injection.

early vitrectomy rather than waiting for the development of detachment involving the macula before operating (44 vs. 28% with conventional management at 4-year follow-up) [18]. These visual benefits are associated with improved quality of life [113]. Anti-VEGF injections might be useful adjuncts to facilitate effective fibrovascular membrane dissection in eyes with aggressive, active vascularity components [105]. However, there is a risk (~5%) of inducing traction retinal detachment within 1–4 weeks of surgery, so in general the case should be scheduled in a timely manner after the injection [107].

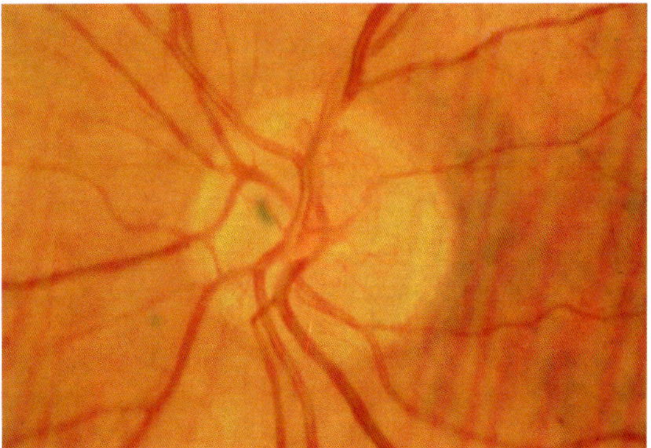

Fig. 21. Standard photograph 10a illustrates the severity of retinal neovascularization at the optic nerve head constituting HR-PDR. Reproduced with permission [15].

Conclusions

Ophthalmological management of patients with diabetes is based on the results of many well-designed scientific studies of natural history and response to different treatment modalities. Strict control of blood glucose and blood pressure is critical for reduction of the incidence and progression of DR. Follow-up of patients with diabetes mellitus is protocol-based and not based solely on the presence of symptoms. (Patients can be asymptomatic, for example, and yet have HR-PDR.) Staging of the level of DR drives the follow-up interval. Staging involves categorizing the patient as having mild, moderate, or severe NPDR vs. PDR. The most common

Table 5. Treatment technique for PRP using conventional laser

Item	Technique
Anesthesia	Topical or subconjunctival/peribulbar (2% lidocaine without epinephrine) Rarely, retrobulbar anesthesia
Spot size	With Rodenstock or panfundus lens: 250 μm With 3- or 4-mirror lens: 500 μm
Spot spacing	1/2 to 1 burn width apart
Duration of laser application	0.05 s preferred Can increase duration if power is maximal and laser uptake is inadequate
Wavelength	Usually argon green Diode or krypton red laser used in setting of significant nuclear sclerosis or VH
Power	Sufficient to create moderate retinal whitening
Number of sessions	2–4
Extent of treatment	From outside the temporal arcades to the equator Bring treatment no closer than 2.5 disc diameters to the macula temporally and no closer than 500 μm to the optic nerve Do not treat closer than 1 disc diameter to areas of traction retinal detachment
Supplemental PRP after 'full' treatment	NV regresses, but <50% with persistent capillary brush border appearance Frequent recurrent VH Development of rubeosis iridis

Table 6. Eyes with initial mild-severe NPDR or early PDR undergoing vitrectomy and/or experiencing severe visual loss at 5-year follow-up in the ETDRS [12, 109]

Assignment	Number/total in study	Percent of overall study
Deferral	154/3,711	4.1
Mild scatter PRP	53/1,868	2.8
Full scatter PRP	36/1,843	2.0

Table 7. Indications for PPV for severe complications of DR

Media opacity
- Nonclearing VH
- Nonclearing subhyaloid hemorrhage
- Rubeosis iridis with VH

Retinal traction
- Severe, progressive fibrovascular proliferation (including anterior hyaloidal fibrovascular proliferation)
- Traction retinal detachment involving the macula
- Traction-rhegmatogenous retinal detachment
- Taut posterior hyaloid face

Ghost cell glaucoma

Fibrinoid syndrome

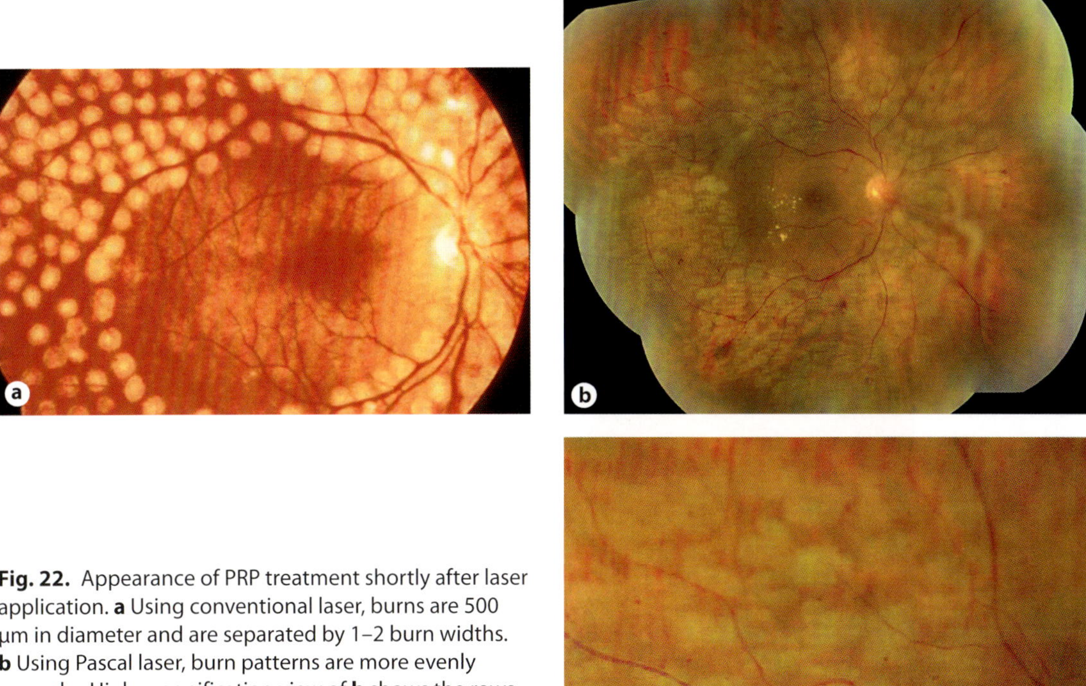

Fig. 22. Appearance of PRP treatment shortly after laser application. **a** Using conventional laser, burns are 500 μm in diameter and are separated by 1–2 burn widths. **b** Using Pascal laser, burn patterns are more evenly spaced. **c** High-magnification view of **b** shows the rows of evenly spaced, lower intensity burns typical of Pascal laser treatment.

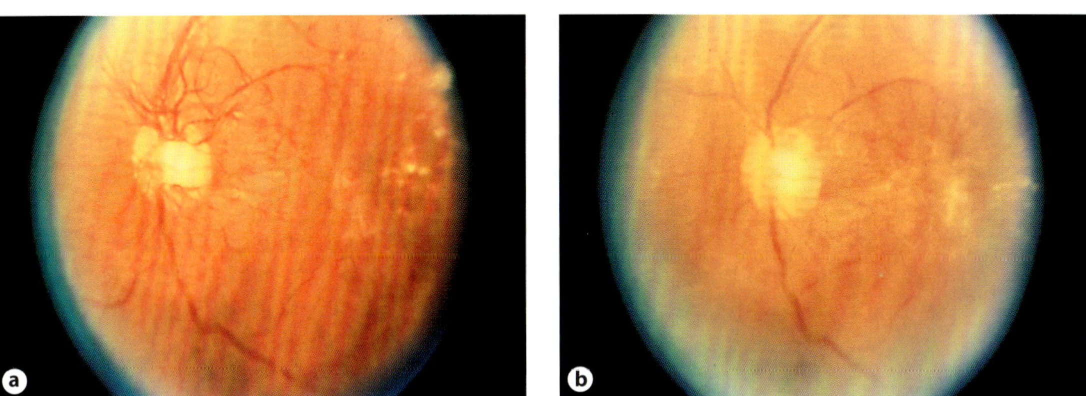

Fig. 23. Regression of retinal neovascularization after PRP typically requires 3 weeks. **a** Appearance of neovascularization at the optic disc before laser treatment. **b** Appearance 3 weeks after laser. Only ghost vessels remain. Occasionally, regression is associated only with loss of the fine capillary network and with persistence of larger, trunk-like vessels and/or fibrous tissue.

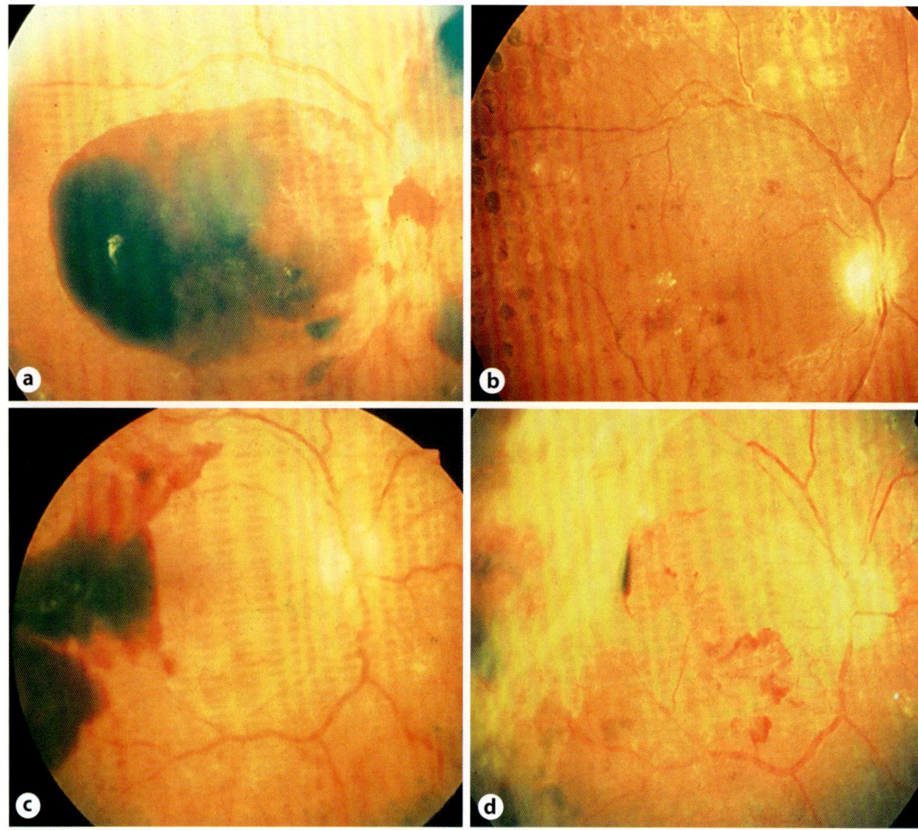

Fig. 24. Development of severe epiretinal fibrosis in an eye with longstanding subhyaloid hemorrhage. **a** Eye with subhyaloid hemorrhage and PDR. **b** Same eye as in **a** but following vitrectomy and membrane peeling. **c** Another eye with subhyaloid hemorrhage and PDR. **d** Same eye after a period of several months of follow-up. Note extensive epiretinal fibrosis in the area of subhyaloid hemorrhage. Courtesy of Dr. Alexander Irvine, University of California, San Francisco.

cause of visual loss in diabetic patients is DME. The results of multicenter, randomized studies indicate that among patients with visual acuity 20/32–20/40 or worse, currently the best visual results for DME are achieved with intravitreal anti-VEGF (e.g. ranibizumab, bevacizumab) injections ± focal laser photocoagulation. This approach also seems to reduce the likelihood of progression of DR. Selected patients also may benefit from intravitreal steroid treatment + focal laser therapy, but there is a relatively higher risk of glaucoma and cataract formation. PRP is currently the most effective treatment for HR-PDR. PRP also should be considered for patients with severe NPDR and early PDR, particularly if follow-up cannot be assured and/or if the patient has type 2 diabetes mellitus. PPV is used to manage severe complications of DR such as nonclearing VH, severe fibrovascular proliferation, and retinal detachment.

References

1 Klein R, Klein BE, Moss SE, Davis MD, DeMets DL: The Wisconsin epidemiologic study of diabetic retinopathy. IX. Four-year incidence and progression of diabetic retinopathy when age at diagnosis is less than 30 years. Arch Ophthalmol 1989;107:237–243.

2 Klein R, Klein BE, Moss SE, Davis MD, DeMets DL: The Wisconsin epidemiologic study of diabetic retinopathy. II. Prevalence and risk of diabetic retinopathy when age at diagnosis is less than 30 years. Arch Ophthalmol 1984;102:520–526.

3 Klein R, Klein BE, Moss SE, Davis MD, DeMets DL: The Wisconsin epidemiologic study of diabetic retinopathy. III. Prevalence and risk of diabetic retinopathy when age at diagnosis is 30 or more years. Arch Ophthalmol 1984;102:527–532.

4 Klein R, Klein BE, Moss SE, Davis MD, DeMets DL: The Wisconsin epidemiologic study of diabetic retinopathy. IV. Diabetic macular edema. Ophthalmology 1984;91:1464–1474.

5 Klein R, Klein BE, Moss SE, Davis MD, DeMets DL: The Wisconsin epidemiologic study of diabetic retinopathy. X. Four-year incidence and progression of diabetic retinopathy when age at diagnosis is 30 years is more. Arch Ophthalmol 1989;107:244–249.

6 Klein R, Klein BE, Moss SE, Cruickshanks KJ: The Wisconsin Epidemiologic Study of diabetic retinopathy. XIV. Ten-year incidence and progression of diabetic retinopathy. Arch Ophthalmol 1994;112:1217–1228.

7 Klein R, Klein BE, Moss SE, Cruickshanks KJ: The Wisconsin Epidemiologic Study of Diabetic Retinopathy: XVII. The 14-year incidence and progression of diabetic retinopathy and associated risk factors in type 1 diabetes. Ophthalmology 1998;105:1801–1815.

8 The Diabetes Control and Complications Trial Research Group: The effect of intensive treatment of diabetes on the development and progression of long-term complications in insulin-dependent diabetes mellitus. N Engl J Med 1993;329:977–986.

9 UK Prospective Diabetes Study (UKPDS): VIII. Study design, progress and performance. Diabetologia 1991;34:877–890.

10 UK Prospective Diabetes Study Group: Tight blood pressure control and risk of macrovascular and microvascular complications in type 2 diabetes: UKPDS 38. BMJ 1998;317:703–713.

11 Early Treatment Diabetic Retinopathy Study research group: Photocoagulation for diabetic macular edema. Early Treatment Diabetic Retinopathy Study report number 1. Arch Ophthalmol 1985;103:1796–1806.

12 Early Treatment Diabetic Retinopathy Study Research Group: Early photocoagulation for diabetic retinopathy. ETDRS report number 9. Ophthalmology 1991;98:766–785.

13 Early Treatment Diabetic Retinopathy Study design and baseline patient characteristics. ETDRS report number 7. Ophthalmology 1991;98:741–756.

14 Photocoagulation treatment of proliferative diabetic retinopathy: the second report of Diabetic Retinopathy Study findings. Ophthalmology 1978;85:82–106.

15 The Diabetic Retinopathy Study Research Group: Four risk factors for severe visual loss in diabetic retinopathy. The third report from the Diabetic Retinopathy Study. Arch Ophthalmol 1979;97:654–655.

16 The Diabetic Retinopathy Study Research Group: Photocoagulation treatment of proliferative diabetic retinopathy. Clinical application of Diabetic Retinopathy Study (DRS) findings, DRS Report Number 8. Ophthalmology 1981;88:583–600.

17 Two-year course of visual acuity in severe proliferative diabetic retinopathy with conventional management. Diabetic Retinopathy Vitrectomy Study (DRVS) report 1. Ophthalmology 1985;92:492–502.

18 The Diabetic Retinopathy Vitrectomy Study Research Group: Early vitrectomy for severe proliferative diabetic retinopathy in eyes with useful vision. Results of a randomized trial–Diabetic Retinopathy Vitrectomy Study Report 3. Ophthalmology 1988;95:1307–1320.

19 Early vitrectomy for severe vitreous hemorrhage in diabetic retinopathy. Four-year results of a randomized trial: Diabetic Retinopathy Vitrectomy Study Report 5. Arch Ophthalmol 1990;108:958–964.

20 Fong DS, Strauber SF, Aiello LP, et al: Comparison of the modified Early Treatment Diabetic Retinopathy Study and mild macular grid laser photocoagulation strategies for diabetic macular edema. Arch Ophthalmol 2007;125:469–480.

21 Chew E, Strauber S, Beck R, et al: Randomized trial of peribulbar triamcinolone acetonide with and without focal photocoagulation for mild diabetic macular edema: a pilot study. Ophthalmology 2007;114:1190–1196.

22 Diabetic Retinopathy Clinical Research Network: A randomized trial comparing intravitreal triamcinolone acetonide and focal/grid photocoagulation for diabetic macular edema. Ophthalmology 2008;115:1447–1449, 1449.e1–1449.e10.

23 Beck RW, Edwards AR, Aiello LP, et al: Three-year follow-up of a randomized trial comparing focal/grid photocoagulation and intravitreal triamcinolone for diabetic macular edema. Arch Ophthalmol 2009;127:245–251.

24 Moss SE, Klein R, Klein BE: The incidence of vision loss in a diabetic population. Ophthalmology 1988;95:1340–1348.

25 Do DV, Shah SM, Sung JU, Haller JA, Nguyen QD: Persistent diabetic macular edema is associated with elevated hemoglobin A1c. Am J Ophthalmol 2005;139:620–623.

26 Krzystolik MG, Filippopoulos T, Ducharme JF, Loewenstein JI: Pegaptanib as an adjunctive treatment for complicated neovascular diabetic retinopathy. Arch Ophthalmol 2006;124:920–921.

27 Zein WM, Noureddin BN, Jurdi FA, Schakal A, Bashshur ZF: Panretinal photocoagulation and intravitreal triamcinolone acetonide for the management of proliferative diabetic retinopathy with macular edema. Retina 2006;26:137–142.

28 Ferris FL 3rd, Davis MD: Treating 20/20 eyes with diabetic macular edema. Arch Ophthalmol 1999;117:675–676.

29 Kang SW, Sa HS, Cho HY, Kim JI: Macular grid photocoagulation after intravitreal triamcinolone acetonide for diffuse diabetic macular edema. Arch Ophthalmol 2006;124:653–658.

30 Gillies MC, Sutter FK, Simpson JM, Larsson J, Ali H, Zhu M: Intravitreal triamcinolone for refractory diabetic macular edema: two-year results of a double-masked, placebo-controlled, randomized clinical trial. Ophthalmology 2006;113:1533–1538.

31 Arevalo JF, Fromow-Guerra J, Quiroz-Mercado H, et al: Primary intravitreal bevacizumab (Avastin) for diabetic macular edema: results from the Pan-American Collaborative Retina Study Group at 6-month follow-up. Ophthalmology 2007;114:743–750.

32 Grigorian R, Bhagat N, Lanzetta P, Tutela A, Zarbin M: Pars plana vitrectomy for refractory diabetic macular edema. Semin Ophthalmol 2003;18:116–120.

33 Grigorian RA, Castellarin A, Bhagat N, Del Priore L, Von Hagen S, Zarbin MA: Use of viscodissection and silicone oil in vitrectomy for severe diabetic retinopathy. Semin Ophthalmol 2003;18:121–126.

34 Bhagat N, Grigorian RA, Tutela A, Zarbin MA: Diabetic macular edema: pathogenesis and treatment. Surv Ophthalmol 2009;54:1–32.

35 Lanzagorta-Aresti A, Palacios-Pozo E, Menezo Rozalen JL, Navea-Tejerina A: Prevention of vision loss after cataract surgery in diabetic macular edema with intravitreal bevacizumab: a pilot study. Retina 2009;29:530–535.

36 Oshima Y, Shima C, Wakabayashi T, et al: Microincision vitrectomy surgery and intravitreal bevacizumab as a surgical adjunct to treat diabetic traction retinal detachment. Ophthalmology 2009;116:927–938.

37 Giacco F, Brownlee M: Oxidative stress and diabetic complications. Circ Res 2010;107:1058–1070.

38 Jardeleza MS, Miller JW: Review of anti-VEGF therapy in proliferative diabetic retinopathy. Semin Ophthalmol 2009;24:87–92.

39 Witmer AN, Vrensen GF, Van Noorden CJ, Schlingemann RO: Vascular endothelial growth factors and angiogenesis in eye disease. Prog Retin Eye Res 2003;22:1–29.

40 Ramasamy R, Vannucci SJ, Yan SS, Herold K, Yan SF, Schmidt AM: Advanced glycation end products and RAGE: a common thread in aging, diabetes, neurodegeneration, and inflammation. Glycobiology 2005;15:16R–28R.

41 Miyamoto K, Khosrof S, Bursell SE, et al: Prevention of leukostasis and vascular leakage in streptozotocin-induced diabetic retinopathy via intercellular adhesion molecule-1 inhibition. Proc Natl Acad Sci USA 1999;96:10836–10841.

42 Kim W, Hudson BI, Moser B, et al: Receptor for advanced glycation end products and its ligands: a journey from the complications of diabetes to its pathogenesis. Ann N Y Acad Sci 2005;1043:553–561.

43 Barber AJ, Lieth E, Khin SA, Antonetti DA, Buchanan AG, Gardner TW: Neural apoptosis in the retina during experimental and human diabetes. Early onset and effect of insulin. J Clin Invest 1998;102:783–791.

44 Han Y, Schneck ME, Bearse MA Jr, et al: Formulation and evaluation of a predictive model to identify the sites of future diabetic retinopathy. Invest Ophthalmol Vis Sci 2004;45:4106–4112.

45 Bearse MA Jr, Adams AJ, Han Y, et al: A multifocal electroretinogram model predicting the development of diabetic retinopathy. Prog Retin Eye Res 2006;25:425–448.

46 Harrison WW, Bearse MA Jr, Ng JS, et al: Multifocal electroretinograms predict onset of diabetic retinopathy in adult patients with diabetes. Invest Ophthalmol Vis Sci 2011;52:772–777.

47 Barber AJ: A new view of diabetic retinopathy: a neurodegenerative disease of the eye. Prog Neuropsychopharmacol Biol Psychiatry 2003;27:283–290.

48 Bek T: A clinicopathological study of venous loops and reduplications in diabetic retinopathy. Acta Ophthalmol Scand 2002;80:69–75.

49 Arend O, Wolf S, Harris A, Reim M: The relationship of macular microcirculation to visual acuity in diabetic patients. Arch Ophthalmol 1995;113:610–614.

50 Klein BE, Moss SE, Klein R, Surawicz TS: The Wisconsin Epidemiologic Study of Diabetic Retinopathy. XIII. Relationship of serum cholesterol to retinopathy and hard exudate. Ophthalmology 1991;98:1261–1265.

51 Brown JC, Solomon SD, Bressler SB, Schachat AP, DiBernardo C, Bressler NM: Detection of diabetic foveal edema: contact lens biomicroscopy compared with optical coherence tomography. Arch Ophthalmol 2004;122:330–335.

52 Browning DJ, McOwen MD, Bowen RM Jr, O'Marah TL: Comparison of the clinical diagnosis of diabetic macular edema with diagnosis by optical coherence tomography. Ophthalmology 2004;111:712–715.

53 Maheshwary AS, Oster SF, Yuson RM, Cheng L, Mojana F, Freeman WR: The association between percent disruption of the photoreceptor inner segment-outer segment junction and visual acuity in diabetic macular edema. Am J Ophthalmol 2010;150:63–67.e1.

54 Forooghian F, Stetson PF, Meyer SA, et al: Relationship between photoreceptor outer segment length and visual acuity in diabetic macular edema. Retina 2010;30:63–70.

55 Davis MD, Bressler SB, Aiello LP, et al: Comparison of time-domain OCT and fundus photographic assessments of retinal thickening in eyes with diabetic macular edema. Invest Ophthalmol Vis Sci 2008;49:1745–1752.

56 Kozak I, Morrison VL, Clark TM, et al: Discrepancy between fluorescein angiography and optical coherence tomography in detection of macular disease. Retina 2008;28:538–544.

57 Harris MI, Klein R, Cowie CC, Rowland M, Byrd-Holt DD: Is the risk of diabetic retinopathy greater in non-Hispanic blacks and Mexican Americans than in non-Hispanic whites with type 2 diabetes? A U.S. population study. Diabetes Care 1998;21:1230–1235.

58 West SK, Munoz B, Klein R, et al: Risk factors for type II diabetes and diabetic retinopathy in a Mexican-American population: Proyecto VER. Am J Ophthalmol 2002;134:390–398.

59 Xie XW, Xu L, Jonas JB, Wang YX: Prevalence of diabetic retinopathy among subjects with known diabetes in China: the Beijing Eye Study. Eur J Ophthalmol 2009;19:91–99.

60 Klein BE, Moss SE, Klein R: Effect of pregnancy on progression of diabetic retinopathy. Diabetes Care 1990;13:34–40.

61 Wu Z, Huang J, Sadda S: Inadvertent use of bevacizumab to treat choroidal neovascularisation during pregnancy: a case report. Ann Acad Med Singapore 2010;39:143–145.

62 Charles S, Flinn CE: The natural history of diabetic extramacular traction retinal detachment. Arch Ophthalmol 1981;99:66–68.

63 Charonis AS, Tsilbary EC: Structural and functional changes of laminin and type IV collagen after nonenzymatic glycation. Diabetes 1992;41(suppl 2):49–51.

64 The relationship of glycemic exposure (HbA1c) to the risk of development and progression of retinopathy in the diabetes control and complications trial. Diabetes 1995;44:968–983.

65 UK Prospective Diabetes Study (UKPDS) Group: Intensive blood-glucose control with sulphonylureas or insulin compared with conventional treatment and risk of complications in patients with type 2 diabetes (UKPDS 33). Lancet 1998;352:837–853.

66 Matthews DR, Stratton IM, Aldington SJ, Holman RR, Kohner EM: Risks of progression of retinopathy and vision loss related to tight blood pressure control in type 2 diabetes mellitus: UKPDS 69. Arch Ophthalmol 2004;122:1631–1640.

67 Schachat AP: A new look at an old treatment for diabetic macular edema. Ophthalmology 2008;115:1445–1446.

68 Cruess AF, Williams JC, Willan AR: Argon green and krypton red laser treatment of diabetic macular edema. Can J Ophthalmol 1988;23:262–266.

69 Akduman L, Olk RJ: Diode laser (810 nm) versus argon green (514 nm) modified grid photocoagulation for diffuse diabetic macular edema. Ophthalmology 1997;104:1433–1441.

70 Ulbig MW, McHugh DA, Hamilton AM: Diode laser photocoagulation for diabetic macular oedema. Br J Ophthalmol 1995;79:318–321.

71 Friberg TR, Karatza EC: The treatment of macular disease using a micropulsed and continuous wave 810-nm diode laser. Ophthalmology 1997;104:2030–2038.

72 Moorman CM, Hamilton AM: Clinical applications of the MicroPulse diode laser. Eye (Lond) 1999;13:145–150.

73 Stanga PE, Reck AC, Hamilton AM: Micropulse laser in the treatment of diabetic macular edema. Semin Ophthalmol 1999;14:210–213.

74 Vujosevic S, Bottega E, Casciano M, Pilotto E, Convento E, Midena E: Microperimetry and fundus autofluorescence in diabetic macular edema: subthreshold micropulse diode laser versus modified early treatment diabetic retinopathy study laser photocoagulation. Retina 2010;30:908–916.

75 Sivaprasad S, Elagouz M, McHugh D, Shona O, Dorin G: Micropulsed diode laser therapy: evolution and clinical applications. Surv Ophthalmol 2010;55:516–530.

76 Ohkoshi K, Yamaguchi T: Subthreshold micropulse diode laser photocoagulation for diabetic macular edema in Japanese patients. Am J Ophthalmol 2010; 149:133–139.

77 Lavinsky D, Cardillo JA, Melo LA Jr, Dare A, Farah ME, Belfort R Jr: Randomized Clinical Trial Evaluating mETDRS versus Normal or High-Density Micropulse Photocoagulation for Diabetic Macular Edema. Invest Ophthalmol Vis Sci 2011:52:4314–4323.

78 Ishida S, Usui T, Yamashiro K, et al: VEGF164-mediated inflammation is required for pathological, but not physiological, ischemia-induced retinal neovascularization. J Exp Med 2003; 198:483–489.

79 Ishida S, Usui T, Yamashiro K, et al: VEGF164 is proinflammatory in the diabetic retina. Invest Ophthalmol Vis Sci 2003;44:2155–2162.

80 Joussen AM, Poulaki V, Qin W, et al: Retinal vascular endothelial growth factor induces intercellular adhesion molecule-1 and endothelial nitric oxide synthase expression and initiates early diabetic retinal leukocyte adhesion in vivo. Am J Pathol 2002;160:501–509.

81 McLeod DS, Lefer DJ, Merges C, Lutty GA: Enhanced expression of intracellular adhesion molecule-1 and P-selectin in the diabetic human retina and choroid. Am J Pathol 1995;147:642–653.

82 Aiello LP, Avery RL, Arrigg PG, et al: Vascular endothelial growth factor in ocular fluid of patients with diabetic retinopathy and other retinal disorders. N Engl J Med 1994;331:1480–1487.

83 Lutty GA, McLeod DS, Merges C, Diggs A, Plouet J: Localization of vascular endothelial growth factor in human retina and choroid. Arch Ophthalmol 1996;114:971–977.

84 Gilbert RE, Vranes D, Berka JL, et al: Vascular endothelial growth factor and its receptors in control and diabetic rat eyes. Lab Invest 1998;78:1017–1027.

85 Qaum T, Xu Q, Joussen AM, et al: VEGF-initiated blood-retinal barrier breakdown in early diabetes. Invest Ophthalmol Vis Sci 2001;42:2408–2413.

86 Robinson GS, Pierce EA, Rook SL, Foley E, Webb R, Smith LE: Oligodeoxynucleotides inhibit retinal neovascularization in a murine model of proliferative retinopathy. Proc Natl Acad Sci USA 1996;93:4851–4856.

87 Nicholson BP, Schachat AP: A review of clinical trials of anti-VEGF agents for diabetic retinopathy. Graefes Arch Clin Exp Ophthalmol 2010;248:915–930.

88 Elman MJ, Aiello LP, Beck RW, et al: Randomized trial evaluating ranibizumab plus prompt or deferred laser or triamcinolone plus prompt laser for diabetic macular edema. Ophthalmology 2010;117:1064–1077.e35.

89 Massin P, Bandello F, Garweg JG, et al: Safety and efficacy of ranibizumab in diabetic macular edema (RESOLVE Study): a 12-month, randomized, controlled, double-masked, multicenter phase II study. Diabetes Care 2010;33:2399–2405.

90 Michaelides M, Kaines A, Hamilton RD, et al: A prospective randomized trial of intravitreal bevacizumab or laser therapy in the management of diabetic macular edema (BOLT study) 12-month data: report 2. Ophthalmology 2010;117:1078–1086.e2.

91 Chung EJ, Roh MI, Kwon OW, Koh HJ: Effects of macular ischemia on the outcome of intravitreal bevacizumab therapy for diabetic macular edema. Retina 2008;28:957–963.

92 Neubauer AS, Kook D, Haritoglou C, et al: Bevacizumab and retinal ischemia. Ophthalmology 2007;114:2096.

93 Michaelides M, Fraser-Bell S, Hamilton R, et al: Macular perfusion determined by fundus fluorescein angiography at the 4-month time point in a prospective randomized trial of intravitreal bevacizumab or laser therapy in the management of diabetic macular edema (Bolt Study): Report 1. Retina 2010;30:781–786.

94 Haller JA, Kuppermann BD, Blumenkranz MS, et al: Randomized controlled trial of an intravitreous dexamethasone drug delivery system in patients with diabetic macular edema. Arch Ophthalmol 2010;128:289–296.

95 Hnik P, Boyer DS, Grillone LR, Clement JG, Henry SP, Green EA: Antisense oligonucleotide therapy in diabetic retinopathy. J Diabetes Sci Technol 2009;3:924–930.

96 Cunningham ET Jr, Adamis AP, Altaweel M, et al: A phase II randomized double-masked trial of pegaptanib, an anti-vascular endothelial growth factor aptamer, for diabetic macular edema. Ophthalmology 2005;112:1747–1757.

97 Lewis H, Abrams GW, Blumenkranz MS, Campo RV: Vitrectomy for diabetic macular traction and edema associated with posterior hyaloidal traction. Ophthalmology 1992;99:753–759.

98 Flaxel CJ, Edwards AR, Aiello LP, et al: Factors associated with visual acuity outcomes after vitrectomy for diabetic macular edema: diabetic retinopathy clinical research network. Retina 2010;30:1488–1495.

99 Haller JA, Qin H, Apte RS, et al: Vitrectomy outcomes in eyes with diabetic macular edema and vitreomacular traction. Ophthalmology 2010;117:1087–1093.e3.

100 Diaz-Llopis M, Udaondo P, Arevalo F, et al: Intravitreal plasmin without associated vitrectomy as a treatment for refractory diabetic macular edema. J Ocul Pharmacol Ther 2009;25:379–384.

101 McDonald HR, Schatz H: Macular edema following panretinal photocoagulation. Retina 1985;5:5–10.

102 Lee SB, Yun YJ, Kim SH, Kim JY: Changes in macular thickness after panretinal photocoagulation in patients with severe diabetic retinopathy and no macular edema. Retina 2010;30:756–760.

103 Shimura M, Yasuda K, Nakazawa T, Kano T, Ohta S, Tamai M: Quantifying alterations of macular thickness before and after panretinal photocoagulation in patients with severe diabetic retinopathy and good vision. Ophthalmology 2003;110:2386–2394.

104 Unoki N, Nishijima K, Kita M, et al: Randomised controlled trial of posterior sub-Tenon triamcinolone as adjunct to panretinal photocoagulation for treatment of diabetic retinopathy. Br J Ophthalmol 2009;93:765–770.

105 Avery RL, Pearlman J, Pieramici DJ, et al: Intravitreal bevacizumab (Avastin) in the treatment of proliferative diabetic retinopathy. Ophthalmology 2006;113:1695.e1–1695.e15.

106 Moradian S, Ahmadieh H, Malihi M, Soheilian M, Dehghan MH, Azarmina M: Intravitreal bevacizumab in active progressive proliferative diabetic retinopathy. Graefes Arch Clin Exp Ophthalmol 2008;246:1699–1705.

107 Arevalo JF, Maia M, Flynn HW Jr, et al: Tractional retinal detachment following intravitreal bevacizumab (Avastin) in patients with severe proliferative diabetic retinopathy. Br J Ophthalmol 2008;92:213–216.

108 Ferris F: Early photocoagulation in patients with either type I or type II diabetes. Tr Am Ophth Soc 1996;94:505–537.

109 Flynn HW Jr, Chew EY, Simons BD, Barton FB, Remaley NA, Ferris FL 3rd, The Early Treatment Diabetic Retinopathy Study Research Group: Pars plana vitrectomy in the Early Treatment Diabetic Retinopathy Study. ETDRS report number 17. Ophthalmology 1992;99:1351–1357.

110 Smiddy WE, Flynn HW Jr: Vitrectomy in the management of diabetic retinopathy. Surv Ophthalmol 1999;43:491–507.

111 Castellarin A, Grigorian R, Bhagat N, Del Priore L, Zarbin MA: Vitrectomy with silicone oil infusion in severe diabetic retinopathy. Br J Ophthalmol 2003;87:318–321.

112 The Diabetic Retinopathy Vitrectomy Study Research Group: Early vitrectomy for severe vitreous hemorrhage in diabetic retinopathy. Two-year results of a randomized trial. Diabetic Retinopathy Vitrectomy Study report 2. Arch Ophthalmol 1985;103:1644–1652.

113 Okamoto F, Okamoto Y, Fukuda S, Hiraoka T, Oshika T: Vision-related quality of life and visual function following vitrectomy for proliferative diabetic retinopathy. Am J Ophthalmol 2008;145:1031–1036.

114 Aiello LP, Gardner TW: Future Therapies for Diabetic Retinopathy. San Francisco, Foundation of the American Academy of Ophthalmology, 2000.

115 Clermont AC, Aiello LP, Mori F, Aiello LM, Bursell SE: Vascular endothelial growth factor and severity of nonproliferative diabetic retinopathy mediate retinal hemodynamics in vivo: a potential role for vascular endothelial growth factor in the progression of nonproliferative diabetic retinopathy. Am J Ophthalmol 1997;124:433–446.

116 Aiello LP, Northrup JM, Keyt BA, Takagi H, Iwamoto MA: Hypoxic regulation of vascular endothelial growth factor in retinal cells. Arch Ophthalmol 1995;113:1538–1544.

117 Skyler JS: Medical Management of Diabetic Retinopathy. San Francisco, American Academy of Ophthalmology, 2000.

Marco A. Zarbin, MD, PhD
Institute of Ophthalmology and Visual Science-New Jersey Medical School
Room 6156, Doctors Office Center
90 Bergen Street
Newark, NJ 07103 (USA)
Tel. +1 973 972 2038, E-Mail zarbin@earthlink.net

Bandello F, Battaglia Parodi M (eds): Surgical Retina.
ESASO Course Series. Basel, Karger, 2012, vol 2, pp 35–45

Nonsurgical Options for the Treatment of Diabetic Macular Edema

Constantin J. Pournaras[a] · Efstratios Mendrinos[a] · Jean-Antoine Pournaras[b]

[a]Vitreo-Retinal Unit, Department of Ophthalmology, Geneva University Hospitals, Geneva, and
[b]Vitreo-Retinal Unit, Jules Gonin Eye Hospital, University of Lausanne, Lausanne, Switzerland

Abstract

Optimum eye care of patients with diabetes requires, first of all, tight glycemic and blood pressure control as well as correction of anemia and hyperlipidemia. There is evidence that tight control of glycemia reduces the risk of development and progression of diabetic retinopathy in both type 1 and type 2 diabetes. Similarly, tight blood pressure control reduces the risk of retinopathy progression, visual loss, and the need for laser treatment in people with type 2 diabetes. Modified focal/grid argon laser photocoagulation is the standard of care in diabetic macular edema (DME) and reduces by 50% the risk of moderate visual loss from clinically significant macular edema. Additional treatments for DME include intravitreal injection of steroids or anti-vascular endothelial growth factor (VEGF) drugs, alone or in combination with laser photocoagulation. Intravitreal injections of triamcinolone acetonide and anti-VEGF agents alone reduce DME and increase visual acuity; however, DME often recurs. Side effects of repeated intravitreal triamcinolone injections include ocular hypertension and cataract formation. Combining intravitreal drugs with laser photocoagulation seems to reduce the amount of residual edema as well as the frequency of injections needed to control edema.

Diabetic macular edema (DME) is defined by retinal thickening involving or threatening the center of the macula, secondary to the intraretinal accumulation of fluid in the macular area. It is mainly caused by the breakdown of the inner blood-retinal barrier and can develop at all stages of diabetic retinopathy (DR), but appears to occur more frequently as the severity of DR increases; in patients with duration of diabetes of 10 years or more, the prevalence of DME is 1.7% in eyes with mild nonproliferative DR and increases to 20.3 and 69.7% in eyes with moderate/severe nonproliferative DR and proliferative DR, respectively. In patients with duration of diabetes of 15 years or more, the prevalence of DME is 6.3% in eyes with mild nonproliferative DR and increases to 63.2 and 74.3% in eyes with moderate/severe nonproliferative DR and proliferative DR, respectively [1].

DME can cause structural retinal changes severe enough to make it the most common cause of visual loss in patients with diabetes. Visual deterioration due to macular edema is usually slow, and only occurs when retinal thickening involves the center of the fovea. In the Early Treatment Diabetic Retinopathy Study (ETDRS), the 3-year risk of moderate visual loss was 33% when thickening initially involved the center of the fovea, and 22% when it did not. Severe visual loss usually results from longstanding DME resulting in degeneration of the photoreceptor-retinal pigment epithelial (RPE)

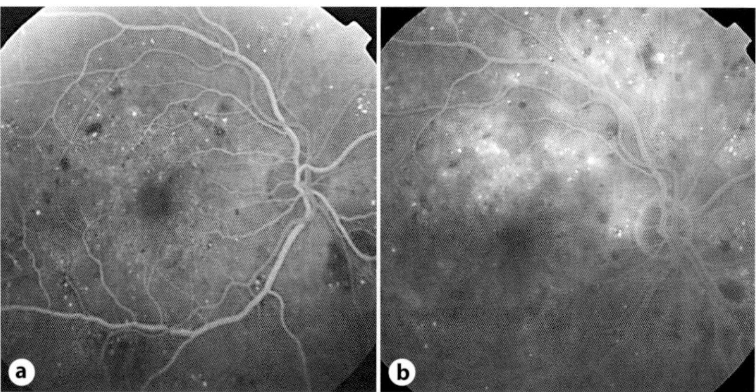

Fig. 1. DME. **a** Early phase fluorescein angiography showing microaneurysms. **b** Late-phase fluorescein angiography showing leakage from microaneurysms and accumulation within small cysts superiorly.

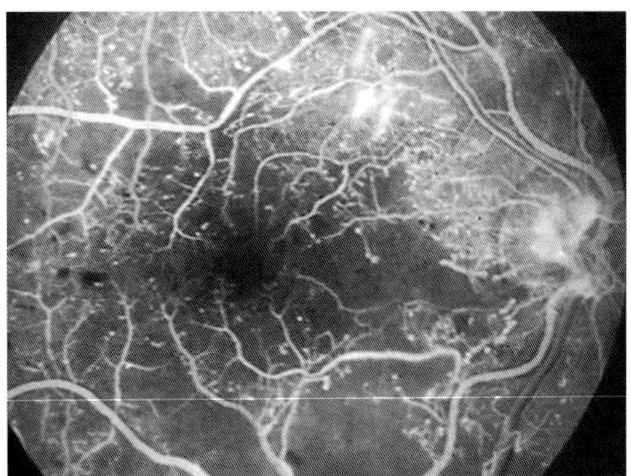

Fig. 2. Ischemic diabetic maculopathy. Fluorescein angiography shows presence of widespread capillary dropout at the macula and new vessels on the disc.

complex and/or combined severe macular capillary closure. Retinal degeneration may also result from the presence of large plaque of hard exudates under the central fovea. Spontaneous fluctuations of DME during the day as well as long-term variations have been reported in several studies [2–4].

Diagnostic Workup

Until recently, the clinical detection and evaluation methods currently used have been limited to slit-lamp biomicroscopy and stereoscopic photography. However, both methods are subjective and insensitive to small changes in retinal thickness.

Fluorescein angiography facilitates the visualization of the breakdown of the inner blood-retinal barrier, demonstrating leakage of fluorescein from the macular capillaries or microaneurysms into the retinal tissue or its accumulation within cystoid spaces (fig. 1). Fluorescein angiography is also useful to identify macular capillary non-perfusion, which may be combined with DME (fig. 2).

Profound change in the diagnosis and management of DME has occurred since the advent of optical coherence tomography (OCT). In the case of DME, OCT demonstrates increased retinal thickness with areas of low intraretinal reflectivity prevailing in the outer retinal layers and loss of foveal depression. OCT seems particularly useful to detect a feature combined with macular edema that is not easily seen on biomicroscopy – serous macular retinal detachment (fig. 3). It is seen in 15% of eyes with DME [5]. OCT may also show disruption in the line of the junction between inner and outer-segment photoreceptors, which is an indicator of poor visual prognosis and seems particularly relevant to analyze the vitreomacular relationship [6–8].

One major advantage of OCT is that it allows measurement of retinal thickness from tomograms by means of computer image processing

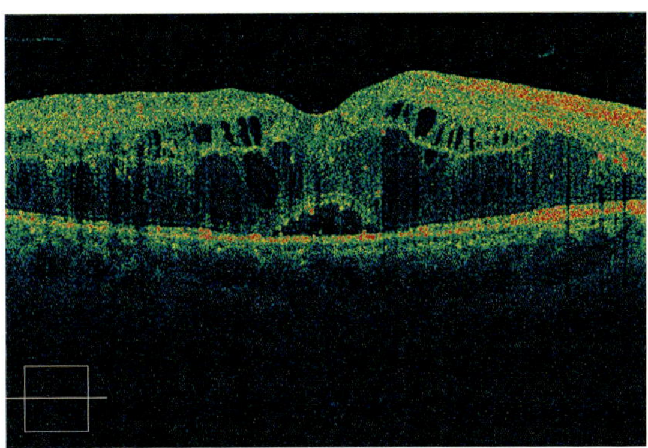

Fig. 3. OCT: serous retinal detachment in cystoid DME. There is diffuse retinal thickening with numerous cystic spaces associated with a shallow elevation of the neuroretina, which is seen as an optically clear space between the retina and the RPE.

techniques allowing the reliability and good reproducibility of such measurements [9–11]. OCT is thus an accurate tool to follow the spontaneous evolution of DME, as well as its response to treatments.

Screening

Timing and frequency of eye examinations in people with diabetes are often individualized. In high-risk patients (e.g. those with long-term diabetes or poor systemic risk-factor control), even in the absence of retinopathy, examination at least once per year is recommended [12]. For children with prepubertal diabetes, beginning retinopathy screening at puberty might be appropriate [13–15]. A comprehensive eye examination might be warranted for pregnant women with non-gestational diabetes during the first trimester, with follow-up throughout pregnancy in the presence of retinopathy. Regular eye examinations might also be appropriate for their positive psychosocial effects on the care of patients with diabetes (e.g. education about risk factors and compliance) [16].

Systemic Therapy

Guidelines for the optimum eye care of patients with diabetes are tight glycemic and blood pressure control as well as anemia, hyperlipidemia, and all causes of intravascular fluid overload (congestive heart failure, renal failure, hypoalbuminemia) [17]. The target glycemia and blood pressure levels for effective prevention of retinopathy development and progression and the potential effect of some hypoglycemic and blood pressure-lowering agents have been established based on numerous well-designed studied.

Glycemic Control

Hyperglycemia instigates a cascade of events that eventually leads to development of DR. The DCCT and the United Kingdom Prospective Diabetes Study (UKPDS) provided strong evidence that tight control of glycemia (glycated hemoglobin, HbA1c, 7%) reduces the risk of development and progression of DR in both type 1 and type 2 diabetes [12]. Although a small risk of initial worsening of retinopathy at the onset of therapy exists, every percent reduction in HbA1c lowers risk of retinopathy by 30–40% [18, 19]. The stability of beneficial effect over time can be achieved as HbA1c is maintained at target values for as long as possible [20].

A recent meta-analysis of three large population-based studies of DR showed a graded relation between the level of glycemia and frequency of retinopathy signs, suggesting that further reduction in glycemic levels might have additional benefits for retinopathy in people with diabetes [21].

The Action in Diabetes and Vascular Disease (ADVANCE) trial and data from the Veterans Affairs Diabetes Trial (VADT) showed aggressive glycemic control did not confirm any beneficial effect on the development or progression of retinopathy in type 2 diabetes [22, 23]. Even more, such aggressive glycemic control could be associated with increased mortality [24]. Although these findings contrast with those from the UKPDS, they could be related to population differences (97% men in VADT), length of follow-up (shorter in VADT), and timing of therapy (later in VADT) [25].

Blood Pressure Control

Epidemiological studies and clinical trials strongly support hypertension as an important modifiable risk factor for DR. In the UKPDS study, tight blood pressure control reduced the risks of retinopathy progression, visual loss, and the need for laser treatment in people with type 2 diabetes [12] (fig. 4). Every 10 mm Hg increase in systolic blood pressure is associated with roughly 10% excess risk of early DR and a 15% excess risk of proliferative retinopathy [26, 27]. A long-term maintenance of blood pressure control leads to a sustainable visual function benefit [28].

Some blood pressure-lowering drugs, such as rennin angiotensin inhibitors, could have benefits beyond their blood pressure-lowering effects. The EURODIAB Controlled Trial of Lisinopril in Insulin-Dependent Diabetes Mellitus (EUCLID) study showed that lisinopril reduced the risk of retinopathy progression by 50% and proliferative retinopathy by 80% [29]. In the Diabetic Retinopathy Candesartan Trials (DIRECT), candesartan reduced risk of retinopathy development by 18–35% in type 1 diabetes, and increased regression of retinopathy by 34% in type 2 diabetes [30, 31].

In the Renin-Angiotensin System Study (RASS), enalapril reduced the risk of retinopathy progression by 65% and losartan by 70% in type 1 diabetes independent of changes in blood pressure during the trial [32]. These data suggest that drugs targeting the renin-angiotensin system might be better than other blood pressure-lowering drugs for reduction of retinopathy risk.

Lipid-Lowering Therapy

Findings indicating an association of the severity of retinopathy with increasing triglycerides and inversely association with HDL cholesterol [33] suggest a potential role of dyslipidemia in the pathogenesis of DR. Fenofibrate, a lipid-modifying agent, reduced the need for laser treatment of vision-threatening DR by 31% in patients with type 2 diabetes [34].

New systemic therapies have been investigated on the basis of their potential roles in the pathogenesis inhibition of DR. For numerous systemic therapeutic strategies focusing on the biochemical pathways underlying DR, such as protein kinase C, formation of advanced glycation end products, erythropoietin, growth hormone and insulin growth factor inhibitors, their effectiveness has not been established [12].

Laser Photocoagulation

Randomized studies have clearly demonstrated the efficacy of laser photocoagulation to prevent vision loss from DME [35–37]. In the ETDRS, eyes with nonproliferative DR and macular edema were randomly assigned to early focal/grid photocoagulation or nonphotocoagulation. After 3 years of follow-up, 24% of the control group lost three lines of the ETDRS visual acuity chart compared with 12% of the treated eye reducing by 50% the risk of moderate visual loss from clinically significant macular edema. In eyes with diffuse DME, more than 15% of patients go on losing vision despite previous laser photocoagulation [37]. In eyes observed with clinically significant DME [35, 38], prompt photocoagulation is highly recommended.

More recently, the Diabetic Retinopathy Clinical Research Network (DRCR.net) showed that about 30% of patients given macular laser gained better vision (≥10 letters) over a 2-year period [39]. As the DRCR.net included a mixture

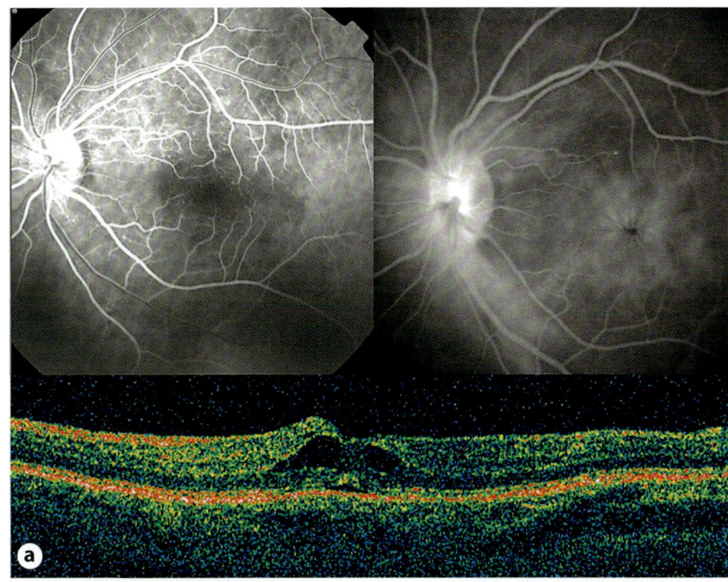

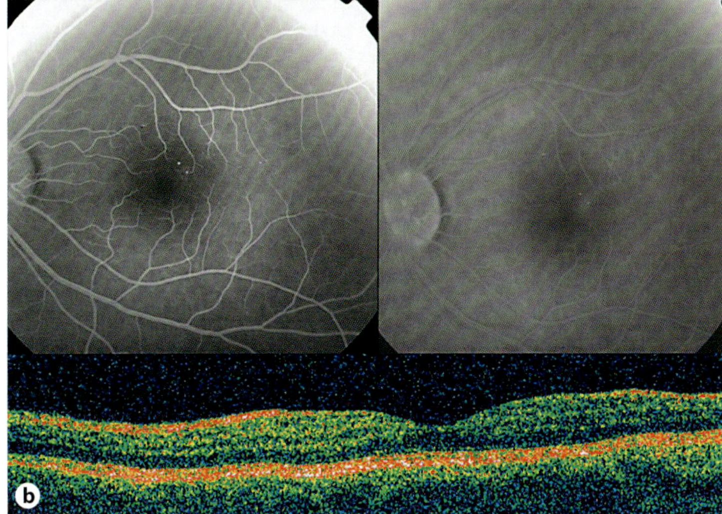

Fig. 4. a Top left: Intermediate-phase fluorescein angiography. There is a dilated capillary bed adjacent to the optic nerve but no microangiopathy at the macula. Top right: Late-phase fluorescein angiography shows diffuse leakage at the macular area with accumulation of the dye within central cysts, and optic nerve head. The presence of diffuse leakage despite the absence of sufficient microvascular abnormalities implicates the presence of breakdown of the inner blood-retinal barrier that can be reversible when systemic risk factors are controlled. Bottom: Time-domain OCT shows central cystoid macular edema. **b** Fluorescein angiography and OCT were repeated when systemic arterial hypertension was treated and optimal hyperglycemia control achieved. No other treatment was applied for the management of this case of DME. Top left: Intermediate-phase fluorescein angiography. There are two microaneurysms at the foveal zone. Top right: Late-phase fluorescein angiography showing minimal leakage from microaneurysms. Note that there is no more diffuse leakage at the macular area or optic nerve head. Bottom: Time-domain OCT shows resolution of previous cystoid macular edema.

of patients with focal or diffuse macular edema, the relative efficacy of laser treatment for specific patterns of macular edema remains unclear, although laser photocoagulation appears to be more effective for focal (fig. 5) than diffuse DME.

Focal or grid macular laser photocoagulation may also be associated with severe side effects such as laser burns to the fovea, enlargement of laser scars over time, choroidal neovascularization, and subretinal fibrosis.

The exact mechanism of action of laser photocoagulation is not known. It may be due to an enhanced proliferation of RPE and endothelial cells leading to a restoration of the blood-retinal barrier [40], or a better oxygenation of the inner

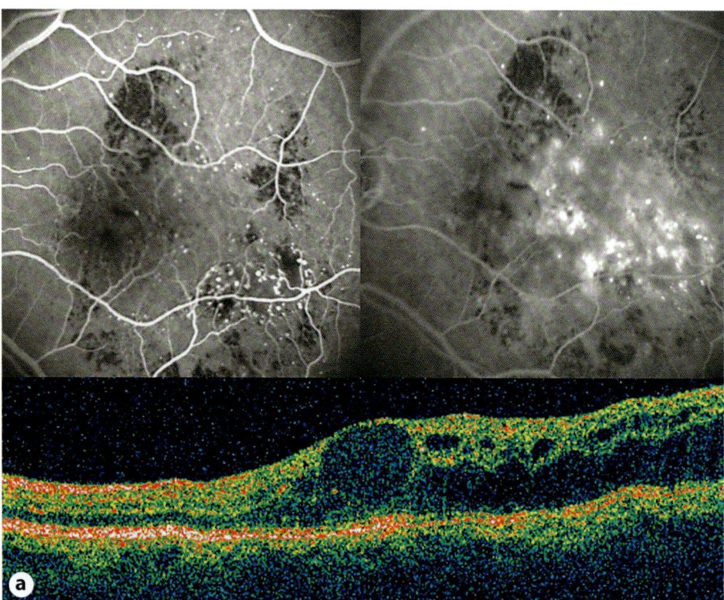

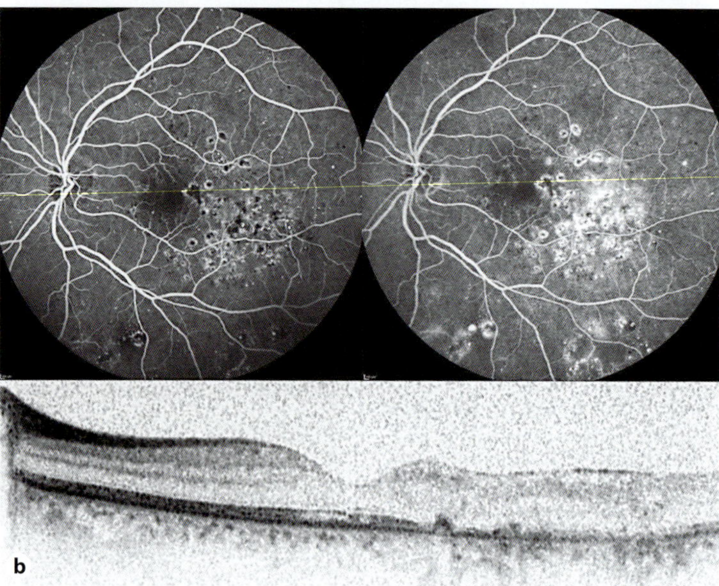

Fig. 5. a Top left: Early-phase fluorescein angiography. There are numerous microaneurysms associated with hard exudates and a zone of capillary dropout. Top right: Late-phase fluorescein angiography showing leakage from the microaneurysms. Bottom: OCT shows a central cyst associated with diffuse retinal thickening temporal to the fovea. **b** Same patient as in figure 5a, 3 months following treatment. Treatment consisted of an intravitreal injection of ranibizumab followed by two consecutive sessions of focal laser on the leaking microaneurysms. Top left: Early phase fluorescein angiography. There are several hypofluorescent spots corresponding to the laser burns. Top right: Late-phase fluorescein angiography. There is absence of leakage. Bottom: OCT shows resolution of DME.

retina from the choroidal circulation after destruction of oxygen-consuming photoreceptors [41, 42]. A retinal vasoconstriction has indeed been observed after grid laser photocoagulation for DME [43, 44], restoring the regulation of the retinal blood flow [45].

Intravitreal Treatments

The drawbacks and side effects of laser photocoagulation have led to the search for alternative treatments for DME. They include intravitreal injection of steroids or anti-vascular endothelial growth factor (VEGF) drugs, combined intravitreal triamcinolone or ranibizumab and laser photocoagulation (fig. 5) and vitrectomy. Steroids act by reducing vascular permeability; indeed, steroids stabilize endothelial tight junctions and increase their numbers. Steroids also suppress inflammation and inhibit the migration of leukocytes. They may also inhibit production of the VEGF [46–48]. Extensive data have established that VEGF is involved in the vascular permeability observed in DR [49, 50]. These data support the use of anti-VEGF therapy for diffuse DME.

Intravitreal Injections of Triamcinolone Acetonide

Several studies have shown the efficacy of intravitreal injections of triamcinolone acetonide to reduce DME temporarily and increase visual acuity (fig. 6) [3, 4, 51–53]. However, recurrence of DME occurs 3–6 months after injection. Side effects of intravitreal injections of triamcinolone acetonide include ocular hypertension in up to 50% of patients, glaucoma requiring surgery in 2%, and cataract surgery in 54% within 2 years of injection [4].

Recently, the DRCR.net comparing the efficacy and safety of 1- and 4-mg doses of preservative-free intravitreal triamcinolone in comparison with focal/grid laser photocoagulation in patients with DME showed that, over a 2- and 3-year period, focal/grid laser photocoagulation is more effective and has fewer side effects than triamcinolone [39, 54].

The few clinical trials on long-acting steroid implants (fluocinolone acetonide or dexamethasone) also reported short-term vision improvements [55, 56].

A recent systematic review reported that although intravitreal triamcinolone improves vision in eyes with refractory diabetic macular edema in the short-term (3 months), the benefits are not long lasting [57]. Nevertheless, intravitreal triamcinolone might have a role as an adjunctive therapy to laser [58].

Intravitreal Injections of Anti-VEGF

Pegaptanib is an anti-VEGF aptamer, binds to VEGF165, sequestering it and preventing VEGF receptor activation. A phase II trial evaluating the efficacy and safety of injections of three doses (0.3, 1, and 3 mg) of pegaptanib versus placebo every 6 weeks has shown interesting results, with better median visual acuity in the group treated with 0.3 mg as compared with sham. The pegaptanib-treated eyes were more likely to show reduction in central retinal thickness, and were deemed less likely to require additional therapy with photocoagulation at week 36 [59].

Ranibizumab, which is a recombinant humanized monoclonal antibody fragment with specificity for all isoforms of human VEGF, is also under investigation for DME.

A phase II trial investigating the efficacy and safety of two concentrations of intravitreal ranibizumab (0.3 and 0.5 mg) in patients with DME with center involvement, compared with sham, showed that at month 12 eyes treated with ranibizumab had a mean ± SD best corrected visual acuity (BCVA) improvement from baseline by 10.3 ± 9.1 letters, and mean central retinal thickness reduction by 194.2 ± 135.1 µm; a gain of ≥10 letters BCVA from baseline occurred in 60.8%, suggesting ranibizumab is effective in improving BCVA and well tolerated in DME [60]. A similar effect of ranibizumab on the visual outcome of DME was also observed in the READ II trial; in addition, when combined with focal or grid laser treatments, the amount of residual edema was reduced, as was the frequency of injections needed to control edema [61].

Combined Intravitreal Triamcinolone or Ranibizumab and Laser Photocoagulation

A study by the DRCR.net [62] evaluated the effect of ranibizumab on diabetic macular edema.

This randomized trial compared sham injection + prompt laser, 0.5 mg ranibizumab + prompt

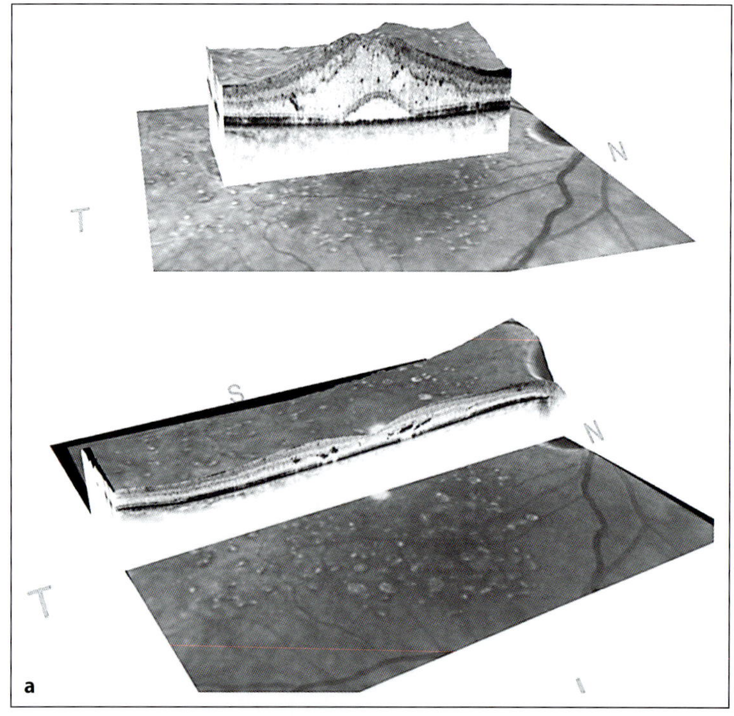

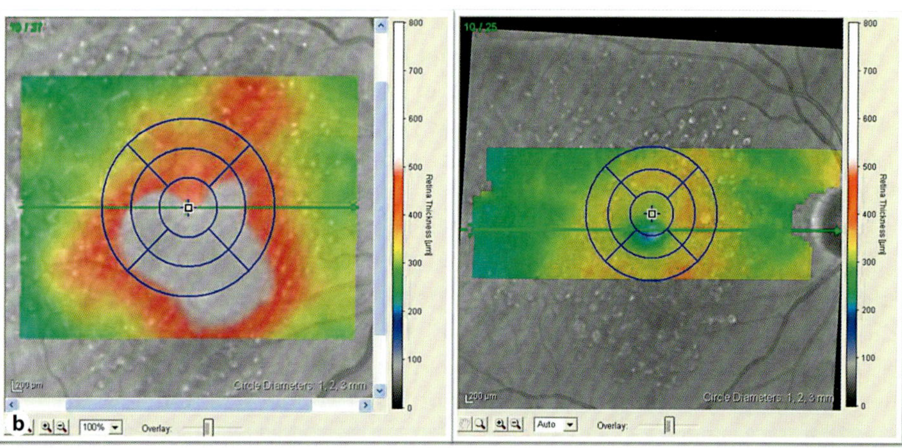

Fig. 6. **a** Top: 3D-OCT (Spectralis) of DME refractive to previous complete laser photocoagulation. OCT shows cystoid macular edema with serous retinal detachment. Visual acuity was 0.2 (Snellen scale). This patient was treated with intravitreal injection of 4 mg of triamcinolone. Bottom: Three weeks after an intravitreal injection of triamcinolone, there is a marked decrease in retinal thickness with restoration of normal foveal profile. Visual acuity improved to 0.6 Snellen. **b** OCT retinal thickness map. Same patient as in figure 6a. Central retinal thickness was 597 μm (left); it decreased to 290 μm (right) 3 weeks following an intravitreal injection of 4 mg of triamcinolone.

laser, 0.5 mg ranibizumab + deferred (≥24 weeks) laser, or 4 mg triamcinolone + prompt laser, in patients with diabetic macular edema. Over the first year, there was an approximate one line extra vision gained over laser therapy in the ranibizumab group. Improvement of vision was twice as frequent in the ranibizumab group (50% for two lines and 30% for three lines or more) as in the laser group (28 and 15%). Importantly, eyes treated with laser and ranibizumab (3–4%) were less likely to have marked visual loss (two line or more) than those treated with laser therapy alone (13%). The favorable visual outcome appears to sustain into the 2nd year, although only about 60% of patients had so far been assessed for 2 years. Furthermore, there were no systemic safety concerns demonstrated.

Another phase III randomized trial compared the effect of intravitreal 0.5 mg ranibizumab with active (same day) laser and laser alone for the treatment of DME at 12 months [RESTORE trial]. There was a mean increase of 6.9 ETDRS letters in the ranibizumab group, 6.4 ETDRS letters in the ranibizumab + laser group and 0.9 ETDRS letters in the laser group. Central macular thickness decreased by 118.7, 128.3 and 61.3 µm, respectively. The results were equally effective for both focal and diffuse DME. At 1 year, no differences were detected between the ranibizumab and ranibizumab + laser arms [63].

Combining intravitreal drugs with laser photocoagulation seems to reduce the amount of residual edema as well as the frequency of injections needed to control edema [61]. In addition, fewer rescue macular laser procedures are necessary in ranibizumab-treated patients [64].

Anti-VEGF therapy alone or in association with laser treatment has promising clinical applications for management of DR; its long-term safety in patients with diabetes was overall similar among the sham and ranibizumab groups. Additional follow-up of patients will provide further long-term guidance on systemic safety.

References

1 Klein R, Klein BE, Moss SE, Davis MD, DeMets DL: The Wisconsin epidemiologic study of diabetic retinopathy. IV. Diabetic macular edema. Ophthalmology 1984;91:1464–1474.
2 Polito A, Del Borrello M, Polini G, Furlan F, Isola M, Bandello F: Diurnal variation in clinically significant diabetic macular edema measured by the Stratus OCT. Retina 2006;26:14–20.
3 Audren F, Erginay A, Haouchine B, Benosman R, Conrath J, Bergmann JF, Gaudric A, Massin P: Intravitreal triamcinolone acetonide for diffuse diabetic macular oedema: 6-month results of a prospective controlled trial. Acta Ophthalmol Scand 2006;84:624–630.
4 Gillies MC, Sutter FK, Simpson JM, Larsson J, Ali H, Zhu M: Intravitreal triamcinolone for refractory diabetic macular edema: two-year results of a double-masked, placebo-controlled, randomized clinical trial. Ophthalmology 2006;113:1533–1538.
5 Otani T, Kishi S, Maruyama Y: Patterns of diabetic macular edema with optical coherence tomography. Am J Ophthalmol 1999;127:688–693.
6 Gaucher D, Tadayoni R, Erginay A, Haouchine B, Gaudric A, Massin P: Optical coherence tomography assessment of the vitreoretinal relationship in diabetic macular edema. Am J Ophthalmol 2005;139:807–813.
7 Lewis H, Abrams GW, Blumenkranz MS, Campo RV: Vitrectomy for diabetic macular traction and edema associated with posterior hyaloidal traction. Ophthalmology 1992;99:753–759.
8 Massin P, Duguid G, Erginay A, Haouchine B, Gaudric A: Optical coherence tomography for evaluating diabetic macular edema before and after vitrectomy. Am J Ophthalmol 2003;135:169–177.
9 Massin P, Vicaut E, Haouchine B, Erginay A, Paques M, Gaudric A: Reproducibility of retinal mapping using optical coherence tomography. Arch Ophthalmol 2001;119:1135–1142.
10 Polito A, Del Borrello M, Isola M, Zemella N, Bandello F: Repeatability and reproducibility of fast macular thickness mapping with stratus optical coherence tomography. Arch Ophthalmol 2005;123:1330–1337.
11 Krzystolik MG, Strauber SF, Aiello LP, Beck RW, Berger BB, Bressler NM, Browning DJ, Chambers RB, Danis RP, Davis MD, Glassman AR, Gonzalez VH, Greenberg PB, Gross JG, Kim JE, Kollman C: Reproducibility of macular thickness and volume using Zeiss optical coherence tomography in patients with diabetic macular edema. Ophthalmology 2007;114:1520–1525.
12 Mohamed Q, Gillies MC, Wong TY: Management of diabetic retinopathy: a systematic review. Jama 2007;298:902–916.
13 Klein BE, Moss SE, Klein R: Is menarche associated with diabetic retinopathy? Diabetes Care 1990;13:1034–1038.

14 Donaghue KC, Fairchild JM, Craig ME, Chan AK, Hing S, Cutler LR, Howard NJ, Silink M: Do all prepubertal years of diabetes duration contribute equally to diabetes complications? Diabetes Care 2003;26:1224–1229.

15 Olsen BS, Sjolie AK, Hougaard P, Johannesen J, Marinelli K, Jacobsen BB, Mortensen HB: The significance of the prepubertal diabetes duration for the development of retinopathy and nephropathy in patients with type 1 diabetes. J Diabetes Complications 2004;18:160–164.

16 Fong DS, Aiello LP, Ferris FL, 3rd, Klein R: Diabetic retinopathy. Diabetes Care 2004;27:2540–2553.

17 Gardner TW, Antonetti DA, Barber AJ, LaNoue KF, Levison SW: Diabetic retinopathy: more than meets the eye. Surv Ophthalmol 2002;47 Suppl 2:S253–262.

18 Early worsening of diabetic retinopathy in the Diabetes Control and Complications Trial. Arch Ophthalmol 1998;116:874–886.

19 White NH, Sun W, Cleary PA, Danis RP, Davis MD, Hainsworth DP, Hubbard LD, Lachin JM, Nathan DM: Prolonged effect of intensive therapy on the risk of retinopathy complications in patients with type 1 diabetes mellitus: 10 years after the Diabetes Control and Complications Trial. Arch Ophthalmol 2008;126:1707–1715.

20 White NH, Sun W, Cleary PA, Tamborlane WV, Danis RP, Hainsworth DP, Davis MD: Effect of prior intensive therapy in type 1 diabetes on 10-year progression of retinopathy in the DCCT/EDIC: comparison of adults and adolescents. Diabetes 2010;59:1244–1253.

21 Wong TY, Liew G, Tapp RJ, Schmidt MI, Wang JJ, Mitchell P, Klein R, Klein BE, Zimmet P, Shaw J: Relation between fasting glucose and retinopathy for diagnosis of diabetes: three population-based cross-sectional studies. Lancet 2008;371:736–743.

22 Patel A, MacMahon S, Chalmers J, Neal B, Billot L, Woodward M, Marre M, Cooper M, Glasziou P, Grobbee D, Hamet P, Harrap S, Heller S, Liu L, Mancia G, Mogensen CE, Pan C, Poulter N, Rodgers A, Williams B, Bompoint S, de Galan BE, Joshi R, Travert F: Intensive blood glucose control and vascular outcomes in patients with type 2 diabetes. N Engl J Med 2008;358:2560–2572.

23 Duckworth W, Abraira C, Moritz T, Reda D, Emanuele N, Reaven PD, Zieve FJ, Marks J, Davis SN, Hayward R, Warren SR, Goldman S, McCarren M, Vitek ME, Henderson WG, Huang GD: Glucose control and vascular complications in veterans with type 2 diabetes. N Engl J Med 2009;360:129–139.

24 Gerstein HC, Miller ME, Byington RP, Goff DC, Jr., Bigger JT, Buse JB, Cushman WC, Genuth S, Ismail-Beigi F, Grimm RH, Jr., Probstfield JL, Simons-Morton DG, Friedewald WT: Effects of intensive glucose lowering in type 2 diabetes. N Engl J Med 2008;358:2545–2559.

25 Cheung N, Mitchell P, Wong TY: Diabetic retinopathy. Lancet 2010;376:124–136.

26 Klein R, Knudtson MD, Lee KE, Gangnon R, Klein BE: The Wisconsin Epidemiologic Study of Diabetic Retinopathy: XXII the twenty-five-year progression of retinopathy in persons with type 1 diabetes. Ophthalmology 2008;115:1859–1868.

27 Gallego PH, Craig ME, Hing S, Donaghue KC: Role of blood pressure in development of early retinopathy in adolescents with type 1 diabetes: prospective cohort study. Bmj 2008;337:a918.

28 Holman RR, Paul SK, Bethel MA, Neil HA, Matthews DR: Long-term follow-up after tight control of blood pressure in type 2 diabetes. N Engl J Med 2008;359:1565–1576.

29 Chaturvedi N, Sjolie AK, Stephenson JM, Abrahamian H, Keipes M, Castellarin A, Rogulja-Pepeonik Z, Fuller JH: Effect of lisinopril on progression of retinopathy in normotensive people with type 1 diabetes. The EUCLID Study Group. EURODIAB Controlled Trial of Lisinopril in Insulin-Dependent Diabetes Mellitus. Lancet 1998;351:28–31.

30 Chaturvedi N, Porta M, Klein R, Orchard T, Fuller J, Parving HH, Bilous R, Sjolie AK: Effect of candesartan on prevention (DIRECT-Prevent 1) and progression (DIRECT-Protect 1) of retinopathy in type 1 diabetes: randomised, placebo-controlled trials. Lancet 2008;372:1394–1402.

31 Sjolie AK, Klein R, Porta M, Orchard T, Fuller J, Parving HH, Bilous R, Chaturvedi N: Effect of candesartan on progression and regression of retinopathy in type 2 diabetes (DIRECT-Protect 2): a randomised placebo-controlled trial. Lancet 2008;372:1385–1393.

32 Mauer M, Zinman B, Gardiner R, Suissa S, Sinaiko A, Strand T, Drummond K, Donnelly S, Goodyer P, Gubler MC, Klein R: Renal and retinal effects of enalapril and losartan in type 1 diabetes. N Engl J Med 2009;361:40–51.

33 Lyons TJ, Jenkins AJ, Zheng D, Lackland DT, McGee D, Garvey WT, Klein RL: Diabetic retinopathy and serum lipoprotein subclasses in the DCCT/EDIC cohort. Invest Ophthalmol Vis Sci 2004;45:910–918.

34 Keech AC, Mitchell P, Summanen PA, O'Day J, Davis TM, Moffitt MS, Taskinen MR, Simes RJ, Tse D, Williamson E, Merrifield A, Laatikainen LT, d'Emden MC, Crimet DC, O'Connell RL, Colman PG: Effect of fenofibrate on the need for laser treatment for diabetic retinopathy (FIELD study): a randomised controlled trial. Lancet 2007;370:1687–1697.

35 Photocoagulation for diabetic macular edema. Early Treatment Diabetic Retinopathy Study report number 1. Early Treatment Diabetic Retinopathy Study research group. Arch Ophthalmol 1985;103:1796–1806.

36 Olk RJ: Modified grid argon (blue-green) laser photocoagulation for diffuse diabetic macular edema. Ophthalmology 1986;93:938–950.

37 Olk RJ: Argon green (514 nm) versus krypton red (647 nm) modified grid laser photocoagulation for diffuse diabetic macular edema. Ophthalmology 1990;97:1101–1112; discussion 1112–1113.

38 Wilkinson CP, Ferris FL, 3rd, Klein RE, Lee PP, Agardh CD, Davis M, Dills D, Kampik A, Pararajasegaram R, Verdaguer JT: Proposed international clinical diabetic retinopathy and diabetic macular edema disease severity scales. Ophthalmology 2003;110:1677–1682.

39 A randomized trial comparing intravitreal triamcinolone acetonide and focal/grid photocoagulation for diabetic macular edema. Ophthalmology 2008;115:1447–1449, 1449 e1441–1410.

40 Wallow IH, Bindley CD: Focal photocoagulation of diabetic macular edema. A clinicopathologic case report. Retina 1988;8:261–269.

41 Stefansson E, Machemer R, de Juan E, Jr., McCuen BW, 2nd, Peterson J: Retinal oxygenation and laser treatment in patients with diabetic retinopathy. Am J Ophthalmol 1992;113:36–38.

42 Pournaras CJ, Tsacopoulos M, Strommer K, Gilodi N, Leuenberger PM: Scatter photocoagulation restores tissue hypoxia in experimental vasoproliferative microangiopathy in miniature pigs. Ophthalmology 1990;97:1329–1333.

43 Gottfredsdottir MS, Stefansson E, Jonasson F, Gislason I: Retinal vasoconstriction after laser treatment for diabetic macular edema. Am J Ophthalmol 1993;115:64–67.

44 Mendrinos E, Mangioris G, Papadopoulou DN, Dosso AA, Pournaras CJ: Retinal vessel analyzer measurements of the effect of panretinal photocoagulation on the retinal arteriolar diameter in diabetic retinopathy. Retina 2010;30:555–561.

45 Grunwald JE, Brucker AJ, Petrig BL, Riva CE: Retinal blood flow regulation and the clinical response to panretinal photocoagulation in proliferative diabetic retinopathy. Ophthalmology 1989;96:1518–1522.

46 Antonetti DA, Wolpert EB, DeMaio L, Harhaj NS, Scaduto RC, Jr.: Hydrocortisone decreases retinal endothelial cell water and solute flux coincident with increased content and decreased phosphorylation of occludin. J Neurochem 2002;80:667–677.

47 Brooks HL, Jr., Caballero S, Jr., Newell CK, Steinmetz RL, Watson D, Segal MS, Harrison JK, Scott EW, Grant MB: Vitreous levels of vascular endothelial growth factor and stromal-derived factor 1 in patients with diabetic retinopathy and cystoid macular edema before and after intraocular injection of triamcinolone. Arch Ophthalmol 2004;122:1801–1807.

48 Edelman JL, Lutz D, Castro MR: Corticosteroids inhibit VEGF-induced vascular leakage in a rabbit model of blood-retinal and blood-aqueous barrier breakdown. Exp Eye Res 2005;80:249–258.

49 Aiello LP, Avery RL, Arrigg PG, Keyt BA, Jampel HD, Shah ST, Pasquale LR, Thieme H, Iwamoto MA, Park JE, et al.: Vascular endothelial growth factor in ocular fluid of patients with diabetic retinopathy and other retinal disorders. N Engl J Med 1994;331:1480–1487.

50 Funatsu H, Yamashita H, Noma H, Mimura T, Yamashita T, Hori S: Increased levels of vascular endothelial growth factor and interleukin-6 in the aqueous humor of diabetics with macular edema. Am J Ophthalmol 2002;133:70–77.

51 Massin P, Audren F, Haouchine B, Erginay A, Bergmann JF, Benosman R, Caulin C, Gaudric A: Intravitreal triamcinolone acetonide for diabetic diffuse macular edema: preliminary results of a prospective controlled trial. Ophthalmology 2004;111:218–224; discussion 224–215.

52 Martidis A, Duker JS, Greenberg PB, Rogers AH, Puliafito CA, Reichel E, Baumal C: Intravitreal triamcinolone for refractory diabetic macular edema. Ophthalmology 2002;109:920–927.

53 Jonas JB, Kamppeter BA, Harder B, Vossmerbaeumer U, Sauder G, Spandau UH: Intravitreal triamcinolone acetonide for diabetic macular edema: a prospective, randomized study. J Ocul Pharmacol Ther 2006;22:200–207.

54 Beck RW, Edwards AR, Aiello LP, Bressler NM, Ferris F, Glassman AR, Hartnett E, Ip MS, Kim JE, Kollman C: Three-year follow-up of a randomized trial comparing focal/grid photocoagulation and intravitreal triamcinolone for diabetic macular edema. Arch Ophthalmol 2009;127:245–251.

55 Haller JA, Kuppermann BD, Blumenkranz MS, Williams GA, Weinberg DV, Chou C, Whitcup SM: Randomized controlled trial of an intravitreous dexamethasone drug delivery system in patients with diabetic macular edema. Arch Ophthalmol 2010;128:289–296.

56 Campochiaro PA, Hafiz G, Shah SM, Bloom S, Brown DM, Busquets M, Ciulla T, Feiner L, Sabates N, Billman K, Kapik B, Green K, Kane F: Sustained ocular delivery of fluocinolone acetonide by an intravitreal insert. Ophthalmology 2010;117:1393–1399 e1393.

57 Yilmaz T, Weaver CD, Gallagher MJ, Cordero-Coma M, Cervantes-Castaneda RA, Klisovic D, Lavaque AJ, Larson RJ: Intravitreal triamcinolone acetonide injection for treatment of refractory diabetic macular edema: a systematic review. Ophthalmology 2009;116:902–911; quiz 912–903.

58 Maia OO, Jr., Takahashi BS, Costa RA, Scott IU, Takahashi WY: Combined laser and intravitreal triamcinolone for proliferative diabetic retinopathy and macular edema: one-year results of a randomized clinical trial. Am J Ophthalmol 2009;147:291–297 e292.

59 Cunningham ET, Jr., Adamis AP, Altaweel M, Aiello LP, Bressler NM, D'Amico DJ, Goldbaum M, Guyer DR, Katz B, Patel M, Schwartz SD: A phase II randomized double-masked trial of pegaptanib, an anti-vascular endothelial growth factor aptamer, for diabetic macular edema. Ophthalmology 2005;112:1747–1757.

60 Massin P, Bandello F, Garweg JG, Hansen LL, Harding SP, Larsen M, Mitchell P, Sharp D, Wolf-Schnurrbusch UE, Gekkieva M, Weichselberger A, Wolf S: Safety and efficacy of ranibizumab in diabetic macular edema (RESOLVE Study): a 12-month, randomized, controlled, double-masked, multicenter phase II study. Diabetes Care 2010;33:2399–2405.

61 Nguyen QD, Shah SM, Khwaja AA, Channa R, Hatef E, Do DV, Boyer D, Heier JS, Abraham P, Thach AB, Lit ES, Foster BS, Kruger E, Dugel P, Chang T, Das A, Ciulla TA, Pollack JS, Lim JI, Eliot D, Campochiaro PA: Two-year outcomes of the ranibizumab for edema of the macula in diabetes (READ-2) study. Ophthalmology 2010;117:2146–2151.

62 Elman MJ, Aiello LP, Beck RW, Bressler NM, Bressler SB, Edwards AR, Ferris FL, 3rd, Friedman SM, Glassman AR, Miller KM, Scott IU, Stockdale CR, Sun JK: Randomized trial evaluating ranibizumab plus prompt or deferred laser or triamcinolone plus prompt laser for diabetic macular edema. Ophthalmology 2010;117:1064–1077

63 Mitchell P, Bandello F, Schmidt-Erfurth U, Lang GE, Massin P, Schlingemann RO, Sutter F, Simader C, Burian G, Gerstner O, Weichselberger A: The RESTORE study: ranibizumab monotherapy or combined with laser versus laser monotherapy for diabetic macular edema. Ophthalmology 2011;118:615–625.

64 Nguyen QD, Brown DM, Marcus DM, Boyer DS, Patel S, Feiner L, Gibson A, Sy J, Rundle AC, Hopkins JJ, Rubio RG, Ehrlich JS: Ranibizumab for Diabetic Macular Edema: Results from 2 Phase III Randomized Trials: RISE and RIDE. Ophthalmology 2012;119:789–801.

Constantin J. Pournaras, MD
Department of Ophthalmology, Vitreo-Retinal Unit, Geneva University Hospitals
22 rue Alcide-Jentzer
CH-12 11 Geneva 14 (Switzerland)
E-Mail constantin.pournaras@hcuge.ch

Bandello F, Battaglia Parodi M (eds): Surgical Retina.
ESASO Course Series. Basel, Karger, 2012, vol 2, pp 46–57

Use of Anti-Vascular Endothelial Growth Factor Drugs for Diabetic Macular Edema

B. Falcomatà[a] · Maurizio Battaglia Parodi[b] · P. Iacono[c] · G. Guarnaccia[a] · F. Bandello[b]

[a]UOC di Oculistica, Azienda Ospedaliera 'Bianchi, Melacrino, Morelli', Reggio Calabria, [b]Department of Ophthalmology, University Vita-Salute, Scientific Institute San Raffaele, Milan, and [c]Fondazione GB Bietti per l'Oftalmologia, IRCCS, Rome, Italy

Abstract

Diabetic macular edema (DME) represents the most common cause of vision loss in patients affected by diabetes mellitus. Diabetic retinopathy has a significant impact on public health and the quality of life of many patients, and thus requires noteworthy consideration. The first line of treatment remains the management of systemic risk factors, but is often insufficient in controlling DME. For 25 years, the focal/grid laser photocoagulation was considered the standard of care for DME. Laser treatment reduces the risk of moderate visual loss by approximately 50%, but it is not associated with remarkable effects on visual improvement. Lately, new approaches in the treatment of DME have been considered; in particular the employment of anti-vascular endothelial growth factor (anti-VEGF) drugs. VEGF is a pluripotent growth factor that functions as a vasopermeability factor and an endothelial cell mitogen, and thereby represents an appealing candidate as a therapeutic target for the treatment of DME. Recent trials have been investigating many anti-VEGF agents in the treatment of DME. The goal of this review is to present the evidence behind the use of anti-VEGF drugs in the treatment of DME.

Diabetic retinopathy is the leading cause of acquired blindness among young adults throughout developed countries [1, 2]. The World Health Organization estimates that about 171 million of persons are affected by diabetes with a likely doubling of the prevalence within 20 years [3].

Diabetic macular edema (DME) is the most common vision-threatening manifestation of diabetic retinopathy. Within 20 years of diagnosis of diabetes, DME affects almost 30% of patients with either type 1 or 2 of the disease [2]. DME is generally defined as retinal thickening or presence of hard exudates within one disc diameter from the center of the macula. Nowadays, we differentiate between center-involved DME and not center-involved DME if the thickening involves the center of the macula [4].

The ETDRS-modified focal/grid laser technique of photocoagulation has been the only treatment for nontractional DME since the mid-1980s. It reduces the risk of moderate vision loss by more than 50% as compared with no treatment. Nevertheless, the visual and functional prognosis in patients with DME is poor, and in spite of the modified focal-grid laser treatment, macular edema is often refractory. In particular, when examining eyes with DME treated with modified focal/grid laser, some vision improvement was demonstrated only in 15% of cases at 3-year follow-up, whereas visual acuity (VA) was unchanged in 61% and reduced in 24% of cases [5, 6]. Furthermore, laser treatment is not without potential complications. That is why we have been searching for better treatments that are able not only to stop vision loss over time but also to restore vision in a greater proportion of patients. Anti-vascular endothelial growth factor (anti-VEGF) drugs seem to fulfill these goals.

In diabetic retinopathy, the alteration of the blood retinal barrier and increased permeability are responsible for the development of DME. VEGF increases the extracellular accumulation of fluid from the intravascular compartment by disrupting the intercellular tight junctions between retinal endothelial cells [7–11]. The observation of increased intraocular VEGF levels in DME led to the hypothesis that VEGF signaling blockade might be beneficial both in restoring normal retinal anatomy and reversing vision loss from macular edema.

The pathway enclosed between VEGF gene transcription and the activation of the VEGF receptor is the object of the new therapeutic approaches based on the use of VEGF antagonists. Pegaptanib, ranibizumab, bevacizumab and VEGF-Trap are molecules able to directly bind the VEGF protein. A new and interesting therapeutic approach is the employment of bevasiranib. This molecule, interfering with messenger RNA, interrupts the synthesis of the VEGF protein. Lastly, rapamycin, employed commonly as an immunosuppressive, anti-inflammatory or antimycotic drug, reduces the activity of the VEGF molecule interfering with the promoting signal, the active synthesis of VEGF and reducing the response of endothelial cells to VEGF. The aim of this review is to present the evidence behind the use of anti-VEGF drugs for the treatment of DME.

Ranibizumab

Ranibizumab (Lucentis) is a high-affinity anti-VEGF Fab specifically designed for ophthalmic use. It binds to and neutralizes all isoforms of VEGF-A and their biologically active degradation products, and has a vitreous elimination half-life of approximately 9 days. Numerous studies confirmed its efficacy in treating DME.

RISE and RIDE were parallel, phase 3, multicenter, double-masked, sham-injection-controlled studies designed to evaluate the efficacy and safety of ranibizumab in patients with vision loss due to DME [12]. Patients were randomized to receive monthly sham injections or intravitreal injections of ranibizumab 0.3 or 0.5 mg. All patients were evaluated monthly for macular laser per protocol-specified criteria. In RISE, 377 patients were randomized to study treatment (sham, n = 127; ranibizumab 0.3 mg, n = 125; ranibizumab 0.5 mg, n = 125). In RIDE, 382 patients were randomized (sham, n = 130; ranibizumab 0.3 mg, n = 125; ranibizumab 0.5 mg, n = 127). In both studies, the median number of injections in the ranibizumab 0.3 mg and 0.5 mg groups was 24. All patients were evaluated monthly for macular laser per protocol-specified criteria, beginning at month 3. Substantially more sham-treated patients received macular laser (70–74% in the sham group vs. 19.7–39.2% in the ranibizumab group). At 24 months, the proportion of patients gaining at least three lines compared to baseline was 18.1, 44.8, and 39.2% in the RISE study and 12.3, 33.6 and 45.7% in the RIDE study in the sham, 0.3 mg ranibizumab, and 0.5 mg ranibizumab groups, respectively. The proportion of patients achieving a VA of at least 20/40 was 37.8, 60 and 63.2% in the RISE study, 34.6, 54.4, and 62.2% in the RIDE study in the sham, 0.3 mg ranibizumab, and 0.5 mg ranibizumab groups, respectively. Two-year data analysis from the two studies showed that treatment with ranibizumab was associated with rapid and statistically significant vision improvements compared with sham.

Additional benefits were noted for other measurements of VA (such as preventing moderate vision loss), and substantial improvements were seen in retinal anatomy (central retinal thickness, CRT). Ranibizumab use in DME patients was associated with low risks of ocular and systemic adverse effects (AEs), and no new significant risks were identified.

Finally, RISE and RIDE evaluated a rigorous monthly treatment regimen, which may generate the best outcomes based on known pharmacokinetics but may not be of use in clinical practice.

The efficacy of a pro re nata (PRN) treatment regimen was investigated in the RESOLVE study. The RESOLVE trial (A Randomized, Double-Masked, Multicenter, Phase 2 Study Assessing the Safety and Efficacy of Two Concentrations of Ranibizumab Compared with Non-Treatment Control for the Treatment of Diabetic Macular Edema with Center Involvement) evaluated the effect of ranibizumab on retinal edema and VA in 151 patients with clinically significant DME. Patients were randomized 1:1:1 to receive ranibizumab monotherapy at a dose of 0.3 mg (n = 51) or 0.5 mg (n = 51) or sham treatment (n = 49) for 3 consecutive months and afterwards on PRN basis for 9 months; retinal photocoagulation was offered after 3 months if disease activity persisted. The mean best-corrected VA (BCVA) increased, and mean CRT decreased continuously over the 12 months of follow-up. The groups receiving 0.3 and 0.5 mg gained, respectively, 11.8 and 8.8 letters [13], and pooled data (including both dosing regimens) showed a gain of 10.3 letters [14]. The RESOLVE study demonstrates the clinical and statistical superiority of ranibizumab loading phase + PRN treatment to sham treatment. Regarding safety, there are no imbalances in the rates of ocular and non-ocular severe AEs or AEs between patients receiving ranibizumab and sham injections. Two cases of endophthalmitis occurred. Also the rate of subjects reporting non-ocular AEs was comparable between the ranibizumab and sham arms.

The role of ranibizumab in DME was investigated in the open-label study READ-1 (Ranibizumab for Edema of the Macula in Diabetes: Phase-1) [15]. Ten patients with chronic DME received intraocular injections of 0.5 mg of ranibizumab at baseline and at 1, 2, 4, and 6 months. Mean and median values of BCVA improved at 7 months by 12.3 and 11 letters, respectively, and foveal thickness showed a significant reduction. Recently, the results of the second phase of the READ study [16, 17] (READ-2; a phase II, prospective, randomized clinical trial conducted at 14 sites in the United States) were reported. The aim of this study was to compare ranibizumab with focal/grid laser, alone or in combination. One hundred and twenty-six patients were randomized to receive 0.5 mg of ranibizumab (n = 42), focal/grid laser photocoagulation (n = 42) or a combination of 0.5 mg of ranibizumab and focal/grid laser (n = 42). At month 6, the group receiving ranibizumab alone showed a significant improvement in mean BCVA compared to patients receiving focal/grid laser. BCVA in the group receiving combined therapy was not statistically different from the other groups. A resolution of 50, 33, and 45% of excess foveal thickening was observed in the three groups, respectively. The 2-year outcomes of READ-2 showed an improvement of BCVA of 7.7, 5.1 and 6.8 letters in groups 1 (n = 33), 2 (n = 34), and 3 (n = 34), respectively. The study reported a single case of severe adverse events. One subject died of a cerebral vascular accident 6 weeks after the first ranibizumab injection. This event was considered unrelated to ranibizumab because of preexistent cardiovascular pathology and because a long period elapsed between injection and vascular event. No statistically significant differences in mean systolic and diastolic blood pressure were found between the groups. Ocular adverse events included vitreous hemorrhages in 8 patients. The visual outcomes of the READ study at month 24 were not significantly different comparing the 3 treatment groups, whereas the anatomic outcomes resulted better with fewer injections of ranibizumab in groups 2 and 3. This suggests that the additional focal/grid laser treatment in groups 2 and 3 helped to reduce persistent or recurrent macular edema and helped to reduce the number of required ranibizumab injections.

The RESTORE study [18] (A 12-month, randomized, double-masked, multicenter, laser-controlled phase III study) included 345 patients affected by DME randomized to three groups: ranibizumab and sham laser (n = 116), ranibizumab and laser photocoagulation (n = 118), or sham injections and laser (n = 111). Ranibizumab/sham was given for 3 months and then on a PRN basis; laser/sham laser was performed at baseline, then PRN at intervals of at least 3 months and in accordance with ETDRS guidelines. After 12 months, a significantly greater proportion of patients had a BCVA letter score ≥15 and BCVA letter score level >73 (20/40 Snellen equivalent) with ranibizumab (22.6 and 53%, respectively) and ranibizumab + laser (22.9 and 44.9%) versus laser (8.2 and 23.6%); no significant differences were detected between ranibizumab monotherapy and ranibizumab associated with laser photocoagulation. All the three groups needed a mean of 7 injections and 2 sessions of laser photocoagulation. The RESTORE study showed that ranibizumab PRN as monotherapy or adjunctive to laser is superior to laser monotherapy in the treatment of vision impairment due to DME, and confirmed that ranibizumab injections are well tolerated and safe. Endophthalmitis did not occur; increased intraocular pressure was reported for 1 patient each in the ranibizumab arms; no increased risk of cardiovascular or cerebrovascular events was documented in this study. Overall, this study has a limited follow-up to allow a real efficacy comparison with laser treatment, the latter being slower in producing its effects.

It is well known that corticosteroids play an important role in reducing DME [19, 20] by decreasing the release of arachidonic acid derivatives such as prostaglandins, responsible for altered retinal vascular permeability, and by inhibiting VEGF production. In order to provide further clarity on the effectiveness of treatments based on administration of steroidal or anti-VEGF drugs in comparison to conventional laser treatment, the DRCRnet designed a randomized, multicenter clinical trial [21, 22]. The study (2 years of follow-up) recruited 691 patients and examined a total of 854 eyes randomized into four groups receiving laser treatment alone (293 eyes), 0.5 mg ranibizumab + prompt laser photocoagulation (187 eyes), 0.5 mg ranibizumab + deferred laser (at least 24 weeks, 188 eyes), intravitreal triamcinolone 4 mg + prompt laser (186 eyes). At 1-year examination, the mean change in the VA letter score with respect to the baseline value showed a statistically significant improvement in the ranibizumab + prompt laser group (+9 ± 11 letters) and ranibizumab + deferred laser group (+9 ± 12), but not in the triamcinolone + prompt laser group (+4 ± 13) compared with the laser group (+3 ± 13). Over the 2 years of follow-up, a different correlation between VA change and retinal thickness was observed in each group. A progressive reduction in mean central subfield thickness (CST) was noted in the laser group during the 24 months of follow-up; however, the mean change in VA did not continue to increase from the 1- to 2-year visit as noted instead during the first year of follow-up. In the triamcinolone + laser group, during the first year of follow-up, an improvement of visual function was associated with a significant reduction in CST, whereas from the 1-year to the 2-year examination the mean CST increased in parallel with a reduction in VA. Ranibizumab groups showed a parallel VA improvement associated with a CST reduction from baseline to the 12-month visit, and following this period the optical coherence tomography (OCT) results remained relatively stable up to the 24-month examination and paralleled the VA outcomes. Intraocular hypertension and cataract surgery were more frequently noted in the triamcinolone + prompt laser group in comparison to groups receiving ranibizumab + laser or laser alone. This trial demonstrates that intravitreal ranibizumab with prompt or deferred laser has superior VA and OCT outcomes compared to laser alone, and shows that intravitreal triamcinolone + prompt laser did not result in superior VA compared with laser alone. Although many subgroup analyses were performed sorting participants by baseline demographic, ocular, and systemic characteristics, the only subgroup analysis that yielded findings that differed from the full cohort was that of eyes that entered the trials pseudophakic. Roughly 1/3 of participants entered the study with a prior history of cataract surgery. In those participants, the triamcinolone + prompt laser-treated patients had vision outcomes that appeared comparable to each of the ranibizumab groups.

Following this result, the DRCR-net proposes the following algorithm for the treatment of the center-involved DME with ranibizumab in clinical practice [23]: start with a series of monthly injections until vision and edema are no longer improving (an increase of approximately 1 line in VA or at least a 10% reduction in the CST on OCT since the last injection) or no longer can improve (VA 20/20 or ME resolved). When an eye is no longer improving, focal/grid laser can be added if there are areas that can be treated (untreated microaneurysms within areas of thickened retina and other areas of thickening without grid laser), and in this case, injections would continue. Injections may be withheld if additional treatment at that visit seemed unlikely to provide any further benefit. After injection has been withheld at a particular visit, it may be resumed if edema recurs or worsens; monthly injections will be performed until vision and edema are no longer improving. If the treatment is not needed at 3 consecutive visits, the follow-up can be extended to 8 weeks. At that point, if the edema did not recur or worsen and no injection was given, follow-up could be extended to 16 weeks. Focal/grid laser generally should be added at any time and repeated after at least 13 weeks if edema persists or is not improving while giving anti-VEGF therapy, and it is believed that additional benefit will be gained by repeating laser.

Less investigated are the other anti-VEGF compounds currently available on the market.

Pegaptanib

Pegaptanib is a pegylated 28-nucleotide RNA aptamer that binds to the $VEGF_{164/165}$ isoform with high affinity. $VEGF_{165}$ levels are present in human eyes affected by DR with increased concentration, and play an active role in promoting angiogenesis and in enhancing vascular permeability.

Macugen Diabetic Retinopathy Study was a randomized, sham-controlled, double-masked, dose-finding phase II trial designed to evaluate the effect of three doses of intravitreal pegaptanib versus sham injection in patients affected by clinically significant DME [24]. One hundred and seventy-two patients were randomized to receive 0.3 mg (n = 44), 1.0 mg (n = 44), 3.0 mg (n = 42) of pegaptanib or sham injection (n = 42) at baseline, at week 6 and week 12. If needed, additional injections were administrated every 6 weeks up to a maximum of three additional injections. Retinal laser photocoagulation could be delivered if the investigators judged it necessary. At the final visit at week 36, the group of patients receiving pegaptanib 0.3 mg was significantly superior to the sham injection, as measured by mean change in VA (+4.7 vs. –0.4 letters, p = 0.04), proportions of patients gaining >10 letters of VA (34 vs. 10%; p = 0.003), change in mean CRT (68 μm reduction vs. 3.7 μm increase; p = 0.02). Moreover, only 25% of patients receiving pegaptanib required retinal photocoagulation in comparison with 40% of patients receiving sham injection (p = 0.04). Patients receiving 1.0 or 3.0 mg did not show a significant improvement compared to 0.3 mg as regards BCVA or CRT changes. Adverse events were noted in all treatment arms; they were transient, procedure related and mild or moderate (such as eye pain, vitreous floaters, eye discharge, conjunctival hemorrhage).

Recently, the results of a sham-controlled, multicenter, parallel-group study were reported [25]. The aim of this study was to demonstrate the efficacy of 0.3 mg pegaptanib intravitreal injection to improve VA more than 10 ETDRS (Early Treatment of Diabetic Retinopathy Study) letters from baseline compared with sham injection. During the study, focal/grid laser photocoagulation was allowed starting at week 18 if necessary. Two hundred and sixty and 207 patients concluded 1 year and 2 years of follow-up, respectively. The authors reported an improvement of VA ≥10 ETDRS letters at week 54 in 36.8% of subjects in the pegaptanib group and in 19.7% of the sham group compared with baseline values. A better VA in the pegaptanib group was also reported at the end of the 2-year follow-up period. Moreover, fewer pegaptanib-treated subjects received laser treatment compared to sham-treated subjects (23.3 vs. 41.7% at week 54, 25.2 vs. 45% at week 102). The incidence of adverse events was lower in pegaptanib group compared with the sham group.

Bevacizumab

Bevacizumab is a full-length recombinant humanized antibody active against all isoforms of VEGF. Short-term effects of bevacizumab for DME in a large randomized phase II clinical trial were initially reported by Diabetic Retinopathy Clinical Research Network [26]. One hundred and nine subjects with DME and Snellen acuity equivalent ranging from 20/32 to 20/320 were prospectively enrolled and randomized into 5 groups: (1) focal photocoagulation at baseline (n = 19), (2) intravitreal injection of 1.25 mg of bevacizumab at baseline and 6 weeks (n = 22), (3) intravitreal injection of 2.5 mg of bevacizumab

at baseline and 6 weeks (n = 24), (4) intravitreal injection of 1.25 mg of bevacizumab at baseline and sham injection at 6 weeks (n = 22), or (5) intravitreal injection of 1.25 mg of bevacizumab at baseline and 6 weeks with photocoagulation at 3 weeks (n = 22).

The BCVA in the groups receiving bevacizumab alone showed a median 1-line improvement at the 3-week visit, which was preserved up to 12 weeks and greater than the change in the group receiving only focal photocoagulation at baseline. A similar trend was observed with regard to CRT; comparing focal photocoagulation versus bevacizumab alone, a greater reduction in CRT was observed in the bevacizumab groups at 3 weeks.

No significant differences among groups receiving bevacizumab 1.25 versus 2.5 mg for changes in BCVA or CRT was observed. Comparing bevacizumab groups with groups receiving combined treatment, no significant differences were observed in reduction of central subfield thickening or improvement in VA.

Lam et al. [27] evaluated the efficacy of two dosing regimens of bevacizumab at 6 months of follow-up. Forty-eight patients were randomized to receive 3-monthly intravitreal injections of bevacizumab 1.25 mg (n = 23) or 2.5 mg (n = 25). At each monthly scheduled visit, a significant mean central foveal thickness reduction was observed in both groups. Similarly, the mean logMAR BCVA showed a statistically significant improvement from baseline to the final visit at 6 months (from 0.63 to 0.52 in the 1.25 mg group; from 0.60 to 0.47 in the 2.5 mg group). No significant difference in BCVA was observed between the two groups. No significant adverse events were reported during the study.

Arevalo et al. [28] reported the results of a retrospective, multicenter, interventional, comparative case series with a long-term follow-up extended to 24 months. The study evaluated 139 eyes receiving bevacizumab intravitreal injection (1.25 mg, n = 74, or 2.5 mg, n = 65). Additional injections were administered if recurrence of macular edema was detected on OCT associated with VA loss. At 1 month, both groups showed a statistically significant improvement in BCVA, and subsequently the gain was preserved up to the examination at 24 months. The 1.25 mg improved from 20/150 to 20/107 at 1 month, and to 20/75 at 24 months. In the 2.5 mg group, the BCVA improved from 20/168 to 20/118 at 1 month to 20/114 at the final visit.

Long-term efficacy of repeated injections of intravitreal bevacizumab 1.25 mg for the treatment of chronic DME was also reported by Kook et al. [29]. The study included 126 patients affected by chronic, diffuse, clinically significant DME in part not responsive to previous treatments including laser photocoagulation (62% focal laser treatment, 38% panretinal laser treatment), triamcinolone intravitreal injection (41%) or vitrectomy (11%). Sixty-seven and 59 patients completed the scheduled visits at 6 and 12 months, respectively. At the 6-month examination, the LogMAR BCVA ranged from the baseline value of 0.82 to 0.74 considering all patients. The mean BCVA of patients who completed the 12-month follow-up improved similarly from 0.82 to 0.74 LogMAR. Mean CRT decreased from 463 to 374 µm after 6 months and to 357 µm after 12 months with a statistically significant difference. This study showed that even in cases with chronic diffuse ischemic DME not responding to other therapy, a successful treatment with repeated intravitreal injections of bevacizumab can be achieved over a long-term follow-up period.

Other studies compared intravitreal bevacizumab treatment with intravitreal triamcinolone or focal retinal photocoagulation in refractory DME or as primary treatment. Paccola et al. [30] designed a randomized, prospective study in order to evaluate the anatomical response and VA outcomes after a single intravitreal injection of triamcinolone acetonide (4 mg) or bevacizumab (1.25 mg) in refractory diffuse DME. The study enrolled 26 patients; at baseline, the LogMAR BCVA was 0.936 and 0.937 in the triamcinolone-group and bevacizumab group, respectively. At 6 months, the BCVA improved to 0.91 and 0.92 without achieving a significant difference; however, interim analysis at 1-month, 2-month and 3-month examination evidenced a significant improvement in the triamcinolone group compared to the bevacizumab group.

A similar prospective and comparative case series was reported by Shimura et al. [31]. The study recruited 14 patients with bilateral long-standing DME; in each patient, one eye was selected to receive a single intravitreal injection of triamcinolone (4 mg) and the other to receive a single intravitreal bevacizumab injection (1.25 mg). LogMAR BCVA in the triamcinolone group improved significantly from 0.64 to 0.33 at one week, and the gain was subsequently preserved up to 12 weeks. At a final observation period of 24 weeks, BCVA decreased to 0.47 but was still significantly different from the baseline value. Similarly, BCVA in the bevacizumab group improved from 0.61 to 0.39 at one week and maintained the initial gain up to 4 weeks. At 12 weeks, BCVA returned to the initial level. No further decrease or improvement was observed in the following 3 months. A statistically significant difference of BCVA was observed in favor of triamcinolone group at 3 and 6 months.

A randomized, three-arm clinical trial comparing intravitreal bevacizumab injection (1.25 mg) alone or in combination with intravitreal triamcinolone acetonide (2 mg) versus macular laser photocoagulation as a primary treatment of DME was published by Soheilian et al. [32]. The bevacizumab group showed a significant BCVA improvement from 0.71 to 0.54 at 6 weeks; the initial gain was maintained in each following visit at 12, 24 and 36 weeks. The patients that underwent combined treatment showed a significant BCVA improvement from 0.73 to 0.60 at 6 weeks. This group showed stability of BCVA at 12 weeks but loss of statistically significant improvement at 6 and 9 months. In the macular photocoagulation group, the BCVA showed a stabilization at 6 weeks in comparison to the baseline value (0.60 vs. 0.55), and similar values were observed at all follow-up evaluations. However, it is important to note that the three groups differed with regard to the baseline VA values. The mean values of central macular thickness (CMT) decreased significantly in all groups only at 6 weeks in comparison to the baseline values, and although the reduction was greater in the bevacizumab group compared to the other 2 groups, no statistically significant difference was registered during follow-up. Recently, the authors categorized the original treatment arms, and the following subgroups were analyzed based on CMT: (1) <250 µm, (2) 250–349 µm, and (3) ≥350 µm [33]. Main outcome measures were changes in VA and CMT at weeks 6, 12, 24, and 36. At 6 weeks, mean VA improvement in the bevacizumab group was significantly greater than in the other groups. With a longer follow-up, however, bevacizumab turned out to be superior to bevacizumab/triamcinolone and macular laser photocoagulation only in the eyes with initial CMT of ≥350 µm, indicating that in the primary treatment of DME, initial CMT may be an important factor in decision making.

Recently, the results of a retrospective, multicenter, interventional comparative case series involving 115 consecutive patients (139 eyes) with DME, receiving primary treatment with 1.25 or 2.5 mg bevacizumab were published [34]. Patients received reinjections whenever there was a recurrence of DME (defined by a decrease in BCVA associated with presence of intraretinal fluid on OCT or fluorescein angiography). In the first month after the initial bevacizumab injection, improvements in BCVA and CMT measurements were recorded, and these significant changes continued throughout the 24-month follow-up. BCVA analysis at 24 months showed that 62 (44.6%) eyes remained stable, 72 (51.8%) eyes improved by two or more ETDRS lines, and 5 (3.6%) eyes had a decrease of two or more ETDRS lines.

The one-year results of a prospective randomized trial have recently been reported [35]. The BOLT study recruited 80 patients (80 eyes) affected by center-involving clinically significant DME and at least one previous macular laser treatment. Subjects were randomized to two groups receiving intravitreal bevacizumab or laser treatment according to ETDRS guidelines. Subjects in the bevacizumab arm underwent an injection at their baseline visit (1.25 mg in 0.05 ml). Patients were reviewed every 6 weeks with an end of the year visit at 52 weeks. After the baseline injection, patients received 2 further injections at 6 and 12 weeks. Additional injections were programmed according to a specific OCT-based retreatment protocol. Subjects in the laser arm underwent modified ETDRS laser treatment at their baseline visit and were reviewed every 4 months with an end of year visit at 52 weeks. Retreatment was performed according to ETDRS guidelines. The primary end point was the difference in ETDRS BCVA at 12 months between the two arms. The bevacizumab group gained a median of 8 ETDRS letters, compared to the laser group which lost 0.5 ETDRS letters (p = 0.0002). Mean CRT change from baseline was –130 and –67 in the bevacizumab and laser groups, respectively (p = 0.06). The median number of treatments was 9 in the bevacizumab arm and 3 in the laser treatment arm.

VEGF Trap

The VEGF Trap-Eye (Regeneron) is a 115-kDa recombinant fusion protein of portions of VEGF receptor 1 and 2 and the Fc region of human IgG which binds all VEGF-A isoforms with higher affinity in comparison to other anti-VEGF substances, including bevacizumab and ranibizumab [36]. Moreover, VEGF Trap-Eye has a longer half-life in the eye after intraocular injection and it binds other members of the VEGF family including placental growth factors 1 and 2, which have been shown to determine excessive vascular permeability. This higher affinity will most likely allow to employ lower doses and to maintain a longer duration of action [37, 38]. A phase I study exploring the safety and bioactivity of a single injection of 4.0 mg VEGF Trap-Eye in subjects with DME demonstrated a reduction in CRT and significant improvement of VA [39].

In the DA VINCI study, 219 diabetic patients with DME were enrolled and assigned to five different groups characterized by different dosing regimens of intravitreal VEGF Trap (monthly injection of 0.5 or 2 mg of VEGF Trap, 3 monthly injections followed by other injections every 8 weeks or on PRN regimen, macular laser photocoagulation alone) [40]. At the 12-month control, the four VEGF Trap groups gained from 9.7 to 13.1 ETDRS letters versus –1.3 letters of the laser group and obtained a reduction in CRT from 165.4 to 227.4 µm, compared with the 58.4 µm of the laser group. Aflibercept was well tolerated, and most common ocular adverse events were typical of those associated with intravitreal injections. Systemic serious adverse events (6 deaths) were not attributed to study drug, and were likely caused by patients' underlying disease.

Bevasiranib

Small interfering RNA molecules are able to inactivate messenger RNA (mRNA) and suppress RNA translation. Bevasiranib is a specific small interfering RNA designed to reduce the levels and activity of VEGF mRNA and may have a role in the treatment of diabetic retinopathy [41–43]. The RACE trial investigated the use of different doses of bevasiranib (0.2, 1.5 or 3.0 mg) [44] administered monthly for 3 months. The study showed a reduction of macular thickness between weeks 8 and 12, and improvement of VA. A phase 3, randomized, double-masked clinical trial evaluating the efficacy of bevasiranib in patients affected by wet AMD was recently terminated. Subjects received bevasiranib either every 8 weeks or every 12 weeks after an initial pre-treatment with 3 injections of ranibizumab compared to ranibizumab given every 4 weeks. Preliminary results after 60 weeks suggest that bevasiranib is efficacious even though slightly inferior to ranibizumab. Average VA remained positive through week 60, and a lower proportion of patients avoided visual loss on the more frequent bevasiranib dosing arm.

Rapamycin

Rapamycin is a macrocyclic antibiotic (produced by *Streptomyces hygroscopicus*) that binds specifically FKBP12; the active complex inhibits the mammalian target of rapamycin (mTOR), a kinase, which integrates growth factor-activated signals including signals that promote angiogenesis mediated by VEGF. Moreover, mTOR is an activator of hypoxia-inducible factor 1a, which upregulates the transcription of VEGF. In hypoxic cells, rapamycin can interfere with HIF-1a activation by increasing the rate of its degradation [45–47]. Therefore, rapamycin may have a meaningful role as therapy for retinal disorders characterized by pathological vascular permeability and proliferation. Preliminary results of application of rapamycin for DME have been presented by Blumenkranz et al. [48] at ARVO Meeting 2008. They show a significant improvement of BCVA and CMT reduction.

Conclusions

VEGF plays a key role in promoting angiogenesis and vascular leakage, and today represents an attractive candidate for a therapeutic target in the treatment and management of diabetic retinopathy. The advent of intravitreal anti-VEGF drugs has opened a new era for the management of DME. While focal/grid laser remains a standard treatment for DME and is supported by evidence provided by large-scale studies, the use of anti-VEGF substances in clinical practice has showed encouraging results. Most of the studies reported in this review were well-designed clinical trials with the objective of demonstrating both the therapeutic effect of anti-VEGF drugs and data regarding their safety. However, only larger trials can consolidate the use of anti-VEGF drugs in the clinical routine with the objective of creating guidelines for the management of DME. Another aspect that must be highlighted is the efficacy of anti-VEGF drugs over longer follow-up periods. Most controlled studies focus on 1- or 2-year results, but long-term results are unavailable. It would be of utmost importance to demonstrate that anti-VEGF drugs are able to provide therapeutic effects over a long period of time, and to compare these effects with those of laser treatment, which is characterized by a slow, but sustained therapeutic effect that most likely is more efficient many years after its employment. The use of combination therapy including anti-VEGF and focal/grid laser treatment has provided encouraging results, and must also be evaluated over a long time span. In particular, the combination of laser application and intravitreal anti-VEGF can reduce the number of injections without a negative effect on visual function in an attempt to lessen the burden of the therapy for both patients and doctors.

Different clinical trials have demonstrated an adequate safety profile for anti-VEGF substances, although a long-term analysis of systemic and ocular side effects is needed. In essence, the anti-VEGF approach has revolutionized the treatment of DME. Nevertheless, the prospect of the large amount of people lining up in retinal practices for monthly intravitreal injections is daunting. Platforms for extended drug delivery will be needed as well as reduced prices of drugs in order to balance the cost and benefits of treatment for this chronic life-long disease. It is likely that the combination treatment with laser photocoagulation becomes the first step for a practical and effective management of DME.

References

1 Kempen JH, O'Colmain BJ, Leske MC, et al: Eye Diseases Prevalence Research Group. The prevalence of diabetic retinopathy among adults in the United States. Arch Ophthalmol 2004;122:552–563.
2 Orchard TJ, Dorman JS, Maser RE, et al: Prevalence of complications in IDDM by sex and duration. Pittsburgh Epidemiology of Diabetes Complications Study II. Diabetes 1990;39:1116–1124.
3 Wild S, Roglic G, Green A, Sicree R, et al: Global prevalence of diabetes: estimates for the year 2000 and projections for 2030. Diabetes Care 2004;27:1047–1053.
4 Bandello F, Parodi MB, Lanzetta P, et al: Diabetic macular edema. Dev Ophthalmol 2010;47:73–110.
5 Early Treatment Diabetic Retinopathy Study Group. Photocoagulation for diabetic macular edema. ETDRS report N°1. Arch Ophthalmol 1985;103:1796–806.
6 Early Treatment Diabetic Retinopathy Study Group: Treatment techniques and clinical guidelines for photocoagulation of diabetic macular edema. ETDRS report N°2. Ophthalmology 1987;94:761–777.
7 Neufeld G, Cohen T, Gengrinovitch S, et al: Vascular endothelial growth factor (VEGF) and its receptors. FASEB J 1999;13:9–22.
8 Grant MB, Afzal A, Spoerri P, et al: The role of growth factors in the pathogenesis of diabetic retinopathy. Expert Opin Investig Drugs 2004;13:1275–1293.
9 Plate KH, Breier G, Weich HA, et al: Vascular endothelial growth factor is a potential tumour angiogenesis factor in human gliomas in vivo. Nature 1992;359:845–848.
10 Shweiki D, Itin A, Soffer D, et al: Vascular endothelial growth factor induced by hypoxia may mediate hypoxia-initiated angiogenesis. Nature 1992;359:843–845.
11 Aiello LP, Avery RL, Arrigg PG, et al: Vascular endothelial growth factor in ocular fluid of patients with diabetic retinopathy and other retinal disorders. N Engl J Med 1994;331:1480–1487.
12 Two pivotal phase III Lucentis studies showed patients with diabetic macular edema experienced significant improvements in vision and fewer developed more advanced retinopathy. www.gene.com. June 28, 2011.

13 Bandello F, De Benedetto U, Knutsson KA, et al: Ranibizumab in the treatment of patients with visual impairment due to diabetic macular edema. Clin Opthalmol 2011;5:1303–1308.

14 Massin P, Bandello F, Garweg JG, et al: Safety and efficacy of ranibizumab in diabetic macular edema (RESOLVE Study): a 12-month, randomized, controlled, double-masked, multicenter phase II study. Diabetes Care 2010;33:2399–2405.

15 Nguyen QD, Tatlipinar S, Shah SM, et al: Vascular endothelial growth factor is a critical stimulus for diabetic macular edema. Am J Ophthalmol 2006;142:961–969.

16 Nguyen QD, Shah SM, Heier JS, et al: READ-2 Study Group. Primary End Point (Six Months) Results of the Ranibizumab for Edema of the mAcula in diabetes (READ-2) study. Ophthalmology 2009;116:2175–2181.e1.

17 Nguyen QD, Shah SM, Khwaja AA, et al: READ-2 Study Group. Two-year outcomes of the ranibizumab for edema of the mAcula in diabetes (READ-2) study. Ophthalmology 2010;117:2146–2151.

18 Mitchell P, Bandello F, Schmidt-Erfurth U, et al: The RESTORE study: ranibizumab monotherapy or combined with laser versus laser monotherapy for diabetic macular edema. Ophthalmology 2011;118:615–625.

19 Massin P, Audren F, Haouchine B, et al: Intravitreal triamcinolone acetonide for diabetic diffuse macular edema: preliminary results of a prospective controlled trial. Ophthalmology 2004;111:218–224.

20 Gillies MC, Sutter FK, Simpson JM, et al: Intravitreal triamcinolone for refractory diabetic macular edema: two-year results of a double-masked, placebo-controlled, randomized clinical trial. Ophthalmology 2006;113:1533–1538.

21 Diabetic Retinopathy Clinical Research Network. Randomized trial evaluating ranibizumab plus prompt or deferred laser or triamcinolone plus prompt laser for diabetic macular edema. Ophthalmology 2010;117:1064–1077.e35.

22 Elman MJ, Bressler NM, Qin H, et al: Expanded 2-year follow-up of ranibizumab plus prompt or deferred laser or triamcinolone plus prompt laser for diabetic macular edema. Diabetic Retinopathy Clinical Research Network. Ophthalmology 2011;118:609–614.

23 Diabetic Retinopathy Clinical Research Network: Rationale for DRCR network treatment protocol for center-involved diabetic macular edema. Ophthalmology 2011;118:e5–e14.

24 Cunningham ET Jr, Adamis AP, Altaweel M, et al: Macugen Diabetic Retinopathy Study Group. A phase II randomized double-masked trial of pegaptanib, an anti-vascular endothelial growth factor aptamer, for diabetic macular edema. Ophthalmology 2005;112:1747–1757.

25 Sultan MB, Zhou D, Loftus J, et al: A phase 2/3, multicenter, randomized, double-masked, 2-year trial of pegaptanib sodium for the treatment of diabetic macular edema. Ophthalmology 2011;118:1107–1118.

26 Diabetic Retinopathy Clinical Research Network, A phase II randomized clinical trial of intravitreal bevacizumab for diabetic macular edema. Ophthalmology 2007;114:1860–1867.

27 Lam DS, Lai TY, Lee VY, et al: Efficacy of 1.25 MG versus 2.5 MG intravitreal bevacizumab for diabetic macular edema: six-month results of a randomized controlled trial. Retina 2009;29:292–299.

28 Arevalo JF, Sanchez JG, Wu L, et al: Pan-American Collaborative Retina Study Group. Primary intravitreal bevacizumab for diffuse diabetic macular edema: the Pan-American Collaborative Retina Study Group at 24 months. Ophthalmology 2009;116:1488–1497.

29 Kook D, Wolf A, Kreutzer T, et al: Long-term effect of intravitreal bevacizumab (avastin) in patients with chronic diffuse diabetic macular edema. Retina 2008;28:1053–1060.

30 Paccola L, Costa RA, Folgosa MS, et al: Intravitreal triamcinolone versus bevacizumab for treatment of refractory diabetic macular oedema (IBEME study). Br J Ophthalmol 2008;92:76–80.

31 Shimura M, Nakazawa T, Yasuda K, et al: Comparative therapy evaluation of intravitreal bevacizumab and triamcinolone acetonide on persistent diffuse diabetic macular edema. Am J Ophthalmol 2008;145:854–861.

32 Soheilian M, Ramezani A, Obudi A, et al: Randomized trial of intravitreal bevacizumab alone or combined with triamcinolone versus macular photocoagulation in diabetic macular edema. Ophthalmology 2009;116:1142–1150.

33 Soheilian M, Ramezani A, Yaseri M, et al: Initial macular thickness and response to treatment in diabetic macular edema. Retina 2011;39:1564–1573.

34 Arevalo JF, Sanchez JG, Lasave AF, et al: Intravitreal bevacizumab (Avastin) for diabetic retinopathy: the 2010 GLADAOF lecture. J Ophthalmol 2011;2011:584238.

35 Michaelides M, Kaines A, Hamilton RD, et al: A prospective randomized trial of intravitreal bevacizumab or laser therapy in the management of Diabetic Macular Edema (BOLT Study). 12 month data: report 2. Ophthalmology 2010;117:1078–1086.

36 Economides AN, Carpenter LR, Rudge JS, et al: Cytokine traps: multi-component, high-affinity blockers of cytokine action. Nat Med 2003;9:47–52.

37 Holash J, Davis S, Papadopoulos N, et al: VEGF-Trap: a VEGF blocker with potent antitumor effects. Proc Natl Acad Sci USA 2002;99:11393–11398.

38 Stewart MW, Rosenfeld PJ: Predicted biological activity of intravitreal VEGF Trap. Br J Ophthalmol 2008;92:667–668.

39 Do DV, Nguyen QD, Shah SM, et al: An exploratory study of the safety, tolerability and bioactivity of a single intravitreal injection of vascular endothelial growth factor trap-eye in patients with diabetic macular oedema. Br J Ophthalmol 2009;93:144–149.

40 Do DV, Schmidt-Erfurth U, Gonzalez VH, et al: The DA VINCI Study: Phase 2 Primary Results of VEGF Trap-Eye in Patients with Diabetic Macular Edema. Ophthalmology 2011;118:1819–1826.

41 Reich SJ, Fosnot J, Kuroki A, et al: Small interfering RNA (siRNA) targeting VEGF effectively inhibits ocular neovascularization in a mouse model. Mol Vis 2003;9:210–216.

42 Shen J, Samul R, Silva RL, et al: Suppression of ocular neovascularization with siRNA targeting VEGF receptor 1. Gene Ther 2006;13:225–234.

43 Singerman LJ: Combination therapy using the small interfering RNA bevasiranib. Retina 2009;29(6 suppl):S49–S50.

44 Singerman LJ: Intravitreal bevasiranib in exudative age-related macular degeneration or diabetic macular edema; in 25th Annu Meet Am Soc Retina Specialists. Indian Wells, December 2007.

45 Sausville EA, Elsayed Y, Monga M, et al:
   Signal transduction-directed cancer
   treatments. Annu Rev Pharmacol Toxi-
   col 2003;43:199–231.
46 Guba M, von Breitenbuch P, Steinbauer
   M, et al: Rapamycin inhibits primary
   and metastatic tumor growth by antian-
   giogenesis: involvement of vascular
   endothelial growth factor. Nat Med
   2002;8:128–135.
47 Sehgal SN: Rapamune (RAPA, rapamycin, sirolimus): mechanism of action
   immunosuppressive effect results from
   blockade of signal transduction and
   inhibition of cell cycle progression. Clin
   Biochem 1998;31:335–340.
48 Blumenkranz MS, Dugel PU, Solley WA,
   et al: A randomized dose-escalation trial
   of locally-administered sirolimus to treat
   diabetic macular edema; in 2008 Annu
   Meet Assoc Res Vision Ophthamol, Fort
   Lauderdale, 2008; v49.
49 ETDRS Research Group: Treatment
   techniques and clinical guidelines for
   photocoagulation of diabetic macular
   edema. Early Treatment Diabetic Retinopathy Study Report Number 2. Early
   Treatment Diabetic Retinopathy Study
   Research Group. Ophthalmology
   1987;94:761–774.

Maurizio Battaglia Parodi, MD
Department of Ophthalmology
University Vita-Salute
Scientific Institute San Raffaele
Via Olgettina 60
IT–20132 Milan (Italy)
E-Mail battagliaparodi.maurizio@hsr.it

Bandello F, Battaglia Parodi M (eds): Surgical Retina.
ESASO Course Series. Basel, Karger, 2012, vol 2, pp 58–64

Proliferative Diabetic Retinopathy: Laser Treatment and Intravitreal Medication

Francesco Bandello · Maurizio Battaglia Parodi · Rosangela Lattanzio · Anders Knutsson

Department of Ophthalmology, University Vita-Salute, Scientific Institute San Raffaele, Milano, Italy

Abstract

Proliferative diabetic retinopathy is characterized by growth of retinal or optic disk vascular proliferation leading to vitreous hemorrhage and scarring. Panretinal photocoagulation treatment is still considered the standard of care for the management of proliferative diabetic retinopathy. The possible advantages related to intravitreal drugs including anti-VEGF and steroids require further studies over long-term follow-up.

Proliferative diabetic retinopathy (PDR) is characterized by the growth of retinal or optic disk vascular proliferation as a consequence of widespread retinal ischemia. The natural course of the new vessels leads to either vitreous hemorrhage or to scarring with consequent tractional retinal detachment. Angle and iris neovascularization development at the anterior segment of the eye can determine the neovascular glaucoma onset.

The risk of PDR is closely related to the duration of diabetes mellitus. Among type 1 diabetic patients, 50% develop PDR after 20 years, and 10% among type 2 diabetics [1]. More recent data show that PDR prevalence is lower than the historically reported figures thanks to the intensive glycemic control and the progress in diagnosis and therapy [2–4]. However, PDR and macular edema (ME) are still the major reasons for visual loss and represent the two major vision-threatening causes in patients affected by diabetes mellitus [5]. Laser treatment can, if timely applied, greatly reduce the probability of vision loss in diabetic retinopathy (DR) [6]. To guarantee a successful laser treatment, risk factors of disease progression such as blood glucose levels [7, 8] and blood pressure [9] must be kept under tight control.

Laser Treatment

The mechanisms of action of laser photocoagulation are not completely understood. Possible mechanisms include: (1) destruction of ischemic retina leading to reduced production of proangiogenetic factors such as VEGF, (2) improved inner retinal oxygenation due to photoreceptors and retinal pigment epithelium (RPE) destruction, (3) release of neovascularization inhibitors from RPE [10–13].

Panretinal photocoagulation (PRP) treatment became a standard of care for DR since

Table 1. PDR high-risk characteristics [16–18]

NVD ≥1/4 to 1/3 disc area in extent
New vessels on or within 1 disc diameter of the optic disc
Any new vessel within 1 disc diameter of the optic disc and associated with vitreous or preretinal hemorrhage
Proliferation elsewhere at least 1/2 disc area in size and associated with vitreous or preretinal hemorrhage

the late 1970s, when the results of the Diabetic Retinopathy Study (DRS) were published [14, 15]. The DRS enrolled patients with PDR or severe nonproliferative DR (NPDR). After 3 years, argon laser photocoagulation decreased the rate of severe visual loss to 13.3%, while untreated eyes had a rate of 26.4%; laser PRP reduced the rate of severe visual loss by 50% and was maintained during a 5-year follow-up period [16]. The DRS also showed that after 2 years, the risk of severe visual loss was 26% for eyes exhibiting high-risk characteristics (table 1) compared to 7% in PDR without those characteristics [17]. Photocoagulation reduced severe visual loss by 50%, and was thus recommended in patients with high-risk PDR.

The Early Treatment Diabetic Retinopathy Study (ETDRS) was designed to address whether treatment at an earlier stage of DR (mild to severe NPDR or early PDR) would be helpful. The results showed that in eyes with mild to moderate NPDR, early photocoagulation benefits were not sufficient to surmount the unwanted side effects [19]. Side effects of laser treatment include scotomas related to the focal burns, reduction of the visual field in the treated area and transient ME, usually associated with a reduction of visual acuity. It has been demonstrated that photocoagulation scars enlarge over time and may eventually be associated with a late reduction of visual acuity. Accidental foveal burns have dramatic effects on vision but fortunately occur rarely. Other complications include choroidal, subretinal, or vitreous hemorrhage and transient elevated intraocular pressure.

Nevertheless, the ETDRS demonstrated that with severe NPDR or early proliferative stages, initiation of PRP before the development of high-risk PDR determined regression of neovascularization in 60% of patients after 3 months, reduced the risk of severe visual loss in 90% of cases, and should therefore be recommended [20]. Furthermore, PRP is particularly effective in reducing severe visual loss in patients with type 2 diabetes [21].

The DRS treatment recommendations for laser therapy are summarized in figure 1 [6]. Laser treatment leads to regression of anterior segment neovascularization, especially when neovascular glaucoma has not yet occurred [22, 23]. Other factors that may favor early treatment include impending pregnancy or cataract surgery, fellow eye status, and poor compliance [24].

Laser treatment should be performed over a period of 4–6 weeks by applying 1,200–2,000 burns, with a size of 500 μm, spacing spots 0.5 burn widths from each other with a 0.1–0.2 s duration. The intensity should be regulated to obtain mild white bleaching, and the treatment area should be from the temporal arcade to the equator and up to 2 disc diameters temporal of the macular center. The area around the optic disc should be spared to avoid central visual defects [25]. A recent study has demonstrated that PRP performed in one or four sittings has the same effects on visual acuity and ME measured by OCT thickness in patients with severe NPDR or early PDR [26].

Recently, new lasers have been developed to increase patient comfort during treatment and

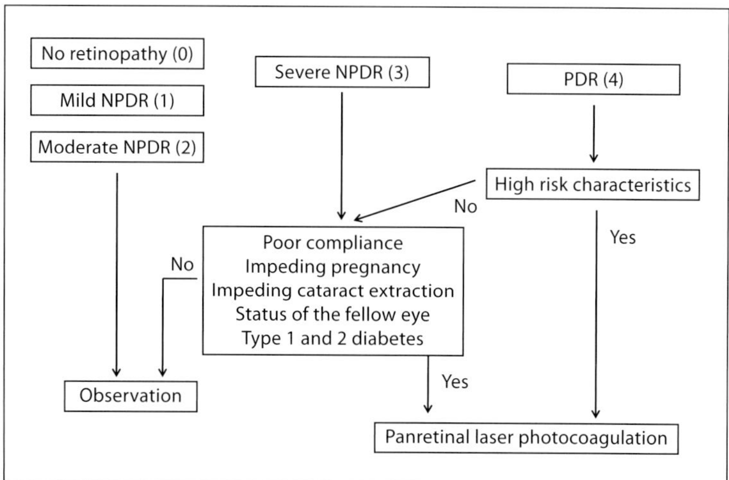

Fig. 1. Treatment recommendations for PRP.

to reduce the treatment time when compared to single-spot photocoagulation. An example is the Pascal® photocoagulator (Pattern Scan Laser, Optimedica Corporation, Santa Barbara, Calif., USA), a frequency-doubled ND:Yag (532 nm) laser system designed to treat using a single spot or a predetermined pattern array of up to 56 spots. Pascal photocoagulation determined less collateral damage, similar regression of retinopathy, reduced treatment time and was less painful for patients compared to a 532-nm solid state green laser (GLX) [27]. Pascal treatment has shown an adequate safety profile [28, 29], and is associated with significantly lower levels of anxiety, headache, pain and photophobia compared to single-spot PRP treatment [30].

The most recently developed system, NAVILAS (ODOS, GmbH, Teltow, Germany), utilizes a scanning slit-based instrument to obtain high-resolution images (infrared, color, fluorescein angiography). The ophthalmologist may then design a treatment strategy based on automated patterns and single spots as appropriate. For treatment, the surgeon activates the laser manually after obtaining a target lock [31].

Intravitreal Medication

Several medications are currently being used in an off-label manner in the treatment of PDR. At present, these medications are administered into the eye by intravitreal injection, and include triamcinolone acetonide and anti-VEGF agents.

Triamcinolone Acetonide

Intravitreal triamcinolone acetonide (IVTA) has been employed in diabetic ME and PDR. For PDR, investigations have suggested an antiangiogenic effect of IVTA. More specifically, IVTA may slow the progression of DR, according to the results of a DRCR.net study. A total of 840 eyes with diabetic ME were enrolled and randomly selected to receive laser therapy (n = 330), 1 mg of triamcinolone acetonide (n = 256), or 4 mg of triamcinolone acetonide (n = 254). The primary end point of the study was progression to PDR or worsening of 2 or more severity levels on reading-center masked evaluation of 7-field fundus photographs, as well as additional eyes that were treated with PRP or that had a vitreous hemorrhage. At 2 years, the cumulative probability of progression of DR was 31% in the laser group, 29% in the 1 mg group,

Bandello · Battaglia Parodi · Lattanzio · Knutsson

and 21% in the 4 mg group (p = 0.64 in the 1 mg group and p = 0.005 in the 4 mg group versus the laser group). These differences were maintained at 3 years, although most eyes in the triamcinolone groups did not receive injections every 4 months during the 2nd year, and less than half received any injections in the 3rd year. Unfortunately, the possible side effects including cataract formation and glaucoma may limit the use of this approach [32]. Moreover, combined therapy with IVTA can be useful in the management of PDR. PRP may induce secondary ME in PDR or exacerbate ME in those with preexisting ME. Corticosteroids have been largely used in the past for the treatment of ME through prostaglandin production inhibition. Several studies have shown that combined IVTA and PRP can lead to reduction of ME associated with complete regression of proliferation [33–35], even though some authors have recently questioned the positive outcomes [36].

Anti-VEGF Drugs
Retinal hypoxia represents the major inducer of VEGF gene transcription, even though VEGF expression is also upregulated by high glucose level, protein kinase C activation, and glycation end products [37]. VEGF is a pluripotent growth factor acting as endothelial cell-specific mitogen and vasopermeability factor, and playing a key role in promoting angiogenesis and vascular leakage [38, 39].

The VEGF molecular family includes five members: placental growth factor, VEGF-A, VEGF-B, VEGF-C and VEGF-D. Each of the different factors may bind to one or more of three VEGF receptors. Moreover, VEGF-A plays the most important role in angiogenesis and vascular permeability. Alternative splicing of VEGF gene produces nine VEGF-A isoforms ($VEGF_{121}$, $VEGF_{145}$, $VEGF_{148}$, $VEGF_{162}$, $VEGF_{165}$, $VEGF_{165b}$, $VEGF_{183}$, $VEGF_{189}$, $VEGF_{206}$), and among them, $VEGF_{165}$ is the most abundantly expressed isoform, and it is considered as the major responsible for DR.

Pegaptanib, bevacizumab, and ranibizumab are the anti-VEGF molecules investigated to treat PDR.

The Macugen Diabetic Retinopathy Study provided information on the ability of pegaptanib sodium to lead to the regression of retinal neovascularization in PDR [40]. Of 16 patients with retinal neovascularization at baseline in the study eye, 13 were assigned to pegaptanib treatment and 3 to sham injections. After 36 weeks, 8 of 13 eyes (62%) under pegaptanib treatment showed regression of neovascularization, as assessed by fundus photography or fluorescein angiography, whereas no regression occurred in the 3 sham-treated eyes. In 3 of 8 eyes with regression, neovascularization progressed at week 52 after the cessation of pegaptanib administration at week 30, suggesting that repeated injections are necessary to control the retinal neovascularization growth.

Gonzalez et al. [41] reported the results of a prospective, randomized, controlled, open-label, exploratory study, designed to compare the efficacy of intravitreal pegaptanib versus PRP in the treatment of active PDR. Twenty subjects were assigned at a 1:1 ratio to receive pegaptanib treatment in one eye every 6 weeks for 30 weeks or to PRP. In 90% of eyes randomized to pegaptanib, retinal neovascularization showed a complete regression by week 3. Moreover, all eyes receiving pegaptanib achieved a complete regression of retinal proliferation by week 12, which was maintained through week 36. In the PRP-treated group, 25% of eyes demonstrated complete regression, 25% showed partial regression, whereas 50% revealed the persistence of active PDR at 9-month examination. Taking into consideration the visual acuity, although the difference was not statistically significant, pegaptanib-treated eyes showed an increase of 5.8 letters, whereas the PRP-treated eyes lost 6.0 letters at week 36.

Intravitreal bevacizumab (IVB) for retinal neovascularization associated with PDR has been addressed by many studies. Avery et al. [42] investigated the biologic effects of IVB in 45 eyes with retinal and iris neovascularization. The patients received IVB in a dose-escalating regimen (6.2 g to 1.25 mg). At 1-week examination, fluorescein angiography disclosed a complete or at least partial reduction in neovascularization leakage. Recurrence was registered in variable time: in a case neovascularization, recurrence was detected after 2 weeks, whereas in other cases no recurrent leakage was registered at last 11-week follow-up. Jorge et al. [43] evaluated in a prospective non-randomized open-label study the effects of IVB in patients affected by active PDR refractory to laser treatment with visual acuity less than 20/40. Each patient received a single 1.5 mg IVB injection. In the 15 patients completing the 12-week follow-up, the mean best corrected visual acuity significantly improved from 0.90 at baseline to 0.76 logMAR at week 1. Visual improvement was preserved up to 12-week examination. At baseline, mean neovascularization leakage area was 27.79 mm^2, whereas at 1-week and 12-week examinations mean neovascularization leakage area significantly decreased to 5.43 and 5.50, respectively.

Additional data on the use of IVB in patients affected by PDR associated with vitreous hemorrhages have been provided by Moradian et al. [44], who prospectively followed up 38 patients for 20 weeks. Mean best corrected visual acuity increased from 1.13 to 0.86 logMAR at 1 week, with a further improvement at 6, 12 and 20 weeks, with a final mean value of 0.53 logMAR. Vitreous hemorrhage resolved significantly at 1-week and at 12-week examinations, with about 50% of patients showing complete resolution. At 20 weeks, only 23% of eyes presented a slight vitreous hemorrhage.

These encouraging results have been confirmed by Huang et al. [45], who evaluated the efficacy of IVB combined with PRP for the treatment of PDR complicated by vitreous hemorrhage. Forty patients underwent IVB (1.25 mg) followed by PRP. An additional injection was administered if no signs of decreased vitreous hemorrhages were noted. Vitreous clear-up time and vitrectomy rate were registered and compared with the control group treated with conventional methods. Vitreous clear-up time in the IVB group was significantly lower than control group (11.9 vs. 18.1 weeks). Similarly, the IVB group required vitrectomy in 10% of patients in comparison to 45% in the control group.

IVB has also been used in combination with pars plana vitrectomy to treat PDR. Ahmadieh et al. [46] randomized 68 eyes with PDR to IVB 1.25 mg or to sham injection 1 week preoperatively, and demonstrated that the incidence of vitreous hemorrhage was significantly reduced in the bevacizumab subgroup.

Even though important results have been obtained with the use of intravitreal ranibizumab for the management of ME, at present there is no reliable trial regarding the effects of ranibizumab on PDR. However, the DRCR.net has designed a prospective, randomized, comparative clinical trial to evaluate the role of ranibizumab or triamcinolone intravitreal injection as adjunctive treatment to PRP for PDR [47].

References

1 Klein R, Klein BEK, Moss SE, Davis MD, DeMets DL: The Wisconsin Epidemiological Study of Diabetic Retinopathy. III. Prevalence and risk of diabetic retinopathy when age at diagnosis is 30 or more years. Arch Ophthalmol 1984;102: 527–532.

2 Hovind P, Tarnow L, Rossing K, Rossing P, Eising S, Larsen N, Binder C, Parving HH: Decreasing incidence of severe diabetic microangiopathy in type 1 diabetes. Diabetes Care 2003;26:1258–1264.

3 Lecaire T, Palta M, Zhang H, Allen C, Klein R, D'Alessio D: Lower-than-expected prevalence and severity of retinopathy in an incident cohort followed during the first 4–14 years of type 1 diabetes: the Wisconsin Diabetes Registry Study. Am J Epidemiol 2006;164: 143–150.

4   Nordwall M, Bojestig M, Arnqvist HJ, Ludvigsson J, Linköping Diabetes Complications Study: Declining incidence of severe retinopathy and persisting decrease of nephropathy in an unselected population of Type 1 diabetes-the Linköping Diabetes Complications Study. Diabetologica 2004;47:1266–1272.

5   Klein R, Klein BE, Moss SE: Visual impairment in diabetes. Ophthalmology 1984;91:1–9.

6   Neubauer AS, Ulbig MW: Laser treatment in diabetic retinopathy. Ophthalmologica 2007;221:95–102.

7   The relationship of glycemic exposure (HbA1c) to the risk of development and progression of retinopathy in the diabetes control and complications trial. Diabetes 1995;44:968–983.

8   The effect of intensive diabetes treatment on the progression of diabetic retinopathy in insulin-dependent diabetes mellitus. The Diabetes Control and Complications Trial. Arch Ophthalmol 1995;113:36–51.

9   Tight blood pressure control and risk of macrovascular and microvascular complications in type 2 diabetes: UKPDS 38. UK Prospective Diabetes Study Group. BMJ 1998;317:703–713.

10 Glaser B: Extracellular modulatory factors and the control of intraocular neovascularization: an overview. Ophthalmology 1988;106:603–607.

11 Glaser B: Retinal pigment epithelial cells release an inhibitor of neovascularization. Arch Ophthalmol 1985;103:1870–1875.

12 Patz A: Retinal neovascularization: early contributions of Professor Michaelson and recent observations. Br J Ophthalmol 1984;68:42–46.

13 Landers M, Stefanson E, Wolbarsht ML: Panretinal photocoagulation and retinal oxygenation. Retina 1982;2:167–175.

14 Preliminary report on effects of photocoagulation therapy. The Diabetic Retinopathy Study Research Group. Am J Ophthalmol 1976;81:383–396.

15 Photocoagulation treatment of proliferative diabetic retinopathy: the second report of diabetic retinopathy study findings. Ophthalmology 1978;85:82–106.

16 Photocoagulation treatment of proliferative diabetic retinopathy: clinical application of Diabetic Retinopathy Study (DRS) findings, DRS Report Number 8. The Diabetic Retinopathy Study Research Group. Ophthalmology 1981;88:583–600.

17 Indications for photocoagulation treatment of diabetic retinopathy: Diabetic Retinopathy Study Report No 14. The Diabetic Retinopathy Study Research Group. Int Ophthalmol Clin 1987;27:239–253.

18 Four risk factors for severe visual loss in diabetic retinopathy. The third report from the Diabetic Retinopathy Study. The Diabetic Retinopathy Study Research Group. Arch Ophthalmol 1979;97:654–655.

19 Early Treatment Diabetic Retinopathy Study Research Group. Early photocoagulation for diabetic retinopathy ETDRS Report Number 9. Ophthalmology 1991;98:766–785.

20 Fundus photographic risk factors for progression of diabetic retinopathy. ETDRS report number 12. Early Treatment Diabetic Retinopathy Study Research Group. Ophthalmology 1991;98:823–833.

21 Ferris F: Early photocoagulation in patients with either type I or type II diabetes. Trans Am Ophthalmol Soc 1996;94:505–537.

22 Pavan PR, Folk JC, Weingeist TA, et al: Diabetic rubeosis and panretinal photocoagulation: a prospective, controlled, masked trial using fluorescein angiography. Arch Ophthalmol 1983;101:882–884.

23 Jacobson D, Murphy RP, Rosenthal AR: The treatment of angle neovascularization with panretinal photocoagulation. Ophthalmology 1979;86:1270–1275.

24 American Academy of Ophthalmology Retina Panel: Preferred Practice Pattern Guidelines. Diabetic Retinopathy. San Francisco, American Academy of Ophthalmology, 2008.

25 Davies N: Altering the pattern of panretinal photocoagulation: could the visual field for driving be preserved? Eye 1999;13:531–536.

26 Diabetic Retinopathy Clinical Research Network, Brucker AJ, Qin H, Antoszyk AN, Beck RW, Bressler NM, et al: Observational study of the development of diabetic macular edema following panretinal (scatter) photocoagulation given in 1 or 4 sittings. Arch Ophthalmol 2009;127:132–140.

27 Nagpal M, Marlecha S, Nagpal K: Comparison of laser photocoagulation for diabetic retinopathy using 532-nm standard laser versus multispot pattern scan laser. Retina 2010;30:452–458.

28 Velez-Montoya R, Guerrero-Naranjo JL, Gonzalez-Mijares CC, Fromow-Guerra J, Marcellino GR, Quiroz-Mercado H, Morales-Cantón V: Pattern scan laser photocoagulation: safety and complications, experience after 1,301 consecutive cases. Br J Ophthalmol 2010;94:720–724.

29 Muqit MM, Sanghvi C, McLauchlan R, Delgado C, Young LB, Charles SJ, Marcellino GR, Stanga PE: Study of clinical applications and safety for Pascal laser photocoagulation in retinal vascular disorders. Acta Ophthalmol 2010, Epub ahead of print.

30 Muqit MM, Marcellino GR, Gray JC, McLauchlan R, Henson DB, Young LB, Patton N, Charles SJ, Turner GS, Stanga PE: Pain responses of Pascal 20 ms multi-spot and 100 ms single-spot panretinal photocoagulation: Manchester Pascal Study, MAPASS report 2. Br J Ophthalmol 2010;94:1493–1498.

31 Kernt M, Cheuteu R, Vounotrypidis E, Haritoglou C, Kampik A, Ulbig MW, Neubauer AS: Focal and panretinal photocoagulation with a navigated laser (NAVILAS®). Acta Ophthalmol 2011;89:e662–e664.

32 Bressler NM, Beck RW, Flaxel CJ, et al: Exploratory analysis of diabetic retinopathy progression through 3 years in a randomized clinical trial that compares intravitreal triamcinolone acetonide with focal/grid photocoagulation. Arch Ophthalmol 2009;127:1566–1571.

33 Zacks DN, Johnson MW: Combined intravitreal injection of triamcinolone acetonide and panretinal photocoagulation for coexisting diabetic macular edema and proliferative diabetic retinopathy. Retina 2005;25:135–140.

34 Zein WM, Noureddin BN, Jurdi FA, et al: Panretinal photocoagulation and intravitreal triamcinolone acetonide for the management of proliferative diabetic retinopathy with macular edema. Retina 2006;26:137–142.

35 Sutter FK, Simpson JM, Gillies MC: Intravitreal triamcinolone for diabetic macular edema that persists after laser treatment. Three-month efficacy and safety results of a prospective, randomized, double-masked, placebo-controlled clinical trial. Ophthalmology 2004;111: 2044–2049.

36 Mirshahi A, Shenazandi H, Lashay A, Faghihi H, Alimahmoudi A, Dianat S: Intravitreal triamcinolone as an adjunct to standard laser therapy in coexisting high-risk proliferative diabetic retinopathy and clinically significant macular edema. Retina 2010;30:254–259.

37 Caldwell RB, Bartoli M, Behzadian MA, et al: Vascular endothelial growth factor and diabetic retinopathy: pathophysiological mechanisms and treatment perspectives. Diabetes Metab Res Rev 2003; 19:442–455.

38 Neufeld G, Cohen T, Gengrinovitch S, et al: Vascular endothelial growth factor (VEGF) and its receptors. FASEB J 1999; 13:9–22.

39 Grant MB, Afzal A, Spoerri P, et al: The role of growth factors in the pathogenesis of diabetic retinopathy. Expert Opin Investig Drugs 2004;13:1275–1293.

40 Adamis AP, Altaweel M, Bressler NM, et al: Macugen Diabetic Retinopathy Study Group. Changes in retinal neovascularization after pegaptanib (Macugen) therapy in diabetic individuals. Ophthalmology 2006;113:23–28.

41 Gonzalez VH, Giuliari GP, Banda RM, et al: Intravitreal injection of pegaptanib sodium for proliferative diabetic retinopathy. Br J Ophthalmol 2009;93:1474–1478.

42 Avery RL, Pearlman J, Pieramici DJ, et al: Intravitreal bevacizumab (Avastin) in the treatment of proliferative diabetic retinopathy. Ophthalmology 2006;113: 1695.e1–1695.e15.

43 Jorge R, Costa RA, Calucci D, et al: Intravitreal bevacizumab (Avastin) for persistent new vessels in diabetic retinopathy (IBEPE study). Retina 2006;26:1006–1013.

44 Moradian S, Ahmadieh H, Malihi M, et al: Intravitreal bevacizumab in active progressive proliferative diabetic retinopathy. Graefes Arch Clin Exp Ophthalmol 2008;246:1699–1705.

45 Huang YH, Yeh PT, Chen MS, et al: Intravitreal bevacizumab and panretinal photocoagulation for proliferative diabetic retinopathy associated with vitreous haemorrhage. Retina 2009;29:1134–1140.

46 Ahmadieh H, Shoeibi N, Entezari M, Monshizadeh R: Intravitreal bevacizumab for prevention of early postvitrectomy hemorrhage in diabetic patients: a randomized clinical trial. Ophthalmology 2009;116:1943–1948.

47 http://clinicaltrials.gov/ct2/show/ NCT00445003.

Prof. Francesco Bandello
Department of Ophthalmology
University Vita-Salute
Scientific Institute San Raffaele
Via Olgettina 60
IT–20132 Milano (Italy)
Tel. +39 0 2 26432648, E-Mail bandello.francesco@hsr.it

Bandello · Battaglia Parodi · Lattanzio · Knutsson

Bandello F, Battaglia Parodi M (eds): Surgical Retina.
ESASO Course Series. Basel, Karger, 2012, vol 2, pp 65–68

Proliferative Diabetic Retinopathy: Surgical Treatment

Anselm Kampik

Augenklinik der LMU, Klinikum der Universität München, München, Germany

Abstract

Proliferative diabetic retinopathy remains one of the major indications for vitreoretinal surgery despite improvement in systemic disease control and pharmacologic and laser surgical options. Improvements in technology have defined clear indications and techniques for surgical treatment of proliferative diabetic retinopathy either by vitrectomy and laser surgery alone or in combination with pharmacologic treatment using anti-VEGF substances or anti-inflammatory agents. The indications and surgical principles are described.

Proliferative diabetic retinopathy (PDR) is the most common blinding disease in the working age group. It is believed that the increase in incidence of diabetes will be exceeding the prognostic increase of 39% of the WHO. Thus, sequelae of diabetes such as diabetic maculopathy as well as PDR will increase in the future. Besides improved systemic treatment of the diabetes syndrome, the advent and the recent improvement in surgical treatment of PDR is and will be an important way to avoid blindness from PDR. The seminal trials on surgical treatment were published between 1976 and 1993 [1–10]. Since then, additional treatment options such as the combination of pharmacologic agents and vitreoretinal microsurgery has added to improve the results of surgery today, even if there are no major randomized trials on this topic during the last 15 years.

Treatment Options and Grading of Proliferative Diabetic Retinopathy

The combination of the information of trials such as the DRS, ETDRS, DRVS, and DCCT have clearly established the indications, techniques, and benefits of (1) photocoagulation, (2) pars plana vitreous surgery, and (3) intensive control of blood sugars for people with diabetes.

The proper indication for surgery in PDR needs knowledge of the surgeon on the clinical findings (judgment on the severity of the disease = grading), the potential risk factors for further progression without intervention, and knowledge on the outcome and risk of each of the possible surgical interventions.

The grading of diabetic retinopathy is derived from the DR and ETDR studies. Most important for any indication for surgical treatment is to distinguish the amount of nonproliferative changes within the retina from proliferative changes at the retina and vitreous (PDR).

PDR is characterized by the presence of newly formed blood vessels arising from the retina or the optic disc, fibrous proliferation on the disk or elsewhere, preretinal or vitreous hemorrhages. In more advanced stages, retinal detachment from tractional and/or additional rhegmatogenous changes may occur. In very severe situations, additional neovascularization at the iris is complicating the situation for treatment.

The most important findings predicting further progression to PDR include intraretinal hemorrhages, venous beading and intraretinal microvascular abnormalities. Systemic hypertension increases the risk for further deterioration.

Proper preoperative evaluation includes biomicroscopic slit lamp examination of the anterior and posterior segment, and indirect ophthalmoscopy. In cases of vitreous hemorrhage, ultrasound examination of the vitreous and the retina is helpful. In cases of combined diabetic macular edema and PDR, fluorescein angiography can give additional information especially on the vascularization of the fovea and perifoveolar area. Optical coherence tomography is especially helpful in detecting the amount of macular changes, often predictive of visual recovery after vitreoretinal surgery, and in evaluating the need of additional anti-VEGF treatment before or at the time of surgery.

Photocoagulation in Proliferative Diabetic Retinopathy

Panretinal laser treatment (PRP) is the proper surgical treatment in most DR stages: severe nonproliferative diabetic retinopathy, mild PDR, and is mandatory in the high-risk PDR. As a rule, PRP is done at its full extent only in those situations where a potential macular edema has been treated before either by intravitreal anti-VEGF and/or focal laser treatment.

In almost all cases in which vitreoretinal surgery is indicated, PRP is applied during the time of surgery by endolaser coagulation.

The benefit of PRP includes a 50% suppression of severe visual loss in all patients with PDR. This benefit increases over 90% if performed in patients approaching high-risk stage and when combined with vitrectomy and glycemic control.

In cases with fibrotic membranes with traction, PRP can worsen the situation. If diabetic macular edema is present, PRP may lead to a worsening of the visual acuity.

Vitreoretinal Microsurgery

During the last 2 years, a new standard using transconjunctival sutureless microincisional vitrectomy has evolved. Either a 23- or a 25-gauge system is used in almost all cases. This can be combined with microphaco technology using a one-step approach for situations in which the lens is already cataractous preventing clear view into the vitreous and the vitreous base during vitreous surgery. Thus aphakia should be avoided in all cases of PDR because of the increased risk of neovascularization of the iris in aphakic patients. Combined phaco-vitrectomy delivers good results and should be preferred to a two-step approach.

The recent knowledge on the combination of pharmacologic treatment and vitreoretinal surgery has helped to improve the outcome and minimize the bleeding during vitrectomy markedly. However, tractional retinal detachment may occur following intravitreal anti-VEGF treatment in patients with severe PDR. Therefore, the interval between preoperative anti-VEGF treatment and vitrectomy should be a few days [11, 12].

Indications for vitrectomy in PDR include primarily these clinical findings:

- severe non clearing vitreous hemorrhage
- tractional retinal detachment ± involvement of the macula
- combined tractional and rhegmatogenous retinal detachment
- severe progressive fibrovascular proliferation

- intense preretinal hemorrhage (subhyaloidal hemorrhage)
- rubeosis iridis (neovascularization of the iris) associated with vitreous hemorrhage
- ghost cell glaucoma
- macular edema in instances with a tractional component

The proper timing for vitrectomy in PDR was for a long time under discussion. With today's options of vitreous technology, surgery can be performed as early as it is needed by the patient. Waiting up to 3 months as it was suggested is no longer necessary and even increases the risk for deterioration especially in those situations in which not enough PRP could be applied.

Before the advent of anti-VEGF treatment, iris neovascularization was considered almost a contraindication for vitreous surgery. Today, anti-VEGF should be applied before vitreous surgery. Usually, 24 h after anti-VEGF treatment, the neovascularization disappears. After that time, vitreous surgery with additional PRP is indicated to prevent reoccurrence of iris neovascularization, which is a response to retinal ischemia either from peripheral retinal detachment or from large areas of avascular retina.

The aim of vitrectomy includes removal of opacities from the vitreous space, and the removal of tractional forces from the retinal surface. By doing this, fibrocellular proliferations on the retinal surface as well as fibrovascular proliferations from the optic disc and elsewhere have to be removed as much as possible. In the presence of macular edema, the removal of fine epimacular membranes should be attempted carefully [13].

Special care should be taken also at the vitreous base where fibrocellular proliferations may frequently be hidden at peripheral remnants of vitreous hemorrhages in the area of the pars plana. The end point of vitreous surgery is achieved as soon as all proliferations and hemorrhages and as much vitreous as possible are removed.

At this time, either a fluid air or fluid perfluorocarbon exchange is performed in order to stabilize the retina and perform PRP via an endolaser probe. Only at this time can the decision be made what kind of intraocular tamponade should be used. The latter is dependent on the situation of the retina and the tendency of recurrent hemorrhage. In cases of pure vitreous hemorrhage as an indication for surgery, balanced salt solution or air is usually sufficient. In cases of retinal detachment without major vascular activity, a gas tamponade is usually the choice. Only in very severe cases should silicone oil be applied to fill the vitreous cavity.

A special group of patients have a combination of diabetic macular edema and PDR which can be approached at the time of vitreoretinal surgery as well. In these situations, it has to be taken into consideration that epiretinal membranes in diabetic retinopathy often have a multilayered appearance. Therefore, in this situation it is advisable to remove not only the epiretinal tissue, but also the internal limiting membrane of the retina in order to relieve all necessary traction and gain the maximum in potential visual recovery [13].

Further advances in surgical management will occur and include better understanding of combined pharmacologic and surgical intervention for PDR.

References

1 Diabetic Retinopathy Study Research Group: Preliminary report on effects of photocoagulation therapy. Am J Ophthalmol 1976;81:383–396.

2 The Diabetic Retinopathy Study Research Group: Photocoagulation treatment of proliferative diabetic retinopathy. Clinical application of Diabetic Retinopathy Study (DRS) findings. DRS Report Number 8. Ophthalmology 1981; 88:583–600.

3 Diabetic Retinopathy Study Research Group: Four risk factors for severe visual loss in diabetic retinopathy: the third report from the Diabetic Retinopathy Study. Arch Ophthalmol 1979;97:654–655.

4 Early Treatment Diabetic Retinopathy Study Research Group: Early photocoagulation for diabetic retinopathy. ETDRS Report Number 9. Ophthalmology 1991;98:766–785.

5 Diabetic Retinopathy Vitrectomy Study Research Group (Appended): Early vitrectomy for severe vitreous hemorrhage in diabetic retinopathy. Arch Ophthalmol 1985;103:1644–1652.

6 The Diabetic Retinopathy Vitrectomy Study Research Group: Early vitrectomy for severe proliferative diabetic retinopathy in eyes with useful vision: results of a randomized trial – Diabetic Retinopathy Vitrectomy Study Report 3. Ophthalmology 1988;95:1307–1320.

7 Diabetic Retinopathy Vitrectomy Study Research Group: Early vitrectomy for severe vitreous hemorrhage in diabetic retinopathy: four year results of the randomized trial. Arch Ophthalmol 1990;108:958.

8 Diabetic Retinopathy Vitrectomy Study Research Group: Early vitrectomy for severe proliferative diabetic retinopathy in eyes with useful vision: clinical application of results of the randomized trial. Ophthalmology 1988;95:1321.

9 The Diabetes Control and Complications Trial Research Group: The effect of intensive treatment of diabetes on the development and progression of long-term complications in insulin-dependent diabetes mellitus. N Engl J Med 1993;329:977–986.

10 Early Treatment Diabetic Retinopathy Study Research Group: Fluorescein angiographic risk factors for progression of diabetic retinopathy. ETDRS Report 12. Ophthalmology 1991;98:834–840.

11 Rizzo S, Genovesi-Ebert F, Di Bartolo E, Vento A, Miniaci S, Williams GA: Injection of intravitreal bevacizumab (Avastin) as a preoperative adjunct before vitrectomy surgery in the treatment of severe proliferative diabetic retinopathy (PDR). Graefes Arch Clin Exp Ophthalmol 2008;246:837–842.

12 Arevalo JF, et al: Tractional retinal detachment following intravitreal bevacizumab (Avastin) in patients with severe proliferative diabetic retinopathy. Br J Ophthalmol 2008;92:213–216.

13 Gandorfer A, Rohleder M, Kampik A: Epiretinal pathology of vitreomacular traction syndrome. Br J Ophthalmol 2002;86:902–909.

Prof. Dr. Anselm Kampik FEBO
Augenklinik der LMU, Klinikum der Universität München, Campus Innenstadt
Mathildenstrasse 8
DE–80336 München (Germany)
Tel. +49 89 5160 3800, E-Mail akampik@med.uni-muenchen.de

Bandello F, Battaglia Parodi M (eds): Surgical Retina.
ESASO Course Series. Basel, Karger, 2012, vol 2, pp 69–80

Complications and Management of Diabetic Vitrectomy

Marco A. Zarbin

Institute of Ophthalmology and Visual Science-New Jersey Medical School, Newark, N.J., USA

Abstract

Potential complications after vitrectomy for complications of diabetic retinopathy are numerous and involve all components of the eye and periocular tissues. They also can involve the systemic health of the patient including severe metabolic disequilibrium and death. Good outcomes can be achieved by avoidance of complications through anticipatory intra- and postoperative decision-making and anticipation, early identification, and appropriately aggressive treatment of postoperative complications. Each of the potential complications and their management are considered in detail.

In general, one seeks to avoid complications through proper intra- and postoperative decision-making. Despite these efforts, complications will occur, particularly if one's practice involves cases with advanced disease. One can achieve satisfactory outcomes despite the occurrence of complications through anticipation, early detection, and appropriately aggressive treatment. Most surgical complications (except progressive nuclear sclerosis) occur within the first 3 months after surgery.

Anticipatory Actions to Prevent Complications

Intraoperative Decisions

In addition to achieving the mechanical objectives of surgery, intraoperative decisions and actions tend to focus on avoiding postoperative complications such as infectious endophthalmitis, severe intraocular pressure (IOP) elevation, retinal detachment, and intraocular hemorrhage. The incidence of endophthalmitis after vitrectomy is 0.05% [1]. Infection prophylaxis often is achieved through the use of topical 5% povidone-iodine (unless the patient is iodine-allergic), a plastic adhesive-backed drape (to keep cilia out of the surgical field), and administration of subconjunctival antibiotics (e.g. cefazolin 100 mg/0.5 ml or vancomycin 50 mg/0.5 ml ± ceftazidime 100 mg/0.5 ml; lower doses are used for children). Intraoperative IOP control is particularly important in patients with advanced glaucoma, severe retinal nonperfusion, or blood dyscrasia such as sickle-cell disease (see 'Postoperative Decisions'). To avoid increased IOP after surgery, adjust the final height of a scleral buckle before closing the sclerotomies, discontinue N_2O ~20 min before the introduction of an intraocular gas bubble (fig. 1), and infuse nonexpansile concentrations of C_3F_8 (13%) or SF_6 (20%) [2, 3]. In addition, one should create an inferior iridectomy if silicone oil tamponade is used in an aphakic eye to avoid postoperative pupillary block glaucoma [4]. Blood-induced glaucoma can occur after vitrectomy, particularly in cases with substantial preoperative vitreous hemorrhage (due to leaching of blood from the peripheral vitreous into the fluid-filled vitreous cavity postoperatively). Thus, one should remove all dispersed blood during surgery and make a reasonable attempt to excise hemorrhagic peripheral vitreous gel.

Postoperative retinal detachment can arise from intraoperative iatrogenic retinal breaks and/or development of new retinal breaks after surgery. Iatrogenic retinal breaks can be associated with passing instruments in and out of the eye, particularly if a trocar system is not used. One can minimize the likelihood of such breaks by minimizing instrument passes and, most importantly, by meticulous peripheral vitreous dissection (to reduce the chance for vitreous to become engaged with the instrument tips, which can cause peripheral vitreoretinal traction) and, in non-trocar cases, ensuring that the sclerotomy is large enough to accommodate the instrument without undue wound (and vitreous base) distortion. The likelihood of breaks developing during membrane dissection can be minimized by identifying the correct cleavage plane between the retina and the fibrovascular tissue, which facilitates the dissection. Identification and excision of the posterior hyaloid face is particularly important in this regard. In some cases, there are numerous adhesions between the fibrovascular proliferation and underlying retina. Bimanual illuminated instrument dissection (with chandelier illumination) can help one minimize retinal traction during development of the cleavage plane as can use of viscodissection [5]. Sometimes, it is best to leave behind rather large islands of fibrovascular tissue once all attachments to peripheral vitreous have been severed, particularly if the macula is

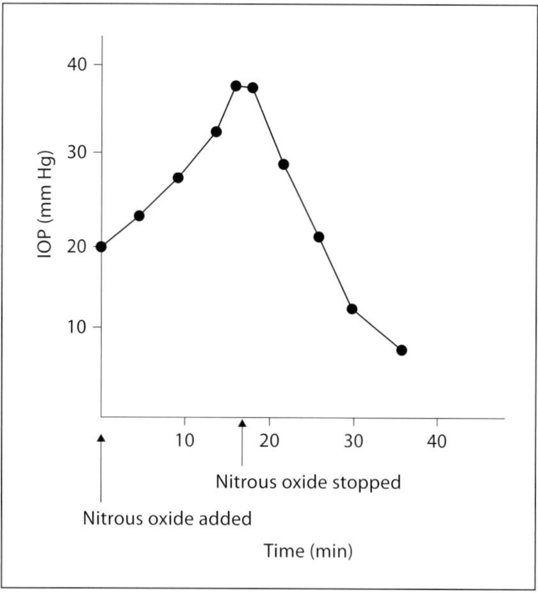

Fig. 1. Diffusion of nitrous oxide into and out of an air-filled eye causes changes in IOP. Reproduced with permission from Smith et al. [2].

not distorted by this tissue and sufficient traction has been relieved to permit retinal reattachment. Development of retinal breaks after surgery often is due to incomplete excision of the posterior vitreous cortex (i.e. posterior hyaloid) and/or fibrovascular tissue with secondary fibrous proliferation and increasing retinal traction (fig. 2).

Selection of the proper retinal tamponade device can help avoid complications such as recurrent retinal detachment, cataract, and postoperative IOP elevation. For example, gas bubbles tamponade inferior retinal breaks better than silicone oil [due to the lower specific gravity of oil (0.963) versus water (1.000 at 4°C)], and gas bubbles require postoperative face-down positioning in phakic eyes (to avoid cataract formation). Gas bubbles expand at high altitude (including airplane cabins, which typically are pressurized at the equivalent of 5,000 feet elevation; Boyle's Law: $PV = k$, where P = pressure, V = volume, and k is a constant provided that the number of

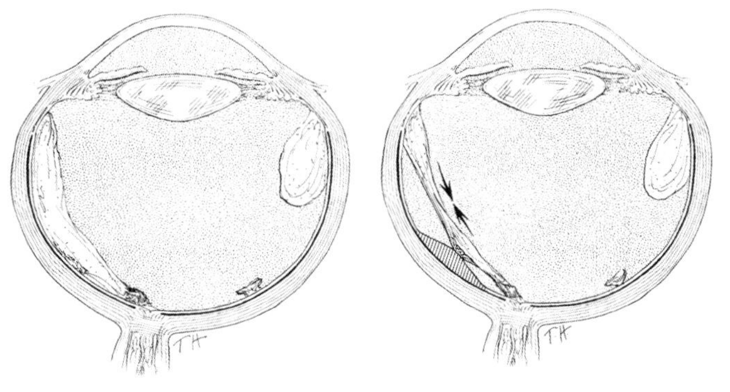

Fig. 2. Incomplete excision of peripheral vitreous (including the posterior hyaloid face) with residual vitreous attachment to fibrovascular proliferation can be associated with tissue contracture and development of a retinal detachment and/or break after surgery. Reproduced with permission from Michels [22].

moles of gas and temperature remain constant). Thus, one might consider placing a scleral buckle to support an inferior retinal break if silicone oil is needed [e.g. a monocular patient (because one cannot see clearly through a gas bubble, silicone oil may be preferred for relatively rapid visual rehabilitation), permanent retinal tamponade is anticipated, or air travel is anticipated].

Postoperative Decisions

Postoperative management of the general health of the patient is of obvious importance. For example, postoperative nausea, emesis, and anorexia can cause dehydration, hyperglycemia, and metabolic acidosis. Diabetic patients must maintain adequate hydration and proper blood glucose control to avoid ketoacidosis. Nausea and vomiting increase the likelihood of intraocular bleeding. Some causes of nausea include: general anesthesia, analgesics (e.g. narcotics), carbonic anhydrase inhibitors, increased IOP, toxic hepatitis, and gastroparesis.

IOP control is achieved typically with topical medications ± acetazolamide (except in patients with sulfa allergies and in patients with advanced renal failure or other contraindications). Special attention to IOP control is needed in patients with advanced glaucoma, poor retinal vascular perfusion, and/or hemoglobinopathy (e.g. sickle-cell trait, sickle-cell disease, thalassemia, or sickle-thalassemia).

If one uses gas tamponade, face-down positioning is critical for maintenance of crystalline lens clarity. Typically, such patients are asked to maintain face-down positioning for 45 min/h during the day and to sleep with the face directed in a downward direction (but not to obstruct breathing) while the bubble occupies 50% or more of the vitreous cavity. Head positioning can also be important to place the gas bubble against the retinal break(s). Also, a rigid shield (supported on the bones of the orbital rim) is used to protect the globe at night (adults) or at all times (e.g. children, mentally incompetent) against accidental trauma. During the day, spectacles can be used to protect the globe in appropriately selected patients.

Intraoperative Recognition and Treatment of Complications

Anterior Segment

Corneal epithelial defect occurs frequently with contact lens viewing systems, particularly in diabetic patients and in eyes with map-dot-fingerprint corneal dystrophy. (Irrigating contact lenses are likely to cause this problem.) Corneal edema can impair one's view of the fundus and

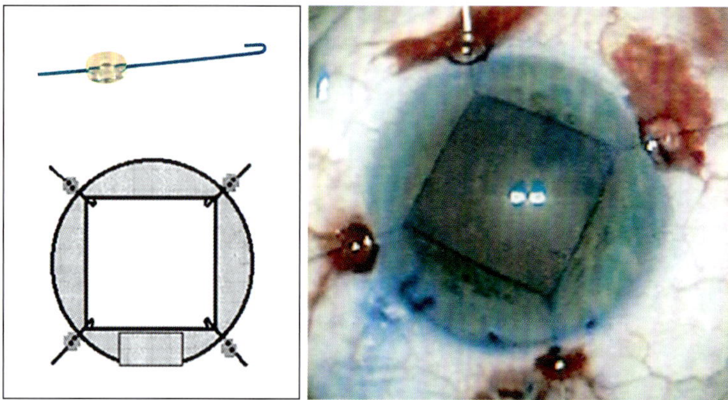

Fig. 3. Flexible iris retractors to manage intraoperative miosis. Reproduced with permission from Oetting and Omphroy [21].

can be treated effectively in most cases with frequent application of sterile topical 6% glycerin. Clearing begins to be evident after 5–10 min of treatment. When intraoperative corneal edema develops, one should check the patient's blood pressure, as, in the author's experience, hypotension can promote stromal edema, especially in diabetic patients. Endothelial striae also can interfere with one's view of the fundus, particularly in a gas-filled aphakic eye. Application of viscoelastic to the endothelial surface is effective therapy. Endothelial striae can be precipitated by phacoemulsification. To avoid this complication, one should maintain occlusion of the fragmatome port with lens material and avoid excessive use of phaco power and suction. Preservation of the anterior capsule during lensectomy and infusion of viscoelastic into the anterior chamber before and, if needed, during the lensectomy also can reduce the incidence of this complication.

Preoperatively, mydriasis is achieved pharmacologically (e.g. phenylephrine 10%, homatropine 5% every 10 min × 6 doses before surgery). Intraoperative miosis can be managed with additional topical medication or with subconjunctival injection of Pierce's solution (0.4% homatropine + 0.5% phenylephrine + procaine; contraindicated in patients with hypertension). Miosis can be managed most readily, however, with flexible iris retractors (fig. 3) [6]. Alternatively, one can excise portions of the iris with the vitrectomy probe (e.g. sphincterotomy).

Inadvertent lens damage occurs in <1% of cases, and can be avoided by maintaining globe infusion to avoid globe collapse (which can cause contact between the irrigation cannula, instruments, and/or chandelier illuminator and the lens), by using retroillumination, and by moving the fiberoptic illuminator to the opposite sclerotomy to avoid 'reaching' across the crystalline lens (fig. 4). Some surgeons feel that use of BSS Plus® (Alcon) and glucose in the infusion bottle helps to avoid intraoperative cataract progression in diabetic eyes. If damage occurs and if it is peripheral and minor, it can be observed. Otherwise, one should excise the lens. Displacement of lens fragments into the vitreous cavity occurs in approximately 20% of cases during pars plana lensectomy with a fragmatome. To avoid this complication, maintain occlusion of the fragmatome tip with lens material at all times, use only the suction needed to aspirate the lens material, and use the fragmatome to excise the nuclear material while using the vitrectomy probe on the suction mode to aspirate the peripheral cortical material. When removing nuclear material from the posterior segment, be sure to excise the vitreous around the displaced nuclear fragments before ultrasonic removal.

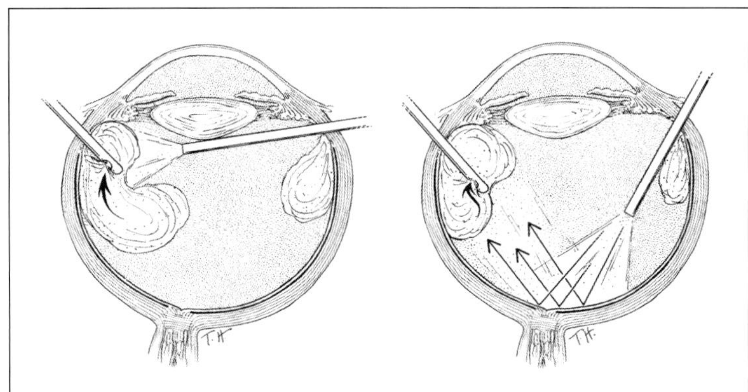

Fig. 4. Illustration of how to avoid lens damage by not 'reaching' across the crystalline lens and using retroillumination. Reproduced with permission from Michels [22].

A pseudophakos can be associated with complications. Droplet condensation on the posterior surface after fluid-air exchange can be managed with application of viscoelastic to the posterior surface, droplet removal (e.g. aspiration with a flute needle), or air-fluid exchange. Adherence of silicone oil droplets to the posterior surface of a silicone lens after silicone oil removal [7] can be managed by application of viscoelastic to the posterior surface, reinfusion of silicone oil, or, as a last resort, removal of the lens.

Intraocular hemorrhage can arise from a variety of sources, including rubeotic vessels, sclerotomies (e.g. uveal bleeding), retinal tears, and retinal blood vessels. Hemorrhage is more frequent among renal dialysis patients (due to coagulopathy associated with uremia as well as use of heparin) and among patients using anticoagulants (e.g. warfarin, clopidogrel bisulfate). Hemorrhage from retinal blood vessels can be managed by: (1) preoperative bevacizumab injection (in selected patients), which can induce substantial regression of the fine blood vessels typically within one week (since it also may be associated with progressive traction retinal detachment) [8, 9], (2) endodiathermize the bleeding vessel (avoid excessive current delivery to the retina/optic nerve), (3) increase the infusion pressure temporarily, (4) infuse intraocular thrombin (100 U/ml;

postoperative hypopyon occurs) [10], and/or (5) perform fluid-air exchange to clear the vitreous cavity and identify bleeding site(s). It may be wise to leave intact small clots on the retinal surface to avoid additional hemorrhage, but one should remove large clots (often with active suction, but sometimes forceps are required to peel adherent clot from the retinal surface), which seem to serve as a stimulus/scaffold for postoperative epiretinal proliferation.

Intraoperative retinal tears can result from direct and/or indirect (traction) retinal damage. Anterior tears usually are located in the meridian of the sclerotomies, and may be due to inadequate uveal incision (associated with vitreous base distortion during instrument insertion), vitreous incarceration with instruments (typically, horizontal scissors, which have a less streamlined profile than vertical scissors or forceps), and/or vitreous prolapse. The use of a trocar system may lower the incidence of peripheral tears. One can attempt to prevent the development of peripheral retinal tears by debriding vitreous from the sclerotomies meticulously and performing a peripheral vitreous dissection (using a prism lens or wide-angle viewing system for visualization of the peripheral vitreous and working at a high cutting rate and low suction). Anterior retinal breaks also can occur in areas of lattice degeneration, in areas of anterior

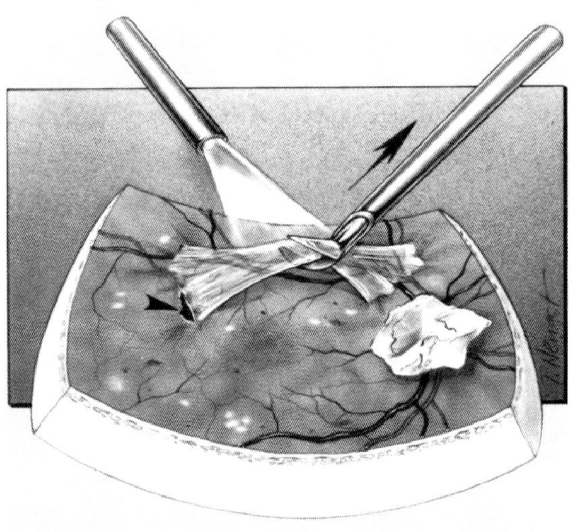

Fig. 5. Development of a retinal tear during membrane dissection due to firm attachment of fibrovascular tissue to underlying ischemic/atrophic retina. Reproduced with permission from Michels et al. [23].

fibrovascular proliferation, and in areas of strong adherence between the hyaloid and the retina.

Iatrogenic posterior retinal tears typically occur during membrane dissection, particularly if the posterior hyaloid is attached to detached, atrophic retina (fig. 5). These breaks can be avoided by: (1) identifying the correct cleavage plane between the fibrovascular tissue and the underlying retina [sometimes facilitated by using a diamond-dusted cannula (Tano [11]) to develop the cleavage plane], and (2) minimizing retinal traction during the dissection (e.g. with bimanual dissection or with use of viscodissection [5]). Retinal breaks also can occur during excision of the posterior hyaloid face, especially if the posterior hyaloid is opaque and the underlying retina is detached. Rarely, posterior retinal breaks can occur during removal of preretinal blood (especially if the underlying retina is detached) or due to a forceful infusion stream. In the former case, if the blood is clotted and adherent to the retina, development of a cleavage plane with a pick or Tano

cannula followed by clot removal with forceps is advised. If the blood is dispersed, one can use passive suction with a flute needle [12] and a low infusion pressure or active, very low suction.

Management of retinal tears requires release of direct relief of surrounding antero-posterior and tangential retinal traction (through meticulous vitrectomy and epiretinal membrane peeling). Rarely, an episcleral buckle (e.g. 5-mm-wide silicone sponge or a solid silicone boat) is placed to offset traction. The retina is then apposed against the retinal pigment epithelium using retinal tamponade (e.g. fluid-gas exchange, especially inferior tears, or air-silicone oil exchange, especially if many tears are present). Retinopexy is then applied. Usually, laser photocoagulation is used, but cryotherapy (transscleral or endocryotherapy) can be used if blood (epi- or subretinal) precludes good laser uptake. One should consider deferring retinopexy to breaks near the optic nerve or fovea once traction is released and tamponade is provided.

Rarely, the retina becomes incarcerated in the sclerotomy. If no posterior retinal break is present, one can take advantage of the specific gravity of perfluoro-n-octane (1.754) and infuse it into the vitreous cavity to force the retina posteriorly and disincarcerate the tissue. (Viscoelastic can be used if perfluoro-n-octane is not available, but a substantial amount will be needed.) Alternatively, if a posterior drainage site is accessible, one can perform a fluid-air exchange to force the retina posteriorly and disincarcerate it. If vitreous is extruded through the sclerotomy site in association with retinal incarceration, it should be excised with the vitrectomy probe or scissors. If retina extrudes through the sclerotomy, it should be repositioned into the vitreous cavity. If that is not possible, the extruded portion should be excised.

Choroidal detachment can arise from inadvertent infusion into the suprachoroidal space or from hypotony with secondary choroidal effusion and hemorrhage. To prevent inadvertent suprachoroidal infusion, one visualizes directly the infusion cannula in the vitreous cavity before turning on the infusion. If a choroidal detachment is present preoperatively, one can drain the effusion through a sclerotomy with simultaneous balanced salt infusion into the anterior chamber (e.g. via a 23-gauge needle), or one can use a 6-mm infusion cannula (vs. 4 mm), which may penetrate into the vitreous cavity if the detachment is not too large. If inadvertent suprachoroidal infusion occurs, one should turn off the infusion immediately, insert an infusion cannula through a different sclerotomy (ideally 180° away), and infuse through the new infusion system while draining suprachoroidal fluid via the original sclerotomy. Hypotony is avoided by ensuring that the sclerotomies are not too large, that sclerotomies are closed with plugs when not occupied with instruments, and that the fluid level in the infusion bottle is never below a critical level.

Optic nerve damage can result from intraoperative ischemia (maintain adequate blood pressure intraoperatively and monitor central retinal artery perfusion constantly via direct visualization), elevated IOP (avoid prolonged periods of elevated infusion pressure, particularly if the blood pressure is low), or electrical damage. The latter is most likely to occur with application of unipolar diathermy (monitor tissue shrinkage during application of diathermy to neovascular tissue emanating from the optic nerve head).

Postoperative Examination, and Recognition and Treatment of Complications

External examination may reveal lid swelling and/or chemosis, which usually are a consequence of face-down positioning and/or placement of a scleral buckle. In these cases, the swelling can be treated with ice packs. Chemosis can occur, even in the absence of a scleral buckle. If the conjunctiva prolapses through the lids, one should treat with aggressive lubrication (e.g. antibiotic ointment), ice packs, and eliminate contact with gauze dressings, which can exacerbate the problem. Lid swelling and erythema can be a sign of drug allergy (e.g. atropine, brimonidine). Swelling occasionally is a sign of orbital cellulitis (a rare complication, generally associated with other signs such as pain, proptosis, limited extraocular motility, and optic neuropathy).

Sclerotomy-associated complications include wound leak, ectasia, and fibrovascular ingrowth. If chemosis occurs with hypotony (i.e. filtering bleb), one should consider the possibility of a leaking sclerotomy, which often can be detected by inspection. This condition is more likely to occur if the sclerotomies have not been sutured. Proper wound construction (biplanar) should render leaking non-sutured sclerotomies an uncommon occurrence. One should verify that the sclerotomies are air-/watertight at the end of the case. If the sclerotomy is leaking, one can close the incision with 7-0 polyglycolic acid sutures in a figure-of-eight pattern. Infusion of air at the end of the case usually allows one to verify that unsutured sclerotomies are airtight and closed adequately. Occasionally, scleral ectasia occurs at the sclerotomy site (e.g. with rheumatoid arthritis). Fibrovascular ingrowth can be associated with vitreous hemorrhage ± peripheral retinal traction ± retinal tear/rhegmatogenous detachment. Fibrovascular ingrowth can be detected with ultrasound biomicroscopy and can be managed with reoperation, direct dissection with release of peripheral retinal traction or release of traction via a scleral buckle, and extensive application of retinopexy locally. Extensive panretinal photocoagulation at the time of initial vitrectomy may help to prevent clinically significant occurrence of this complication, which is sometimes associated with severe ischemia and anterior hyaloidal proliferation.

Corneal epithelial defect (with associated degrees of stromal edema) probably is the most frequent postoperative abnormality observed with slit lamp examination. The condition usually resolves spontaneously during the first week after surgery. It is wise to continue topical antibiotic therapy until the defect is healed completely. If the epithelial defect persists by week 1 after surgery, additional treatment (e.g. bandage contact lens or antibiotic ointment) is indicated. Generally, firm attachment between the epithelium and Bowman's membrane requires 6–12 weeks in diabetic patients. Rarely, corneal epithelial defects persist (neurotrophic) or corneal ulcer develops. Management of these conditions is beyond the scope of this chapter, but usually involves the expertise of a corneal surgeon. Mild corneal edema is often present in the setting of an epithelial defect or after lensectomy, and usually it resolves within 2–12 weeks.

Iris-related complications include fibrous pupillary membrane, posterior synechiae, and/or a widely dilated, fixed pupil. Fibrous pupillary membrane can be managed with frequent topical application of corticosteroids or intracameral injection of tissue plasminogen activator (TPA) using a short 30-gauge needle attached to a tuberculin syringe (5 µg in 0.05 ml). It may be wise to wait 48–72 h after surgery before injecting TPA to avoid TPA-induced anterior chamber bleeding. Fibrous pupillary membranes that become thick and organized are uncommon, but can be excised using intraocular forceps and the vitrectomy probe via limbal incisions. Posterior synechiae can be lysed with short-acting mydriatics (e.g. 2.5% phenylephrine) or, if needed, using an iris sweep through limbal incisions in the minor procedure room. A widely dilated, fixed pupil can result from excessive sphincter excision or may be a manifestation of retroiridal epiciliary fibrous tissue proliferation in aphakic eyes [13].

Posterior subcapsular cataract is often present if a large gas bubble fills the vitreous cavity, particularly if the patient has not maintained strict face-down positioning. If rigorous face-down positioning is instituted within the first 24 h after surgery, this condition can reverse substantially, even completely.

Rarely, slit lamp examination reveals signs of infectious endophthalmitis such as hypopyon.

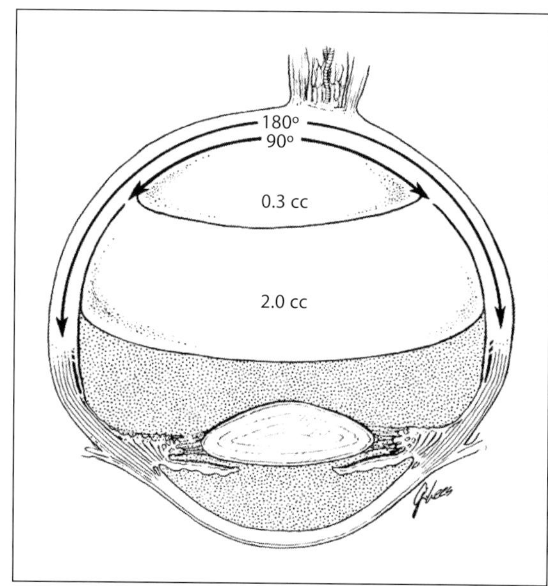

Fig. 6. Surface area tamponade by intraocular gas bubble. Reproduced with permission from Michels [22].

Associated symptoms typically include pain and decreased visual acuity. It is important to gently retract the lower lid in order to visualize clearly the inferior anterior chamber, as the hypopyon may occasionally be rather small. Gonioscopy can aid in visualizing a small hypopyon. Treatment of endophthalmitis is beyond the scope of this chapter but has been reviewed elsewhere [14]. Hypopyon can be a sign of noninfectious inflammation, e.g. following intraoperative use of thrombin to control bleeding. Treatment of noninfectious inflammation usually involves frequent application of topical corticosteroids and occasionally the use of intracameral TPA (e.g. to lyse fibrin pupillary membranes). Finally, one should assess the size of the gas or silicone oil bubble. At minimum, the bubble must be large enough to tamponade all retinal breaks. Small bubbles have a relatively large surface area of tamponade (fig. 6). With the patient gazing straight ahead, a 50% bubble occupies the superior 50% of the vitreous cavity as viewed through a 5-mm-diameter pupillary aperture.

Fundus examination may reveal an unexpected retinal detachment, which can signify an untreated iatrogenic retinal break or inadequate relief of traction around a previously identified retinal break. Rhegmatogenous retinal detachment arising from an intraoperative retinal break usually arises within 2 weeks of surgery. (New retinal breaks after surgery can arise within 2–12 months of vitrectomy.) If the gas bubble does not fill the vitreous cavity, one can position the patient such that one views the fundus through the fluid phase, which often affords the clearest view. As noted earlier, retinal breaks typically occur at the posterior margin of the vitreous base in the meridians of the sclerotomies (iatrogenic) and in areas of unrelieved or newly developed tangential retinal traction. Recurrent retinal detachment can be treated with additional surgery in the operating room. Occasionally, one can treat the break in the office with the indirect laser photocoagulation or cryotherapy followed by head positioning that places the tamponade device over the break. The latter approach is most likely to be effective if there is no residual traction around the margins of the break. If there is traction, one should treat with repeat vitrectomy and full relief of traction (direct dissection and/or, less commonly, scleral buckle) and retinal tamponade. Residual subretinal fluid associated with traction retinal detachment or with rhegmatogenous detachment and adequately closed retinal breaks usually shows definite signs of absorption during the first week after surgery.

Postoperative vitreous hemorrhage occurs in ~20% of eyes with severe proliferative diabetic retinopathy. Some causes of postoperative vitreous hemorrhage include retina tear, retinal neovascularization, fibrovascular ingrowth from a sclerotomy, rubeosis iridis (aphakia), and anterior hyaloidal fibrovascular proliferation. Since extensive panretinal photocoagulation is applied intraoperatively, eyes with postoperative vitreous hemorrhage usually are observed for 6–8 weeks for

spontaneous resolution (unless the patient is one eyed) and are followed with serial B-scan echography to identify retinal detachment. Presence of retinal detachment or strong suspicion of an untreated retinal tear mandates prompt intervention. If rubeosis iridis is present, one would consider intervention within one month after surgery (sooner if glaucoma or extensive neovascularization in the anterior chamber angle is present), and one probably would provide intravitreal bevacizumab (1.25 mg/0.05 ml) or ranibizumab (0.5 mg/0.05 ml) to induce prompt regression of the rubeosis iridis (and also of persistent posterior retinal neovascularization).

Anterior hyaloidal fibrovascularization is uncommon, but most often occurs after phakic vitrectomy with scleral buckle for severe proliferative diabetic retinopathy, and is difficult to treat [15]. Typically, the patient presents with postoperative vitreous hemorrhage and develops progressive peripheral retinal detachment. The anterior hyaloid vessels can be visualized in the pupillary space at the slit lamp in severe cases (fig. 7). Ultrasound biomicroscopy can facilitate diagnosis. The condition usually progresses to phthisis bulbi without intervention. Therapy may involve repeat vitrectomy, lensectomy, direct dissection, endodiathermy of the vessels, provision of full panretinal photocoagulation if not done previously, intravitreal injection of an anti-vascular endothelial growth factor agent, and possibly silicone oil infusion to compartmentalize the eye (i.e. restrict water-soluble, diffusible vasoactive factors to the thin fluid phase between the retina and silicone oil bubble).

Increased IOP immediately after surgery can be associated with an open or closed anterior chamber angle. Blood-induced, open-angle glaucoma (typically in aphakic eyes) may be associated with a small hyphema (fig. 8). Patients often respond to medical management while the blood clears. In unresponsive cases, vitreous washout is done, usually in the operating room, but it can be done in the office under subconjunctival

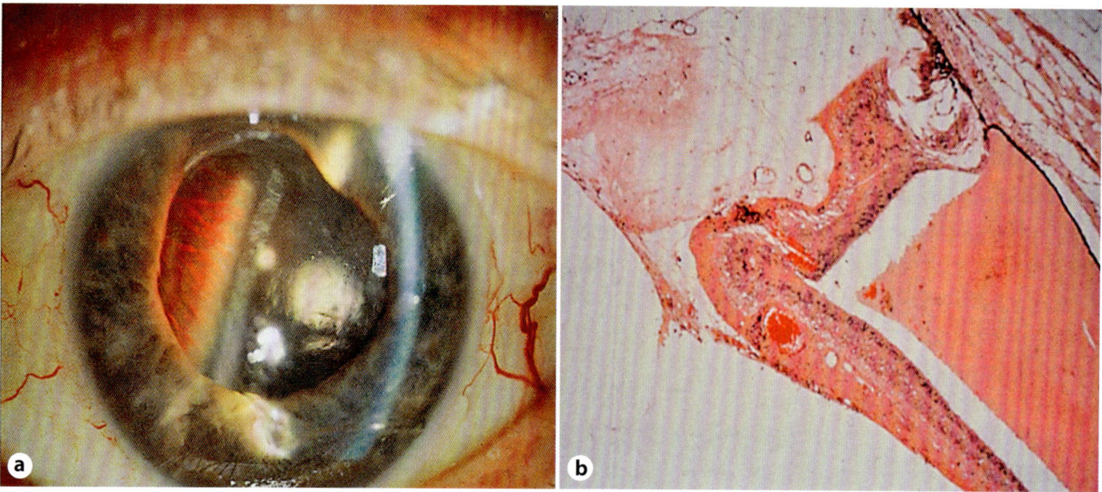

Fig. 7. Anterior hyaloidal fibrovascular proliferation in an eye with severe proliferative diabetic retinopathy. Note the presence of abnormal vessels behind the intraocular lens (**a**) and the presence of anterior dragging of the retina onto the pars plana in histological section (**b**). Reproduced with permission from Eliott et al. [24].

anesthesia (e.g. via fluid-air exchange) in properly selected patients. With the patient sterilely prepped at the slit lamp, one can infuse air using a 5/8th inch 30-gauge needle through the pars plana (superiorly) while draining fluid (passively or using active suction) via a separate needle inferiorly. A bubble (oil or gas) can cause pupillary block (typically with supine positioning), or the vitreous cavity can be overfilled. Treatment could include medical therapy, peripheral iridotomy (in phakic eyes), or, if a pupillary membrane is present, intracameral TPA. (Fibrin pupillary membrane can cause pupillary block in aphakic eyes even in the absence of a bubble in the vitreous cavity.) In aphakic eyes with a vitreous bubble (oil or gas), one also can treat with prone head positioning and/or removal of gas (using a 5/8th inch 30-gauge needle attached to a tuberculin syringe inserted through the pars plana). In the case of silicone-filled eyes, one can restore patency of the inferior iridectomy using YAG laser (sometimes difficult immediately after surgery) or by enlarging the iridectomy using a 5/8th-inch 30-gauge needle. Although removal of silicone oil in the

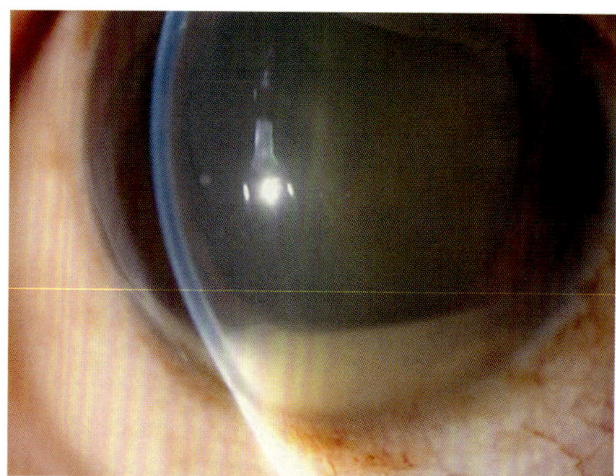

Fig. 8. Blood-induced glaucoma due to vitreous hemorrhage. The hemorrhage is chronic and the blood is dehemoglobinized, leading to a resemblance to a small hypopyon. Note that corneal edema, usually present with hypopyon, is absent.

office can be done, it is usually difficult to remove enough without causing patient discomfort unless it is low viscosity oil (e.g. 1,000 cSt). Oil removal in the operating room or in a fully equipped minor procedure room is easier. An encircling scleral buckle can cause ciliary body edema and secondary angle closure glaucoma. If medical therapy fails, cutting the scleral buckle can be effective. As noted earlier, ascent to an altitude of >5,000 feet with a bubble >10% of the vitreous cavity volume can cause increased IOP. Topical or subconjunctival corticosteroids can cause glaucoma, but usually several weeks of therapy are needed to induce ocular hypertension. It is important to note that patients with severe diabetic retinopathy can develop no light perception in association with moderate IOP elevation (e.g. ≥25 mm Hg) [16]. Paracentesis and IOP lowering to ≤10 mm Hg can restore vision.

Causes of hypotony after diabetic vitrectomy include retinal detachment, cyclitic membrane formation (often associated with retrodisplacement of the iris in aphakic eyes and treated with vitrectomy, epiciliary dissection, and, in some eyes, silicone oil infusion) [13], cyclodialysis cleft (detected on gonioscopy and by the typical shallow choroidal detachment evident on B-scan echography), or a leaking sclerotomy.

In addition to pupillary block glaucoma, intravitreal silicone oil can be associated with open-angle glaucoma [17]. Often, gonioscopy of such eyes will reveal numerous tiny emulsified silicone oil bubbles occupying the superior anterior chamber angle. This migration of oil from the posterior to the anterior chamber can occur even in phakic eyes. Silicone can be associated with additional complications such as bullous keratopathy (with cornea-silicone touch), cataract, refractive change (~6 dpt due to its refractive index of 1.44), posterior (peri-silicone) epiretinal proliferation, and, perhaps, retinal toxicity (the vitreous cavity normally is a sink for K^+ ions) [18]. The surface tension and specific gravity render silicone oil suboptimal for tamponading inferior retinal breaks.

Fibrinoid syndrome is a rare condition that can occur in patients with severe diabetic retinopathy with or without vitreous surgery. It is characterized by massive fibrin deposition in the vitreous cavity with subsequent development of traction retinal detachment, fibrin organization, rubeosis iridis, and hypotony. As a postoperative complication, it tends to occur in patients with severe retinal ischemia, extensive/prolonged surgery, and/or extensive cryotherapy or laser photocoagulation. Treatment includes topical corticosteroids (systemic steroids can be effective but usually are not well tolerated in diabetic patients), intravitreal TPA (≤25 µg), vitrectomy, and silicone oil infusion [19].

Scleral buckle infection is an uncommon complication, but may occur somewhat more often in diabetic patients. Therapy involves treatment with systemic and/or topical antibiotics and buckle removal. Occasionally, one can treat an exposed buckle with a pericardial graft.

Phthisis bulbi is an uncommon complication of diabetic vitrectomy (<5% of eyes), and may be associated with a series of findings, e.g. hypotony, cyclitic membrane formation, retinal detachment, epi- and/or subretinal fibrosis, fibrinoid syndrome, rubeosis iridis, anterior hyaloid fibrovascular proliferation, each of which may be treatable if intervention is done early. For untreatable cases, topical atropine 1% and prednisolone acetate 1% can provide symptomatic relief. Unresponsive cases may obtain relief (usually temporary) with retrobulbar alcohol injection [0.5 ml 2% lidocaine, then 2 ml ethanol-2% lidocaine (3:1 mixture), then 0.5 ml 2% lidocaine all through the same 1 1/2-inch 25-gauge needle in the muscle cone]. Definitive treatment of phthisical eyes with intractable pain is enucleation.

Sympathetic ophthalmia is a rare complication of diabetic vitrectomy (0.01%), and probably is more likely to occur after trauma (0.06%) [20]. One should rule out infectious causes of intraocular inflammation, enucleate the inciting eye if it is blind (for diagnosis), and treat initially with systemic corticosteroids. One may add steroid-sparing agents (e.g. cyclosporine, azathioprine) later, and may augment treatment with local steroids (e.g. subconjunctival, intravitreal sustained delivery) if necessary.

Conclusions

Potential complications after vitrectomy for complications of diabetic retinopathy are numerous, and involve all components of the eye and periocular tissues. They also can involve the systemic health of the patient, including severe metabolic disequilibrium and death. Good outcomes can be achieved by avoidance of complications through anticipatory intra- and postoperative decision-making and anticipation, early identification, and appropriately aggressive treatment of postoperative complications.

References

1 Aaberg TM Jr, Flynn HW Jr, Schiffman J, Newton J: Nosocomial acute-onset postoperative endophthalmitis survey. A 10-year review of incidence and outcomes. Ophthalmology 1998;105:1004–1010.

2 Smith RB, Carl B, Linn JG Jr, Nemoto E: Effect of nitrous oxide on air in vitreous. Am J Ophthalmol 1974;78:314–317.

3 Abrams GW, Edelhauser HF, Aaberg TM, Hamilton LH: Dynamics of intravitreal sulfur hexafluoride gas. Invest Ophthalmol 1974;13:863–868.

4 Ando F: Intraocular hypertension resulting from pupillary block by silicone oil. Am J Ophthalmol 1985;99:87–88.

5 Grigorian RA, Castellarin A, Fegan R, et al: Epiretinal membrane removal in diabetic eyes: comparison of viscodissection with conventional methods of membrane peeling. Br J Ophthalmol 2003;87:737–741.

6 de Juan E Jr, Hickingbotham D: Flexible iris retractor. Am J Ophthalmol 1991;111:776–777.

7 Kusaka S, Kodama T, Ohashi Y: Condensation of silicone oil on the posterior surface of a silicone intraocular lens during vitrectomy. Am J Ophthalmol 1996;121:574–575.

8 Avery RL, Pearlman J, Pieramici DJ, et al: Intravitreal bevacizumab (Avastin) in the treatment of proliferative diabetic retinopathy. Ophthalmology 2006;113:1695.e1–1695.e15.

9 Arevalo JF, Maia M, Flynn HW Jr, et al: Tractional retinal detachment following intravitreal bevacizumab (Avastin) in patients with severe proliferative diabetic retinopathy. Br J Ophthalmol 2008;92:213–216.

10 Thompson JT, Glaser B, Michels RG, De Bustros S: The use of intravitreal thrombin to control hemorrhage during vitrectomy. Ophthalmology 1986;93:279–282.

11 Lewis JM, Park I, Ohji M, Saito Y, Tano Y: Diamond-dusted silicone cannula for epiretinal membrane separation during vitreous surgery. Am J Ophthalmol 1997;124:552–554.

12 Charles S: Vitreous Microsurgery, ed 1. Baltimore, Williams and Wilkins, 1981.

13 Zarbin MA, Michels RG, Green WR: Dissection of epiciliary tissue to treat chronic hypotony after surgery for retinal detachment with proliferative vitreoretinopathy. Retina 1991;11:208–213.

14 Kresloff MS, Castellarin AA, Zarbin MA: Endophthalmitis. Surv Ophthalmol 1998;43:193–224.

15 Lewis H, Abrams GW, Williams GA: Anterior hyaloidal fibrovascular proliferation after diabetic vitrectomy. Am J Ophthalmol 1987;104:607–613.

16 Kangas TA, Bennet SR, Flynn HW Jr, Murray TG, Rubsamen PE, Han DP, Mieler WF, Williams DF, Abrams GW: Reversible loss of light perception after vitreoretinal surgery. Am J Ophthalmol 1995;120:751–756.

17 Valone J Jr, McCarthy M: Emulsified anterior chamber silicone oil and glaucoma. Ophthalmology 1994;101:1908–1912.

18 Winter M, Eberhardt W, Scholz C, Reichenbach A: Failure of potassium siphoning by Muller cells: a new hypothesis of perfluorocarbon liquid-induced retinopathy. Invest Ophthalmol Vis Sci 2000;41:256–261.

19 Castellarin A, Grigorian R, Bhagat N, Del Priore L, Zarbin MA: Vitrectomy with silicone oil infusion in severe diabetic retinopathy. Br J Ophthalmol 2003;87:318–321.

20 Gass JD: Sympathetic ophthalmia following vitrectomy. Am J Ophthalmol 1982;93:552–558.

21 Oetting TA, Omphroy LC: Modified technique using flexible iris retractors in clear corneal cataract surgery. J Cataract Refract Surg 2002;28:596–598.

22 Michels RG: Vitreous Surgery. St Louis, Mosby, 1981.

23 Michels RG, Wilkinson CP, Rice TA: Retinal Detachment. St. Louis, Mosby, 1990.

24 Eliott D, Lee MS, Abrams GW: Proliferative diabetic retinopathy: Principles and techniques of surgical treatment; in Ryan SJ, Hinton DR, Schachat AP, Wilkinson CP (ed): Retina, ed 4. Philadelphia, Mosby, vol 3, chapter 142, 2006.

Marco A. Zarbin, MD, PhD
Institute of Ophthalmology and Visual Science-New Jersey Medical School
Room 6156, Doctors Office Center
90 Bergen Street
Newark, NJ 07103 (USA)
Tel. +1 973 972 2038, E-Mail zarbin@earthlink.net

Bandello F, Battaglia Parodi M (eds): Surgical Retina.
ESASO Course Series. Basel, Karger, 2012, vol 2, pp 81–90

Diabetic Macular Edema: Cases and Diagnostics

Constantin J. Pournaras[a] · Jean-Antoine Pournaras[b] · Efstratios Mendrinos[a]

[a]Vitreo-Retinal Unit, Department of Ophthalmology, Geneva University Hospitals, Geneva, and
[b]Vitreo-Retinal Unit, Jules Gonin Eye Hospital, University of Lausanne, Lausanne, Switzerland

Abstract

Diabetic macular edema (DME) is the most common cause of visual impairment in patients with diabetes mellitus. It is characterized by the presence of increased retinal thickness with or without hard exudates. The pathogenesis is complex and multifactorial. DME may be focal or diffuse. Ischemia may also be present. Other than slit-lamp biomicroscopy and stereoscopic photography, fluorescein angiography (FA) and optical coherence tomography (OCT) are integrate part of the diagnosis and follow-up of patients with DME. Combination of information that is obtained by FA and OCT allows for appropriate management of DME. FA is useful for evaluating the severity of the dysfunction in the blood-retinal barrier and the detection of retinal ischemia; however, it does not reliably quantify the degree of fluid accumulation in the retina. OCT can detect early changes in retinal thickness despite normal findings on slit-lamp biomicroscopy. Diffuse retinal thickening, cystoid macular edema, serous retinal detachment and vitreomacular interface abnormalities can be seen by OCT in DME.

Diabetic macular edema (DME) is the most common cause of visual impairment in patients with diabetes mellitus. The pathogenesis of DME is complex and multifactorial. It occurs mainly as a result of disruption of the blood-retinal barrier (BRB), which leads to increased accumulation of fluid within the intraretinal layers of the macula. Altered vitreomacular interface may also contribute significantly to the progression of macular edema. Other factors such as hypoxia, altered blood flow, retinal ischemia, and inflammation are also associated with the progression of DME. Inflammatory processes, such as increased vascular endothelial growth factor levels, endothelial dysfunction, leukocyte adhesion, decreased pigment epithelium-derived factor levels, and increased protein kinase C production, that cause breakdown of the BRB and increase vascular permeability are upregulated within the diabetic retinal vasculature [1].

The clinical detection and evaluation methods currently used have, until recently, been limited to slit-lamp biomicroscopy and stereoscopic photography. Routine slit-lamp biomicroscopy can provide information that is useful in the clinical diagnosis of DME. However, early detection of macular thickening is hard to estimate using this technique, and both slit-lamp biomicroscopy and stereoscopic photography are subjective and insensitive to small changes in retinal thickness. Fluorescein angiography (FA) is useful for evaluating the severity of the dysfunction in the BRB and the detection of retinal

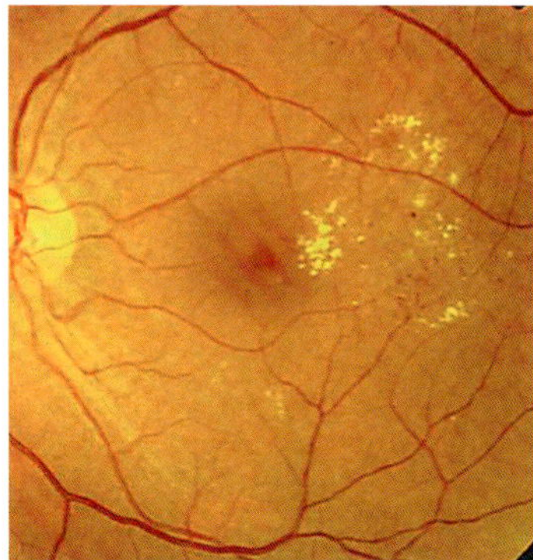

Fig. 1. CSME. Hard exudates within 500 μm of the macular center and retinal thickening at this area. Note the circinate pattern of hard exudates around the microaneurysms.

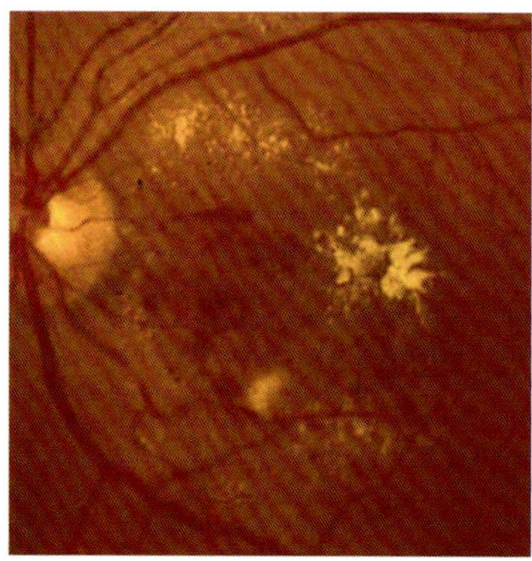

Fig. 2. CSME. Hard exudates at the foveal zone and retinal thickening.

ischemia; however, it does not reliably quantify the degree of fluid accumulation in the retina. Recently, several novel imaging techniques for the objective assessment of DME have been developed. One of the most promising of these new modalities is optical coherence tomography (OCT).

Epidemiology

The incidence of DME has been studied in the Wisconsin Epidemiologic Diabetic Retinopathy Study [2, 3]. The results of this study demonstrated a higher 4- and 10-year DME incidence in diabetic patients with early onset (8.2 and 20%, respectively) and in those with late onset and taking insulin (8.4 and 26%, respectively) compared to those not taking insulin (2.9 and 14%, respectively). Risk factors that contribute to the progression of DME include increasing levels of hyperglycemia, diabetes duration, severity of DR at baseline, diastolic blood pressure, and the presence of gross proteinuria. The UK Prospective Diabetes Study Group clearly demonstrated the beneficial effect of tight blood pressure control on DME in type 2 diabetic patients as it showed, at 9 years of follow-up, a 47% reduced risk of visual loss due to reduced incidence of macular edema [4]. Lastly, several studies found a correlation between elevated rate of serum lipids and the amount of lipid exudates [5, 6]. It is strongly recommended that in all patients with DME, maximum care should be given to normalize elevated blood glucose, lipids and decrease elevated blood pressure.

Clinical Description and Classification

DME is diagnosed stereoscopically as retinal thickening in the macula using fundus contact lens biomicroscopy. The Early Treatment Diabetic Retinopathy Study defined that the following characteristics indicate clinically significant macular edema (CSME; fig. 1, 2): (1) thickening of the retina (as seen either by slit lamp biomicroscopy or by stereo fundus photography) at or within 500 μm of the center of the macula; (2) hard exudates at or within 500 μm of the center of the macula, associated with the thickening of the adjacent retina (but not residual hard exudates remaining after disappearance of retinal

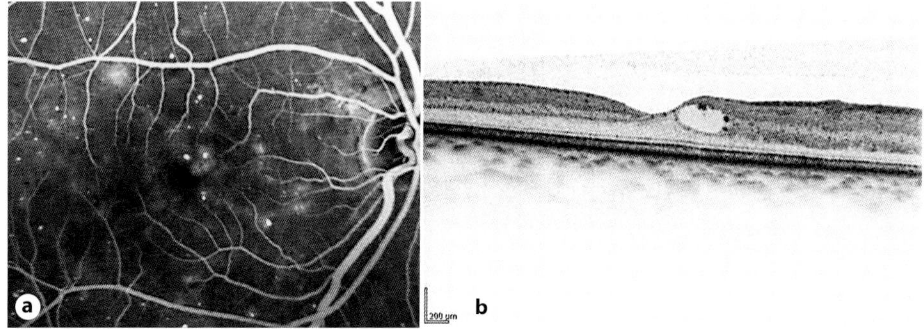

Fig. 3. Focal DME. **a** Fluorescein angiography showing leakage from microaneurysms located within the macular center. Note the accumulation of fluorescein in a central cyst surrounding two microaneurysms. **b** Corresponding macular SD-OCT shows a juxtafoveal cyst. The hyperreflective spots at the border of the cyst represent the microaneurysms.

thickening), and (3) a zone, or zones, of retinal thickening one disc area or larger size, any part of which is within one disc diameter of the center of the macula [7].

Twenty-four percent of eyes with CSME and 33% of eyes with center-involving CSME will have a moderate visual loss (15 or more letters on the ETDRS chart) within 3 years if untreated [7, 8].

CSME is further classified into focal or diffuse, depending on the leakage pattern seen on FA. In focal CSME, discrete points of retinal hyperfluorescence are present on the FA due to focal leakage of microaneurysms (fig. 3). The discrete leaking microaneurysms are thought to cause retinal thickening. Commonly, these leaking microaneurysms are surrounded by circinate rings of hard exudates. The exudates are lipoprotein deposits in the outer retinal layers. In diffuse DME, areas of diffuse leakage are noted on the FA due to intraretinal leakage from a dilated retinal capillary bed (fig. 4). There may be associated cystoid macular edema (CME). CME results from a generalized breakdown of the inner BRB with fluid accumulation, primarily in the outer plexiform layer. Furthermore, focal DME is responsive to focal laser photocoagulation, whereas diffuse DME represents a more challenging clinical situation and

is refractory to laser photocoagulation in many cases [9, 10].

Diagnosis with Imaging Modalities

The traditional methods of evaluating macular diseases, such as slit-lamp biomicroscopy and stereo fundus photography, are relatively insensitive in determining small changes in retinal thickness. Several additional diagnostic techniques for ocular imaging are available.

Fluorescein Angiography
FA is a standard method used to evaluate patients with DME that is sensitive for qualitative detection of fluid leakage. Leakage on the FA does not equate to clinical retinal thickening or edema since extracellular edema requires that the rate of fluid ingress into the retina exceed the rate of fluid clearance from the retina. Once a patient is diagnosed with CSME, an angiogram is usually performed to identify the treatable leaking lesions and to evaluate ischemic areas. Ischemic maculopathy is diagnosed when capillary nonperfusion is seen on the FA (fig. 5). There is initially a rupture of the perifoveal capillary ring with enlargement of the foveal avascular zone.

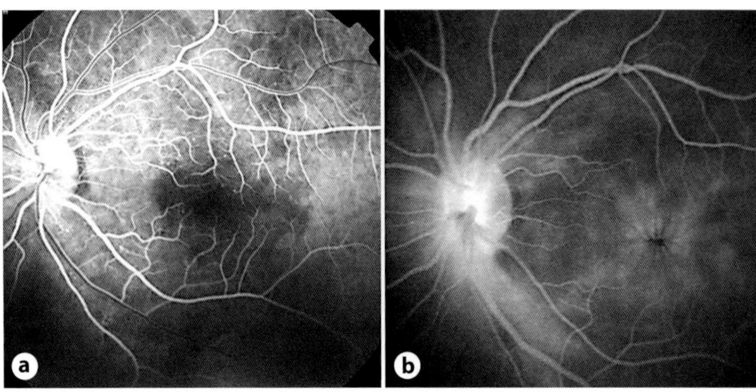

Fig. 4. Diffuse DME. **a** Intermediate-phase FA. There is a dilated capillary bed adjacent to the optic nerve but not any microangiopathy at the macula. **b** Late-phase FA shows diffuse leakage at the macular area with accumulation of the dye within central cysts, and optic nerve head. The presence of diffuse leakage despite the absence of sufficient microvascular abnormalities implicates the presence of breakdown of the inner BRB that can be reversible when systemic risk factors are controlled.

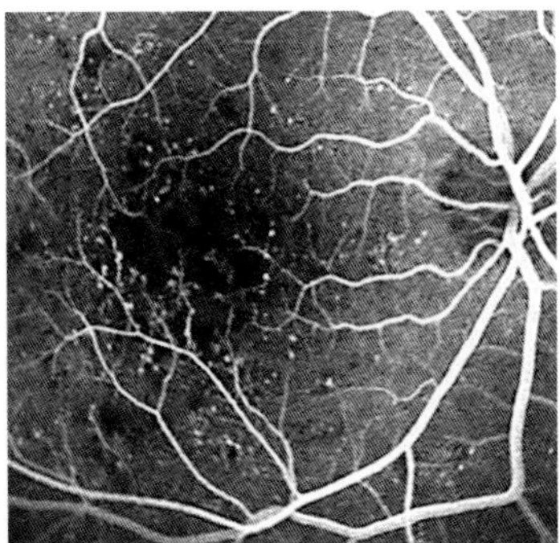

Fig. 5. Ischemic diabetic maculopathy. FA shows presence of capillary dropout at the foveal area with enlargement and irregularity of the foveal avascular zone.

This finding, which can be evaluated only by FA, usually explains a disproportionate decrease in visual acuity when compared to ophthalmoscopic findings.

FA leakage in DME can be categorized into three different types: (1) focal leakage: well-defined focal area of leakage from microaneurysms or dilated capillaries (fig. 3); (2) diffuse leakage: presence of widespread leakage from intraretinal microvascular abnormalities, retinal capillary bed (fig. 4); (3) diffuse cystoid leakage: diffuse leakage and pooling of dye in the cystic spaces of the macula in the late phase of the angiogram (fig. 6) [11]. It is important to evaluate

the FA pattern when managing patients with DME as diffuse leakage from the capillary bed with not yet established microvascular abnormalities usually indicates functional changes that are reversible when optimal control of hyperglycemia and increased arterial blood pressure is achieved.

Optical Coherence Tomography
The historical gold standard tests for diagnosis of DME, such as fundus stereophotography or biomicroscopy, are less sensitive than OCT in the detection of DME [12]. In a systematic review of the literature that compared OCT with gold standard tests concluded that OCT performs well compared with the gold standard tests, and can be used to diagnose and initiate therapy for central DME [13].

Optical Coherence Tomography Patterns in Diabetic Macular Edema

Several authors have proposed classification of DME based on OCT findings: diffuse retinal thickening, CME, serous retinal detachment, and vitreomacular interface abnormality (VMIA). Diffuse retinal thickening is usually defined as sponge-like swelling of the retina with a generalized, heterogeneous, mild hyporeflectivity

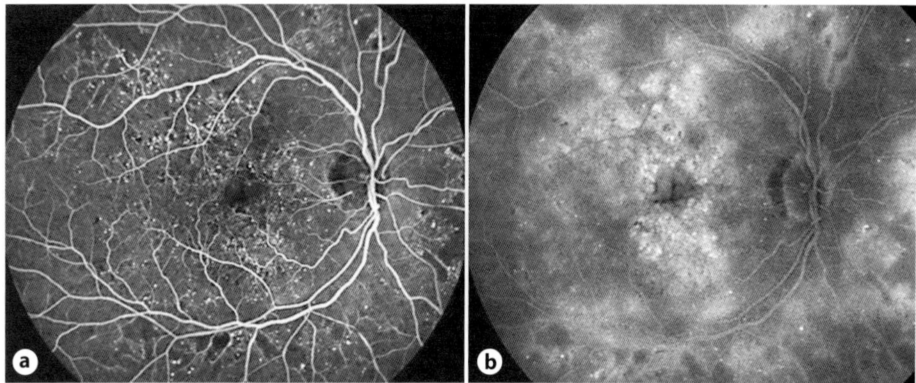

Fig. 6. Cystoid DME. **a** Intermediate-phase FA. There are several microaneurysms and areas of capillary dropout outside the posterior pole. **b** Late-phase FA showing areas of diffuse leakage and pooling of dye in the cystic spaces of the macula.

compared with normal retina (fig. 7). Diffuse retinal thickening is reported to be present in 88–100% of eyes with DME. Diffuse retinal thickening alone (without any features of the other patterns) is present in 36–42% [14, 15]. CME was identified by the presence of intraretinal, round or oval cystoid areas of low reflectivity, which were typically separated by highly reflective septae (fig. 8). CME is typically identified in 44–47% of eyes with DME [14, 15]. OCT seems to be particularly useful for detecting a feature that is found in DME and that is not easily seen on biomicroscopy: serous retinal detachment (fig. 9). This appears as a shallow elevation of the retina, with an optically clear space between the retina and the retinal pigment epithelium (RPE), and a distinct outer border of the detached retina. It was seen in 15% of eyes with DMO in the study by Otani et al. [14]. VMIAs include the presence of epiretinal membranes, vitreomacular traction or both. An epiretinal membrane can be manifested on OCT by the presence of a macular pseudohole, a hyperreflective band along the inner aspect of the retina, or a visible hyperreflective membrane tuft or edge (fig. 10). Vitreomacular traction was identified

by a hyperreflective band that is in apposition with the inner surface of the retina at discrete site(s) and elevated above the surface of the retina elsewhere (fig. 11). VMIAs appear to occur in 14–16% of eyes with DME [15, 16]. In eyes with persistent DME (defined by this study as at least one prior focal laser treatment), VMIAs may be found in up to 52–67% on OCT [17]. OCT seems particularly relevant to the analysis of the vitreomacular relationship. Indeed, OCT is much more accurate than biomicroscopy in determining the status of the posterior hyaloids when it is only slightly detached from the macular surface. In some cases of DMO, the posterior hyaloid on OCT is thick and hyperreflective; it is partially detached from the posterior pole and taut over it, but remains attached to the disc and to the top of the raised macular surface, on which it exerts a traction, indicating an obvious vitreomacular traction [18–20]. In these cases, vitrectomy is beneficial [18, 19].

Small, hyperreflective foci have been identified in patients with DME. These foci can be less than 30 µm in diameter and cannot be identified on fundus biomicroscopy, FA, or infrared imaging. They were characterized by the same amount

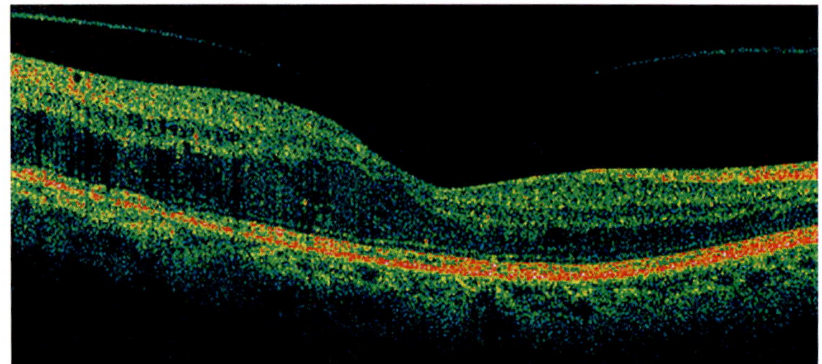

Fig. 7. OCT: diffuse retinal thickening with a heterogeneous mild hyporeflectivity compared with normal retina.

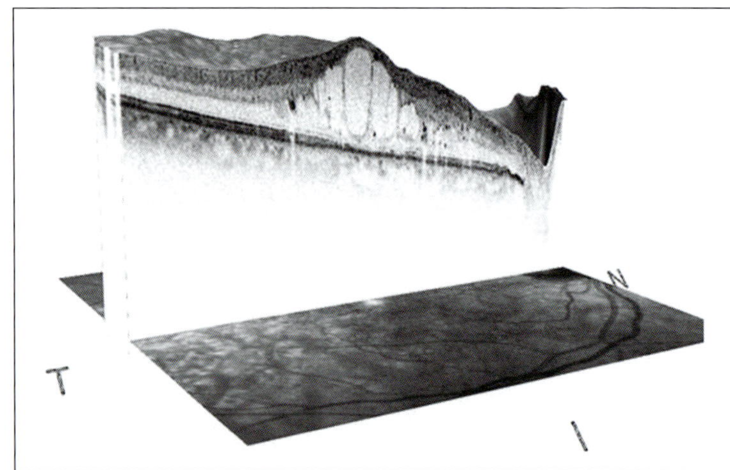

Fig. 8. SD-OCT: CME characterized by the presence of intraretinal, round and oval cystoid areas of low reflectivity, separated by highly reflective septae.

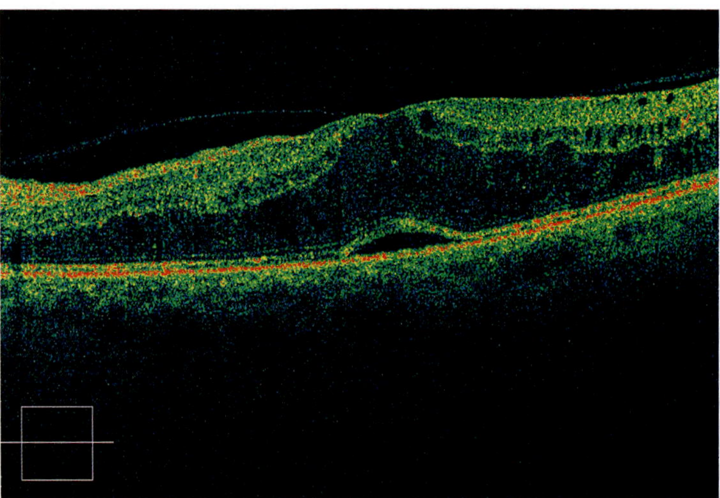

Fig. 9. OCT: serous retinal detachment in DME. There is diffuse retinal thickening with some cystic spaces associated with a shallow elevation of the neuroretina, which is seen as an optically clear space between the retina and the RPE.

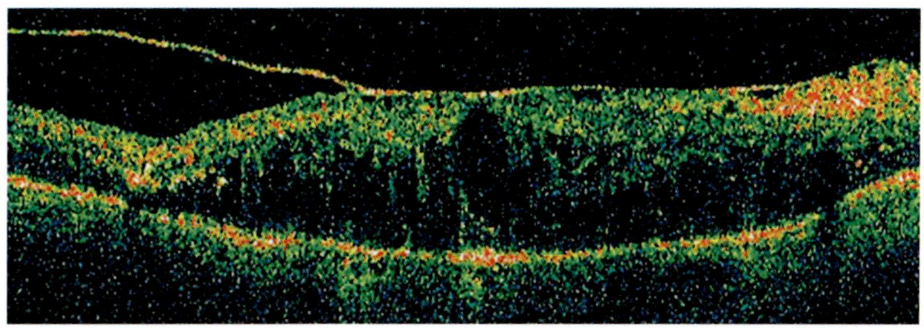

Fig. 10. Epiretinal membrane manifested on OCT by the presence of a hyperreflective band along the inner aspect of the retina. There is associated CME and a shallow serous retinal detachment.

Fig. 11. OCT: vitreomacular traction in DME. Note the presence of diffuse retinal thickening associated with a hyperreflective band that is in apposition with the inner surface of the retina at the central area and elevated above the surface of the retina elsewhere. Vitrectomy is indicated in this case.

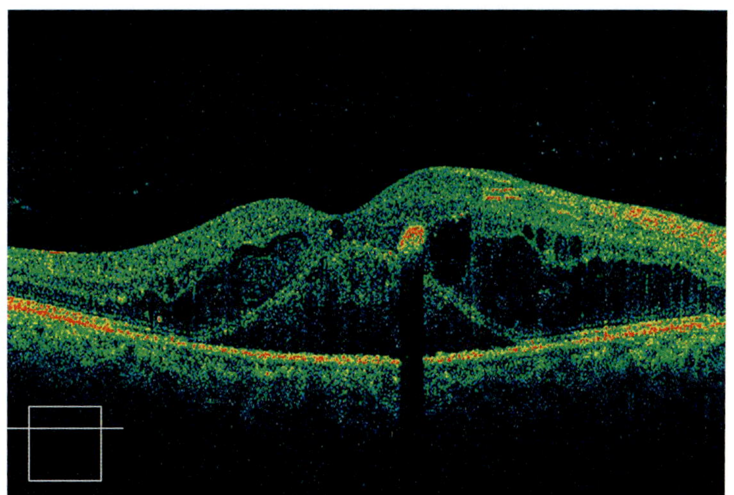

Fig. 12. OCT: hard exudate in DME. Note the presence of a spot of high reflectivity with low-reflective area behind it in the outer retinal layer, corresponding to a hard exudate.

of hyperreflectivity as the accumulated dots in an area of hard exudates; thus, they may represent tiny intraretinal protein, and/or lipid deposits acting as precursors of hard exudates [21]. Hard exudates are detected as spots of high reflectivity with low-reflective areas behind them, and are found primarily in the outer retinal layers (fig. 12).

Spectral-domain OCT (SD-OCT) has enabled us to analyze the integrity of the outer retinal layers in DME. These include the external

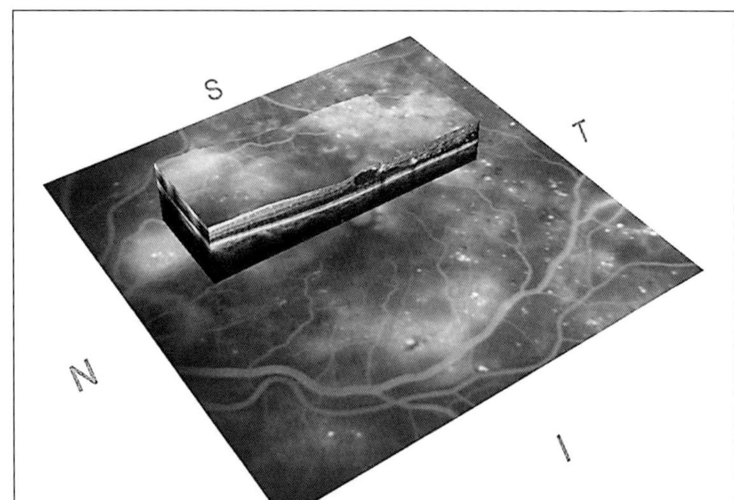

Fig. 13. Combination of FA with 3-D SD-OCT in DME. For each area of the macula as seen in FA, there is a corresponding imaging on OCT at the area that was selected to be scanned. Note that OCT shows a central cyst at the area that corresponds to CME on FA.

limiting membrane, the photoreceptor inner segment (IS), the outer segment (OS), the RPE, and Bruch's membrane. First reports point towards the importance of the integrity of the external limiting membrane, the photoreceptor IS and the OS as a prognostic feature of visual improvement after treatment for DME [22]. Loss of inner retinal layers on SD-OCT is highly specific for capillary nonperfusion on FA [23]. In contrast to the loss of retinal layers seen in areas with photocoagulation scars, areas of capillary nonperfusion had an intact IS/OS junction. Retinal edema on SD-OCT is highly variable in areas of capillary nonperfusion.

Finally, OCT can accurately and reliably quantify macular retinal thickening in both clinically significant DME and non-clinically significant DME [24] and can detect early changes in retinal thickness despite normal findings on slit-lamp biomicroscopy [25].

Conclusion

DME is one of the most significant causes of new blindness and severe visual impairment in patients with diabetes, which can result in reduced quality of life. Assessment of retinal thickness is important for treatment and follow-up of patients with DME. Therefore, the need for objective and quantitative assessments of DME is increasingly acknowledged. Ocular coherence tomography has added another quantitative dimension in the assessment of DME and could lead to better visual outcomes via earlier detection and more targeted therapeutic approaches. It provides valuable information on the retinal morphological changes associated with DME and can monitor the response to treatment. It is particularly valuable in analyzing the vitreomacular interface and in detecting localized sub-foveal serous detachments that are not detectable on biomicroscopy or in FA. FA is essential for the detection of areas of macular ischemia, allows precise localization of microvascular abnormalities and defines the leakage pattern which gives valuable information from a prognostic and therapeutic point of view. Arguably, combination of FA with OCT is the state of the art in the management of DME (fig. 13, 14).

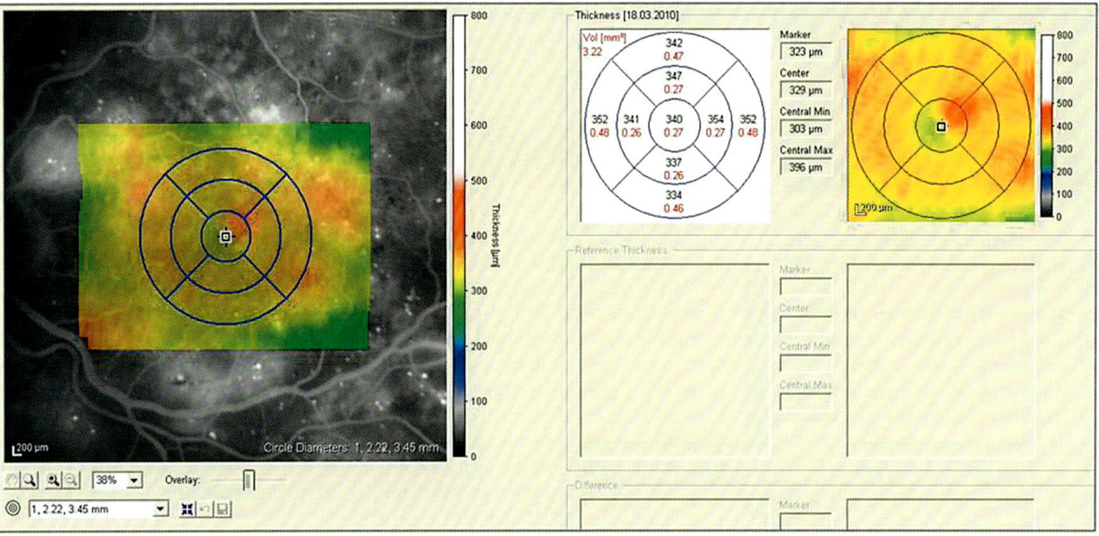

Fig. 14. Macular thickness OCT map and FA in DME. Note the correspondence between areas of increased retinal thickness on the OCT map and areas of leakage in the fluorescein angiogram.

References

1 Bhagat N, Grigorian RA, Tutela A, Zarbin MA: Diabetic macular edema: pathogenesis and treatment. Surv Ophthalmol 2009;54:1–32.
2 Klein R, Klein BE, Moss SE, Cruickshanks KJ: The Wisconsin Epidemiologic Study of Diabetic Retinopathy. XV. The long-term incidence of macular edema. Ophthalmology 1995;102:7–16.
3 Klein R, Moss SE, Klein BE, Davis MD, DeMets DL: The Wisconsin epidemiologic study of diabetic retinopathy. XI. The incidence of macular edema. Ophthalmology 1989;96:1501–1510.
4 Tight blood pressure control and risk of macrovascular and microvascular complications in type 2 diabetes. UKPDS 38. UK Prospective Diabetes Study Group. BMJ 1998;317:703–713.
5 Chew EY, Klein ML, Ferris FL 3rd, et al: Association of elevated serum lipid levels with retinal hard exudate in diabetic retinopathy. Early Treatment Diabetic Retinopathy Study (ETDRS) Report 22. Arch Ophthalmol 1996;114:1079–1084.
6 Klein BE, Moss SE, Klein R, Surawicz TS: The Wisconsin Epidemiologic Study of Diabetic Retinopathy. XIII. Relationship of serum cholesterol to retinopathy and hard exudate. Ophthalmology 1991;98:1261–1265.
7 Photocoagulation for diabetic macular edema. Early Treatment Diabetic Retinopathy Study report number 1. Early Treatment Diabetic Retinopathy Study research group. Arch Ophthalmol 1985;103:1796–1806.
8 Ferris FL 3rd, Podgor MJ, Davis MD: Macular edema in Diabetic Retinopathy Study patients. Diabetic Retinopathy Study Report Number 12. Ophthalmology 1987;94:754–760.
9 Focal photocoagulation treatment of diabetic macular edema. Relationship of treatment effect to fluorescein angiographic and other retinal characteristics at baseline: ETDRS report No. 19. Early Treatment Diabetic Retinopathy Study Research Group. Arch Ophthalmol 1995;113:1144–1155.
10 Lee CM, Olk RJ: Modified grid laser photocoagulation for diffuse diabetic macular edema. Long-term visual results. Ophthalmology 1991;98:1594–1602.
11 Kang SW, Park CY, Ham DI: The correlation between fluorescein angiographic and optical coherence tomographic features in clinically significant diabetic macular edema. Am J Ophthalmol 2004;137:313–322.
12 Browning DJ, McOwen MD, Bowen RM Jr, O'Marah TL: Comparison of the clinical diagnosis of diabetic macular edema with diagnosis by optical coherence tomography. Ophthalmology 2004;111:712–715.
13 Virgili G, Menchini F, Dimastrogiovanni AF, et al: Optical coherence tomography versus stereoscopic fundus photography or biomicroscopy for diagnosing diabetic macular edema: a systematic review. Invest Ophthalmol Vis Sci 2007;48:4963–4973.
14 Otani T, Kishi S, Maruyama Y: Patterns of diabetic macular edema with optical coherence tomography. Am J Ophthalmol 1999;127:688–693.
15 Kim BY, Smith SD, Kaiser PK: Optical coherence tomographic patterns of diabetic macular edema. Am J Ophthalmol 2006;142:405–412.

16 Kim NR, Kim YJ, Chin HS, Moon YS: Optical coherence tomographic patterns in diabetic macular oedema: prediction of visual outcome after focal laser photocoagulation. Br J Ophthalmol 2009; 93:901–905.

17 Ghazi NG, Ciralsky JB, Shah SM, Campochiaro PA, Haller JA: Optical coherence tomography findings in persistent diabetic macular edema: the vitreomacular interface. Am J Ophthalmol 2007; 144:747–754.

18 Massin P, Duguid G, Erginay A, Haouchine B, Gaudric A: Optical coherence tomography for evaluating diabetic macular edema before and after vitrectomy. Am J Ophthalmol 2003;135:169–177.

19 Lewis H, Abrams GW, Blumenkranz MS, Campo RV: Vitrectomy for diabetic macular traction and edema associated with posterior hyaloidal traction. Ophthalmology 1992;99:753–759.

20 Massin P, Girach A, Erginay A, Gaudric A: Optical coherence tomography: a key to the future management of patients with diabetic macular oedema. Acta Ophthalmol Scand 2006;84:466–474.

21 Bolz M, Schmidt-Erfurth U, Deak G, Mylonas G, Kriechbaum K, Scholda C: Optical coherence tomographic hyperreflective foci: a morphologic sign of lipid extravasation in diabetic macular edema. Ophthalmology 2009;116:914–920.

22 Wolf S, Wolf-Schnurrbusch U: Spectral-domain optical coherence tomography use in macular diseases: a review. Ophthalmologica 2010;224:333–340.

23 Yeung L, Lima VC, Garcia P, Landa G, Rosen RB: Correlation between spectral domain optical coherence tomography findings and fluorescein angiography patterns in diabetic macular edema. Ophthalmology 2009;116:1158–1167.

24 Schaudig UH, Glaefke C, Scholz F, Richard G: Optical coherence tomography for retinal thickness measurement in diabetic patients without clinically significant macular edema. Ophthalmic Surg Lasers 2000;31:182–186.

25 Brown JC, Solomon SD, Bressler SB, Schachat AP, DiBernardo C, Bressler NM: Detection of diabetic foveal edema: contact lens biomicroscopy compared with optical coherence tomography. Arch Ophthalmol 2004;122:330–335.

Constantin J. Pournaras, MD
Department of Ophthalmology, Vitreo-Retinal Unit, Geneva University Hospitals
22 rue Alcide-Jentzer
CH-12 11 Geneva 14 (Switzerland)
E-Mail constantin.pournaras@hcuge.ch

Bandello F, Battaglia Parodi M (eds): Surgical Retina.
ESASO Course Series. Basel, Karger, 2012, vol 2, pp 91–98

Retinal Venous Occlusions: Diagnosis and Choice of Treatment

Jose Garcia-Arumi · Josep Badal · Miguel Zapata · Ana Boixadera · Vicente Martinez Castillo

Instituto de Microcirugía Ocular, Barcelona, Spain

Abstract

Retinal vascular occlusive disorders constitute one of the major causes of blindness and impaired vision, and yet there is marked controversy on their pathogeneses, clinical features and particularly their management. Different medical and surgical approaches that rely on evidence-based medicine are set out in this chapter.

Central Retinal Vein Occlusion

Introduction

Central retinal vein occlusion (CRVO) is the third most common blinding vascular retinal disorder after diabetic retinopathy and branch retinal vein occlusion (BRVO) [1, 2]. Among patients with CRVO, 34% develop capillary nonperfusion and retinal ischemia. Iris neovascularization and neovascular glaucoma may occur in 45–85% of the eyes affected by ischemic CRVO and only in 5% of the nonischemic eyes [2, 3]. The main known risk factors of CRVO are hypertension and open-angle glaucoma [2–5].

The pathogenesis of CRVO is still not very well understood. It is thought to be a compartment syndrome, since in a 1.5-mm-diameter area, the central retinal artery, the central retinal vein, and the optic nerve coexist. Thrombotic occlusion is thought to develop as the result of an increase in the arterial diameter, changes in the scleral ring, and the presence of anatomical anomalies and possible systemic factors, which together cause a decrease in the venous lumen, increased turbulence, damage to endothelium and thrombus formation. This is supported by histologic studies that localize the thrombus in the lamina cribosa in most or all cases [6, 7].

It is clear from the Central Vein Occlusion Study [8] that, when left to follow its natural course, the vision in patients with CRVO will most likely worsen or remain unchanged and that those patients with poor vision initially have little hope of significant spontaneous recovery. There is no known effective treatment for CRVO. Numerous treatments are available, including panretinal laser photocoagulation (PRP), grid macular laser photocoagulation, chorioretinal anastomosis (CRA) via high-intensity laser photocoagulation, and intraocular injections of drugs, with varying degrees of effectiveness and complication rates. One surgical procedure that has been developed is termed radial optic neurotomy (RON). PRP has only been effective in managing neovascular complications, and grid macular laser photocoagulation only decreases macular edema without increasing the final VA [1, 8, 9].

Pharmacologic Treatment
Recombinant Tissue Plasminogen Activator
Thrombolytic agents have been proposed as a treatment against a suspected thrombus in the central retinal vein. Recombinant tissue plasminogen activator (r-tPA) is a synthetic fibrinolytic agent that converts plasminogen to plasmin and destabilizes intravascular thrombi. Recombinant tissue plasminogen activator, as therapy against CRVO, has been administered by several routes: systemic [10, 11], intravitreal [12–15], and by endovascular cannulation of retinal vessels, which involves cannulation of retinal vessels, either through a neuroradiologic or a vitreoretinal approach, and delivery of minute quantities of r-tPA directly to the occluded vessels to release the suspected thrombus [16, 17]. Bynoe and Weiss [18] have reported their technique of pars plana vitrectomy (PPV) followed by cannulation of a branch vein and, with the aid of a stabilization arm, injecting a bolus (average 3.4 ml) of 200 µg/ml r-tPA towards the optic nerve head. This was a pilot study with no more evidence data suggesting benefit from this technique.

Intraocular Corticosteroids
The role of corticosteroids has been explored in CRVO with particular interest to improve visual acuity by reducing macular edema. The exact mechanism of action of corticosteroids in modulating retinal edema is unknown, but it is believed that a combination of anti-inflammatory effects with modulation of cytokine and growth factor production and stabilization of the blood-retinal barrier with reduction in vascular permeability may be involved. There is little evidence for using oral corticosteroids to treat macular edema from CRVO. Several reports from intravitreal triamcinolone for CRVO macular edema have been published [19] showing initial improvement but with no longer benefit after one year. High incidence of cataract (63%) and glaucoma (30%) has also been reported as complications from intravitreal triamcinolone.

The most important study in this area is the SCORE study report 5 [20]. The first multicenter, randomized clinical trial with 271 participants. The study compares the efficacy and safety of 1- and 4-mg doses of preservative-free intravitreal triamcinolone with observation in eyes with vision loss associated with macular edema secondary to perfused CRVO. Retreatment was done if necessary every 4 months. With a mean of 2.2 injections, at month 12 gain in visual acuity was found in 7, 27 and 26% of the patients, respectively. More eyes in the 4-mg triamcinolone group (35%) initiated IOP-lowering medication through 12 months compared with the 1-mg triamcinolone (20%) and observation groups (8%). Among eyes that were phakic at baseline, the estimate through month 12 of new-onset lens opacity or progression of an existing opacity in the observation group was 18% compared with 26 and 33% for the 1- and 4-mg triamcinolone groups, respectively.

This study concludes that intravitreal triamcinolone is superior to observation for treating vision loss associated with macular edema secondary to CRVO. The 1-mg dose has a safety profile superior to that of the 4-mg dose.

There is currently a phase III study for intravitreal dexamethasone drug delivery system comparing 350 µg, 700 µg and sham injection with 1,267 patients involved. Dexamethasone is a potent, water-soluble corticosteroid that can be delivered to the vitreous cavity by the dexamethasone intravitreal implant (DEX implant; OZURDEX, Allergan, Inc., Irvine, Calif., USA). A DEX implant is composed of a biodegradable copolymer of lactic acid and glycolic acid containing micronized dexamethasone. The drug-copolymer complex gradually releases the total dose of dexamethasone over a series of months after insertion into the eye through a small 22-gauge pars plana puncture using a customized applicator system.

The percentage of eyes with a 15-letter improvement in BCVA was significantly higher in both DEX implant groups compared with sham at days 30–90, but not significant at 180 days. The percentage of DEX implant-treated eyes with intraocular pressure of 25 mm Hg peaked at 16% at day 60 (both doses), and was not different from sham by day 180. There was no significant between-group difference in the occurrence of cataract or cataract surgery [21]. Additionally, several modes of delivery are being evaluated in the preclinical and clinical trial setting to determine safety and efficacy. The Iluvien sustained-release fluocinolone acetonide device (Alimera Sciences) is an injectable, non-biodegradable, intravitreal insert designed for sustained release of the corticosteroid fluocinolone acetonide for up to 36 months. The drug is injected through a 25-gauge inserter needle. There are two intravitreal triamcinolone acetonide implants under study: the I-vation (SurModics Inc.) and the Verisome delivery system (Icon Biosciences Inc.). The Cortiject implant (NOVA63035, Novagali Parma) is a preservative- and solvent-free emulsion that contains a tissue-activated proprietary corticosteroid prodrug that is activated at the level of the retina once released. For several years, repeated intravitreal injections of non-FDA-approved triamcinolone acetonide have been used for this disease. These new sustained-release delivery systems may provide better side effect profiles and reduce the need for repeated intravitreal injections.

Anti-Vascular Endothelial Growth Factor Drugs
Following CRVO, subsequent hypoxia leads to upregulation of vascular endothelial growth factor (VEGF), resulting in increased retinal capillary permeability and leakage of fluid and blood into the intraretinal space. In addition, VEGF is a key promoter of angiogenesis, potentially contributing to the development of the neovascularization associated with CRVO. Antiangiogenic drugs may decrease vascular permeability and also the macular edema. Bevacizumab has been the most

studied drug in this disease. Good safety and effectiveness in short-term outcomes with this drug have been reported. Main limitations of this treatment modality are its short-term effectiveness and high recurrence rate [22–24].

Ranibizumab is the other drug studied for CRVO. In a prospective study (CRUISE study) [25], 392 participants were evaluated in 3 groups (0.3, 0.5 mg or sham injection every month). At 6 months, gain in visual acuity was found in 46.2, 47.9 and 16.9% of the patients, respectively. In a dose-ranging, double-masked, multicenter, phase 2 trial, subjects with CRVO for 6 months' or less duration were randomly assigned to receive pegaptanib sodium (0.3 and 1 mg) or sham injections every 6 weeks for 24 weeks. At week 30, 36% of subjects treated with 0.3 mg of pegaptanib sodium and 39% treated with 1 mg gained 15 or more letters from baseline versus 28% sham-treated subjects [26]. The main problem of these drugs arises from the deal of what will happen when injections get stopped. In a recent review from the Cochrane database, the authors conclude that ranibizumab and pegaptanib sodium have shown promise in the short-term treatment of nonischemic CRVO macular edema. However, effectiveness and safety data from larger randomized clinical trials with a follow-up beyond 6 months are not yet available. There are no randomized clinical trials on anti-VEGF agents in ischemic CRVO macular edema. The use of anti-VEGF agents to treat this condition therefore remains experimental [27].

Vitrectomy
PPV techniques are used to address complications of CVO and, in investigational studies, to attempt to alter the natural course of the disease. Eyes with non-clearing vitreous hemorrhage from secondary retinal neovascularization may require surgical evacuation. At the time of vitrectomy, clearing of the hemorrhage can be combined with removal of epiretinal membranes and removal of fibrovascular proliferations, if present, and the placement of complete endolaser PRP [28]. Although

this technique may prevent or aid in regression of anterior segment neovascularization, visual outcomes may be limited due to the extent of underlying retinal nonperfusion [29].

In order to improve oxygenation of the fovea and the fluid exchange with the vitreous cavity, some authors suggest peeling the internal limiting membrane (ILM) [30].

Radial Optic Neurotomy

Opremcak et al. [31] proposed combining PPV with transvitreal incision of the nasal scleral ring in order to release pressure on the central retinal vein at the level of the scleral outlet. The procedure addresses the 'compartment syndrome' that may exist in these eyes where the central retinal artery, central retinal vein and optic nerve traverse through a 1.5-mm-diameter area. Previous attempts at external decompression of the orbital portion of the optic nerve by optic nerve sheath fenestration and sectioning of the posterior scleral ring have not been validated as effective treatments for CRVO [32, 33]. RON is performed by PPV followed by use of a 25-gauge microvitreoretinal blade to incise the lamina cribosa and adjacent retina. Care is taken to avoid major retinal vessels, and a radial incision orientation is used to avoid transecting nerve fibers. Intraoperative hemorrhage is typically controlled by transient elevation of intraocular pressure. In the initial retrospective report of 11 eyes by Opremcak et al. [31], successful RON was performed with no complications. There was clinical improvement in retinal hemorrhages and venous congestion [31]. Garcia-Arumi et al. [34] reported, in a prospective interventional trial, successful RON surgery in 14 eyes. Overall, 57% gained one line of distance visual acuity, and visual recovery was significantly related to reduction in macular edema. Six (43%) developed a postoperative CRA at the RON site with a trend towards better final acuity compared to those without anastomosis formation (20/60 vs. 20/110). The CRA seen at RON sites may allow for more active drainage of retinal edema and hemorrhage compared to laser-induced CRA. When evaluating the effectiveness of RON for CRVO in patients <50 years of age versus those >50 in 43 patients [35], better functional results were observed in younger patients (50 vs. 30% gained 15 letters), although functional improvement remained limited in those with low baseline VA. In patients with hemicentral retinal vein occlusion, RON seems to be a potential treatment in selected patients, probably because of the more rapid appearance of chorioretinal collateral vessels, which promote faster resolution of macular edema. In a study of 13 patients, Garcia-Arumi et al. [36] report gain of 2 or more Snellen lines of vision in 69.2% of patients, and in 4 patients (30.8%) VA improved by 4 or more Snellen lines.

In 2006, Opremcak et al. [37] reported on 117 patients with CRVO and severe loss of vision (≤20/200) treated with PPV and RON. Anatomic improvement of CRVO was found in 95% of patients. Visual acuity improved in 71% of patients, with an average of 2.5 lines of vision gained. Subgroup analyses suggested that older age, female sex, duration of CRVO, presence of afferent pupillary defect, absence of perfusion by angiography, and development of anterior segment neovascularization were associated with poorer visual outcomes.

Finally, there is a surgical multicentric clinical trial in process with 83 patients involved evaluating the role of RON in CRVO (ROVO study). At 12 months' follow-up, there was an improvement of >3 lines logMAR in 11.8% of the placebo group, 25% of the triamcinolone group and 48.6% of the RON group.

Branch Retinal Vein Occlusion

Introduction

The majority of the venous lesions in BRVO occur downstream from the arteriovenous crossing site. Changes in rigidity of the artery associated to hypertension induce a vein compression producing turbulence, endothelial cell damage and thrombus formation [38].

Retinal vein occlusion is the second retinal vascular disorder. Until recently, treatment was focused on the vascular proliferative complications, and laser photocoagulation was the only treatment proved. The BRVO Study demonstrated that grid photocoagulation improves macular edema and vision in patients with macular edema secondary to BRVO, but with preserved foveal vascularization [39], this improvement was only 1.3 ETDRS lines at 3 years.

Macular edema is the main cause of decrease in visual acuity in BRVO. The approaches to the management of BRVO are addressed to reperfuse the thrombosed vein, to reduce the permeability of the macular vascular net improving the edema and to increase the vitreoretinal fluid exchange of oxygen and protecting factors.

Pharmacologic Treatment
Recombinant Tissue Plasminogen Activator
Intravitreal tissue plasminogen activator has been used alone [40] and in combination with sheathotomy [41] for BRVO. Results are encouraged, but actually there are not comparative studies with other treatments. Potential benefits of plasminogen activator include the thrombus resolution.

Intraocular Corticosteroids
The exact mechanism of macular edema development from BRVO has not been elucidated, but breakdown of the blood-retinal barrier is thought to play a role. Potential role of corticosteroids are the decrease in vascular permeability and the stabilization of this blood-retinal barrier.

The most important study in this area is the SCORE study [42], the first multicenter, randomized clinical trial with 411 participants. The study compares the efficacy and safety of 1- and 4-mg doses of preservative-free intravitreal triamcinolone with standard care (grid photocoagulation in eyes without dense macular hemorrhage and deferral of photocoagulation until hemorrhage clears in eyes with dense macular hemorrhage) for eyes with vision loss associated with macular edema secondary to BRVO. Despite good initial results with triamcinolone, conclusions are that there is no difference in visual acuity at 12 months for the standard care group compared with the triamcinolone groups. Intraocular pressure-lowering medication was initiated in more eyes through 12 months in the 4-mg triamcinolone group (41%) compared with the 1-mg triamcinolone (7%) and standard care (2%) groups. Among eyes that were phakic at baseline, the estimate of new-onset lens opacity or progression of an existing opacity based on clinical assessment through month 12 in the standard care group was 13% compared with 25 and 35% in the 1- and 4-mg triamcinolone groups, respectively. At this point, use of intravitreal triamcinolone is not recommended in macular edema secondary to BRVO.

As stated in CRVO, there is a phase III study for intravitreal dexamethasone drug delivery system (DEX implant; OZURDEX, Allergan Inc.) comparing 350 µg, 700 µg and sham injection in 1,267 patients with CRVO or BRVO. Gain in visual acuity was set at days 30–90 but not significant at day 180. Mean BCVA slowly improved over the course of the study among BRVO eyes treated with sham, but gradually declined to below baseline levels among CRVO eyes treated with sham [21].

Anti-Vascular Endothelial Growth Factor Drugs
VEGF is elevated in vitreous of patients with BRVO and plays an important role in the pathogenesis of macular edema secondary to BRVO [43]. At this point, antiangiogenic drugs may decrease vascular permeability and also the macular edema. Bevacizumab has been the most studied drug in this disease. We can find short series of cases and retrospective comparative studies concluding good safety and effectiveness in short-term outcomes with this drug. Large and prospective studies report that limitations of this treatment modality are its short-term effectiveness and high recurrence rate [44]. In a prospective, randomized, sham injection-controlled, double-masked, multicenter clinical trial evaluating the efficacy of

ranibizumab for BRVO, the percentage of patients who gained ≥15 letters in BCVA at month 6 was 55.2% (0.3 mg) and 61.1% (0.5 mg) in the ranibizumab groups and 28.8% in the sham group [45]. Pegaptanib sodium studies suggest improvement of visual acuity at week 54 in both 0.3 mg and 1 mg doses [46].

Vitrectomy

There is evidence that PPV and posterior hyaloid dissection may increase oxygenation of the macula and in some cases vitreomacular attachment itself may contribute to the development of macular edema [47]. Despite the lack of large clinical trials, recently pars PPV has been demonstrated to improve perifoveal microcirculation and visual prognosis in BRVO patients with macular edema [48]. In order to improve oxygenation of the fovea and anatomic and functional outcomes of vitrectomy, some authors proposed the peeling of the ILM. Short series of cases have found good outcomes with this technique [49]. In a nonrandomized, comparative study, Arai et al. [50] did not find any difference between PPV with and without ILM peeling for BRVO, and concluded that there is no additional benefit in removing the ILM for BRVO-associated macular edema.

Sheathotomy

Few years after histological changes in BRVO were described [38], Osterloh and Charles published the first report of sheathotomy for BRVO. In 1998, Kumar et al. [51] described again the venous narrowing at the crossing site as the main cause for BRVO, and suggested that removal of the compressive factor by sectioning the adventitial sheath (sheathotomy) may be an effective treatment for BRVO. Surgical technique consists in a PPV with posterior hyaloid dissection. Arteriovenous crossing must be dissected with special forceps and scissors. At this point, the experience of the surgeon plays an important role because small tractions may break the vein. Potential benefits of sheathotomy include the mechanic decompression of the venule and thrombus release that sometimes we can appreciate during the surgery. Successful decompressive surgery is usually followed by disappearance of collateral vessels at the BRVO blockage site, which is a clinical marker for intravascular reperfusion, and resolution of hemorrhages and macular edema. Mester and Dillinger [52] with 43 patients and Garcia-Arumi et al. [41] with 40 patients reported good visual results in patients treated with sheathotomy. At the elaboration of this review, we could find over 25 references of sheathotomy for BRVO, more than 320 patients studied. In 18 references sheathotomy was safe and effective, and in 7 references this technique had the same result as vitrectomy alone. At this point, no randomized controlled study evaluating the benefit of sheathotomy has been published.

As medical research progresses, the selection of options from which we have to choose for patients with retinal vein occlusions widens and improves. We have shifted over from no FDA-approved pharmacologic drugs for retinal vein occlusion treatment to the anti-VEGF drugs that show excellent data. The main downsides are, for anti-VEGF drugs the need for repeated injections, and for corticosteroids the side effects of cataract and increased intraocular pressure. Combination of treatments may offer the best approach, but hard evidence supporting it is still lacking.

In addition, sustained drug delivery to the posterior segment as a therapeutic option is increasing. Current experience suggests that use of these devices will continue increasing over time.

However, when treating macular edema secondary to retinal vein occlusion, we are still unable to address the primary mechanism of the disease: the vein occlusion. We believe that surgery remains a good treatment option for patients with very recent and edematous occlusion and poor visual acuity as reperfusion of the vein is the best approach to treat the macular edema and avoid ischemic complications.

References

1 The Central Vein Occlusion Study Group: Baseline and early natural history report: the Central Vein Occlusion Study. Arch Ophthalmol 1993;111:1087–1095.
2 The Eye Disease Case-Control Study Group: Risk factors for central retinal vein occlusion. Arch Ophthalmol 1996;114:545–554.
3 Rath EZ, Frank RN, Shin DH, Kim C: Risk factors for central retinal vein occlusion: a case controlled study. Ophthalmology 1992;99:509–514.
4 Hayreh SS, Zimmerman MB, Podhajsky P: Incidence of various types of retinal vein occlusion and their recurrence and demographic characteristics. Am J Ophthalmol 1994;117:429–441.
5 Hayreh SS, Zimmerman MB, McCarthy MJ, Podhajsky P: Systemic diseases associated with various types of retinal vein occlusion. Am J Ophthalmol 2001;131:61–77.
6 Green WR, Chan CC, Hutchins GM, Terry JM: Central vein occlusion: a prospective histological study of 29 eyes in 28 cases. Trans Am Ophthalmol Soc 1981;89:371–422.
7 Hayreh SS: Pathogenesis of occlusion of the central retinal vessels. Am J Ophthalmol 1971;72:998–1011.
8 The Central Vein Occlusion Study Group: Natural history and clinical management of central retinal vein occlusion. Arch Ophthalmol 1997;115:486–491.
9 The Central Vein Occlusion Study Group: Evaluation of grid pattern photocoagulation for macular edema in central vein occlusion: the Central Vein Occlusion Study Group N report. Ophthalmology 1995;102:1434–1444.
10 Hattenbach LO, Steinkamp G, Scharrer I, et al: Fibrinolytic therapy with low-dose recombinant tissue plasminogen activator in retinal vein occlusion. Ophthalmologica 1998;212:394–398.
11 Hattenbach LO, Wellermann G, Steinkamp GW, et al: Visual outcome after treatment with low-dose recombinant tissue plasminogen activator or hemodilution in ischemic central retinal vein occlusion. Ophthalmologica 1999;213:360–366.

12 Lahey JM, Fong DS, Kearney J: Intravitreal tissue plasminogen activator for acute central retinal vein occlusion. Ophthalmic Surg Lasers 1999;30:427–434.
13 Glacet-Bernard A, Kuhn D, Vine AK, et al: Treatment of recent onset central retinal vein occlusion with intravitreal tissue plasminogen activator: a pilot study. Br J Ophthalmol 2000;84:609–613.
14 Elman MJ, Raden RZ, Carrigan A: Intravitreal injection of tissue plasminogen activator for central retinal vein occlusion. Trans Am Ophthalmol Soc 2001;99:219–221, discussion 22–23.
15 Ghazi NG, Noureddine BN, Haddad RS, et al: Intravitreal tissue plasminogen activator in the management of central retinal vein occlusion. Retina 2003;23:780–784.
16 Weiss JN: Treatment of central retinal vein occlusion by injection of tissue plasminogen activator into a retinal vein. Am J Ophthalmol 1998;126:142–144.
17 Paques M, Vallee JN, Herbreteau D, et al: Superselective ophthalmic artery fibrinolytic therapy for the treatment of central retinal vein occlusion. Br J Ophthalmol 2000;84:1387–1391.
18 Bynoe LA, Weiss JN: Retinal endovascular surgery and intravitreal triamcinolone acetone for central vein occlusion in young adults. Am J Ophthalmol 2003;135:382–384.
19 Gregori NZ, Rosenfeld PJ, Puliafito CA, et al: One-year safety and efficacy of intravitreal triamcinolone acetonide for the management of macular edema secondary to central retinal vein occlusion. Retina 2006;26:889–95.
20 Ip MS, Scott IU, Van Veldhuisen PC, Oden NL, Bodi BA, Fisher M, Singerman LJ, Tolentino M, Chan CK, Gonzalez VH, SCORE Study Research Group: A randomized trial comparing the efficacy and safety of intravitreal triamcinolone with observation to treat vision loss associated with macular edema secondary to central retinal vein occlusion: the Standard Care vs Corticosteroid for Retinal Vein Occlusion (SCORE) study report 5. Arch Ophthalmol 2009;127:1101–1114.

21 Haller JA, Bandello F, Belfort R Jr, Blumenkranz MS, Gillies M, Heier J, Loewenstein A, Yoon YH, Jacques ML, Jiao J, Li XY, Whitcup SM, Ozurdex Geneva Study Group: Randomized, sham-controlled trial of dexamethasone intravitreal implant in patients with macular edema due to retinal vein occlusion. Ophthalmology 2010;117:1134–1146.
22 Rosenfeld PJ, Fung AE, Puliafito CA: Optical coherence tomography findings after an intravitreal injection of bevacizumab (Avastin) for macular edema from central retinal vein occlusion. Ophthalmic Surg Lasers Imaging 2005;36:336–339.
23 Iturralde D, Spaide RF, Meyerle CB: Intravitreal bevacizumab (Avastin) treatment of macular edema in central retinal vein occlusion: a short-term study. Retina 2006;26:279.
24 Wu L, Martínez-Castellanos MA, Quiroz-Mercado H, Pan American Collaborative Retina Group (PACORES): Twelve-month safety of intravitreal injections of bevacizumab (Avastin): results of the Pan-American Collaborative Retina Study Group (PACORES). Graefes Arch Clin Exp Ophthalmol 2008;246:81–87.
25 Brown DM, Campochiaro PA, Singh RP, Li Z, Gray S, Saroj N, Rundle AC, Rubio RG, Murahashi WY, CRUISE Investigators: Ranibizumab for macular edema following central retinal vein occlusion: six-month primary end point results of a phase III study. Ophthalmology 2010;117:1124–1133.e1
26 Wroblewski JJ, Wells JA, Adamis AP, Buggage RR, Cunningham ET Jr, Goldbaum M, Guyer DR, Katz B, Altaweel MM: Pegaptanib in central retinal vein occlusion study group. Pegaptanib sodium for macular edema secondary to central retinal vein occlusion. Arch Ophthalmol 2009;127:374–380.
27 Braithwaite T, Nanji AA, Greenbert PB: Anti-vascular endothelial growth factor for macular edema secondary to central retinal vein occlusion. Cochrane Database Syst Rev 2010;CD007325.

28 Lam HD, Blumenkranz MS: Treatment of central retinal vein occlusion by vitrectomy with lysis of vitreopapillary and epipapillary adhesions, subretinal peripapillary tissue plasminogen activator injection, and photocoagulation. Am J Ophthalmol 2002;134:609–611.

29 Yeshaya A, Treister G: Pars plana vitrectomy for vitreous hemorrhage and retinal vein occlusion. Ann Ophthalmol 1983;15:615–617.

30 Furino C, Ferrari TM, Boscia F, Cardascia N: Combined radial optic neurotomy, internal limiting membrane peeling, and intravitreal triamcinolone acetonide for central retinal vein occlusion. Ophthalmic Surg Lasers Imaging 2005;36:422–425.

31 Opremcak EM, Bruce RA, Lomeo MD, et al: Radial optic neurotomy for central retinal vein occlusion: a retrospective pilot study of 11 consecutive cases. Retina 2001;21:408–415.

32 Dev S, Buckley EG: Optic nerve sheath decompression for progressive central retinal vein occlusion. Ophthalmic Surg Lasers 1999;30:181–184.

33 Vasco-Posada J: Modification of the circulation in the posterior pole of the eye. Ann Ophthalmol 1972;4:48–59.

34 Garcia-Arumi J, Boixadera A, Martinez-Castillo V, et al: Chorioretinal anastomosis after radial optic neurotomy for central retinal vein occlusion. Arch Ophthalmol 2003;121:1385–1391.

35 Garcia-Arumi J, Boixadera A, Martínez-Castillo V, et al: Radial optic neurotomy in central retinal vein occlusion: comparison of outcome in younger vs older patients. Am J Ophthalmol 2007;143:134–140.

36 Garcia-Arumi J, Boixadera A, Martínez-Castillo V, et al: Radial optic neurotomy for management of hemicentral retinal vein occlusion. Arch Ophthalmol 2006;124:690–695.

37 Opremcak ME, Rehmar AJ, Ridenour CD, et al: Radial optic neurotomy for central retinal vein occlusion. Retina 2006;26:297–305.

38 Frangieh GT, Green WR, Barraquer-Somers E, et al: Histopathologic study of nine branch retinal vein occlusions. Arch Ophthalmol 1982;100:1132–1140.

39 The Branch Vein Occlusion Study Group: Argon laser photocoagulation for macular edema in branch vein occlusion. Am J Ophthalmol 1984;98:271–282.

40 Murakami T, Takagi H, Kita M, Nishiwaki H, Miyamoto K, Ohashi H, Watanabe D, Yoshimura N: Intravitreal tissue plasminogen activator to treat macular edema associated with branch retinal vein occlusion. Am J Ophthalmol 2006;142:318–320.

41 García-Arumí J, Martinez-Castillo V, Boixadera A, Blasco H, Corcostegui B: Management of macular edema in branch retinal vein occlusion with sheathotomy and recombinant tissue plasminogen activator. Retina 2004;24:530–540.

42 Scott IU, Ip MS, VanVeldhuisen PC, Oden NL, Blodi BA, Fisher M, Chan CK, Gonzalez VH, Singerman LJ, Tolentino M, SCORE Study Research Group: A randomized trial comparing the efficacy and safety of intravitreal triamcinolone with standard care to treat vision loss associated with macular edema secondary to branch retinal vein occlusion: the Standard Care vs Corticosteroid for Retinal Vein Occlusion (SCORE) study report 6. Arch Ophthalmol 2009;127:1115–1128.

43 Campochiaro PA, Hafiz G, Shah SM, et al: Ranibizumab for macular edema due to retinal vein occlusions: implication of VEGF as a critical stimulator. Mol Ther 2008;16:791–799.

44 Prager F, Michels S, Kriechbaum K, Georgopoulos M, Funk M, Geitzenauer W, Polak K, Schmidt-Erfurth U: Intravitreal bevacizumab (Avastin) for macular oedema secondary to retinal vein occlusion: 12-month results of a prospective clinical trial. Br J Ophthalmol 2009;93:452–456.

45 Campochiaro PA, Heier JS, Feiner L, Gray S, Saroj N, Rundle AC, Murahashi WY, Rubio RG, BRAVO Investigators: Ranibizumab for macular edema following branch retinal vein occlusion: six-month primary end point results of a phase III study. Ophthalmology 2010;117:1102–1112.

46 Wroblewski JJ, Wells JA, Gonzales CR: Pegaptanib sodium for macular edema secondary to branch retinal vein occlusion. Am J Ophthalmol 2010;149:147–154.

47 Takahashi M, Hikichi T, Akiba J, et al: Role of the vitreous and macular edema in branch retinal vein occlusion. Ophthalmic Surg Lasers 1997;28:294–299.

48 Noma H, Funatsu H, Sakata K, Mimura T, Hori S: Macular microcirculation before and after vitrectomy for macular edema with branch retinal vein occlusion. Graefes Arch Clin Exp Ophthalmol 2010;248:443–445.

49 Raszewska-Steglinska M, Gozdek P, Cisiecki S, Michalewska Z, Michalewski J, Nawrocki J: Pars plana vitrectomy with ILM peeling for macular edema secondary to retinal vein occlusion. Eur J Ophthalmol 2009;19:1055–1062.

50 Arai M, Yamamoto S, Mitamura Y, Sato E, Sugawara T, Mizunoya S: Efficacy of vitrectomy and internal limiting membrane removal for macular edema associated with branch retinal vein occlusion. Ophthalmologica 2009;223:172–176.

51 Kumar B, Yu DY, Morgan WH, et al: The distribution of angioarchitectural changes within the vicinity of the arteriovenous crossing in branch retinal vein occlusion. Ophthalmology 1998;105:424–427.

52 Mester U, Dillinger P: Vitrectomy with arteriovenous decompression and internal limiting membrane dissection in branch retinal vein occlusion. Retina 2002;22:740–746.

Jose Garcia-Arumi, MD
Instituto de Microcirugía Ocular
c/ Josep Maria Lladó n° 3
ES–08022 Barcelona (Spain)
Tel. +34 93 2531500, E-Mail 17215jga@comb.es

Bandello F, Battaglia Parodi M (eds): Surgical Retina.
ESASO Course Series. Basel, Karger, 2012, vol 2, pp 99–104

Rhegmatogenous Retinal Detachment: Clinical Preoperative and Postoperative Handling

Naomi Fischer · Anat Loewenstein

Department of Ophthalmology, Tel Aviv Medical Center, Sackler Faculty of Medicine, Tel-Aviv University, Tel-Aviv, Israel

Abstract

Successful rhegmatogenous retinal detachment surgery depends on appropriate handling. Preoperative
management of both ocular and systemic conditions is
paramount in maximizing successful surgery with optimal visual recovery. Optimal postoperative management
aims to maximize retinal reattachment result whilst preventing and minimizing complications. Patient education and understanding of their ocular management plan
improves compliance and relieves anxiety, enabling best
possible outcome.

Copyright © 2012 S. Karger AG, Basel

Preoperative Handling

Goals

The preoperative handling goals of rhegmatogenous retinal detachment are to maximize the
chance of successful surgery with optimal visual recovery. Simultaneous medical conditions
must be managed to prevent complications
due to surgery and anesthesia. Coexisting ocular problems need to be dealt with to maximize
outcome.

Preoperative Head Positioning and Activity

Placing the break in a dependent position encour-
ages retinal flattening. It enables vitreous gel to
cover the break so that vitreous cavity fluid can
no longer enter the subretinal space, and existing
subretinal fluid (SRF) can be absorbed by the retinal pigment epithelium.

Maximizing Pupil Dilation

Pupil dilation must be optimal to facilitate evaluation of the retina and enable intraoperative visualization. Potent topical mydriatics should be
administered several times every 10–15 min immediately prior to surgery (phenylephrine 10%
and tropicamide 1%). In the presence of heavily
pigmented irides or intraocular inflammation,
some people advocate adjuvant subconjunctival
mydriasis (0.2 ml 0.5% phenylephrine hydrochloride, 0.4% homatropine hydrobromide and 1%
procaine hydrochloride in an isotonic solution). It
should be remembered that 10% phenylephrine is
contraindicated in severe systemic hypertension
as well as certain types of arrhythmia, and topical
2.5% phenylephrine should be used instead. The
topical non-steroidal anti-inflammatory drug
flurbiprofen sodium 0.03% (Ocufen) may prevent
prostaglandin-mediated intraoperative miosis (1
drop q 30 min 2 h prior to surgery). However, in
a double-masked trial, it was shown to be ineffective in maintaining intraoperative dilation in
scleral buckling surgery [1].

Prevention of Ocular Infection
There is a lack of efficacy data regarding the use of prophylactic antibiotics. Povidone-iodide has been shown to reduce the incidence of endophthalmitis [2]. Surgical drapes should cover the ocular adnexa immediately prior to surgery.

Management of Coexisting Ocular Problems
Factors Interfering with Optimal Fundus Visibility
Adequate visualization is necessary to identify and treat all retinal breaks and to monitor retina status throughout the surgery. Ab externo retinal surgery requires adequate pupillary size and clarity of the ocular media.

Corneal Opacification
This may range from mild epithelial edema to scarring for previous surgery or trauma. Mild epithelial clouding may occur due to topical pharmacologic agents. Eyelids should be kept closed immediately after drop administration to limit damage. High intraocular pressure should be managed to limit secondary corneal edema.

Anterior Chamber and Lens Opacities
Anterior chamber opacities and cataract/subluxated lens are generally managed intra- rather than preoperatively. Preoperative posterior capsulotomy for secondary posterior intraocular lens opacities may be extremely helpful in maximizing visualization.

Opacification of the Vitreous Gel
Mild vitreous hemorrhage and retinal cell clumping require no preoperative management. Severe vitreous opacity affects retinal detachment surgery choice.

Intraocular Inflammation
Mild inflammation is common, and does not require preoperative treatment. Severe inflammation may be accompanied by hypotony and choroidal detachment with a worse prognosis [3]. It should be treated with topical steroids and atropine sulfate. If there are posterior synechiae, topical or subconjunctival active mydriasis should be administered. Increased intraocular pressure also has a worse prognosis [3], and should be managed with anti-glaucomatous medication prior to surgery.

Existing Ocular Infections
Preexisting infectious conjunctivitis and blepharitis should be managed with topical antibiotics and hygiene.

Preoperative Anesthetic Management and Evaluation
Anesthetic risk needs to be evaluated preoperatively and managed accordingly, especially if there is evidence of significant systemic disease and potential adverse drug reactions [4]. Local anesthesia can be considered for short procedures (<2 h), and in most cases sedation with monitored anesthesia care can be used. Preoperative laboratory test recommendations are based on the patient's age and gender. Additional examinations are performed in the case of specific diseases, and drug use is revealed by careful patient history taking and examination [5–7]. A recent study suggests that preoperative testing can be omitted in a selected group of patients undergoing ambulatory surgery with no increased risk of perioperative complications [8]. There are no recent data regarding mortality associated with ophthalmologic operations. In the past, mortality has been reported in 0.1% of 47,000 ophthalmologic procedures [9]. It is twice as common in retinal detachment surgery, probably because of greater use of general anesthesia and increased risk of pulmonary embolism due to postoperative bed rest. Patients must be assessed by an anesthesiologist and specialist physician where appropriate. Management of diseases such as congestive heart failure, COPD, urinary retention (e.g. BPH), diabetes (keep blood glucose 150–250 mg/ml prior to surgery), adrenal insufficiency

(intravenous hydrocortisone on day of surgery), anemia (consider blood transfusion with hematocrit <30), sickle cell disease and hypertension must be maximized to enable surgery and postoperative care. Electrolyte imbalances must be corrected prior to surgery. Recent myocardial infarction and infection carry an increased mortality risk. If possible, alternatives such as pneumatic retinopexy should be considered. Sedatives in anxious patients can be considered. Some anesthesiologists advocate using anti-muscarinic anesthetic agents in young children due to increased risk of bradycardia (oculocardiac reflex). Medications that interfere with anesthetic agents must be known, and they or the anesthetic agent must be adjusted accordingly. Hepatotoxic anesthetics should be avoided in patients with liver disease, and patients with myotonic dystrophy should not receive succinylcholine anesthesia as it may prolong muscle contraction and interfere with respiration. Patients with previous malignant hyperthermia or family history require special anesthetic precautions [4].

Topical Ocular Medication-Anesthesia Reactions
It is important to be aware that topical ocular medications may interact with anesthesia or cause systemic side effects. Timolol (beta-blocker reducing aqueous humor secretion) may cause bradycardia, heart block, CHF, exacerbation of asthma. Phenylephrine hydrochloride is a powerful sympathomimetic alpha receptor agonist which may exacerbate hypertension. Although rarely used today, the antiglaucomatous echothiophate iodide (acetylcholinesterase inhibitor), can interact with succinylcholine anesthesia and cause prolonged apnea. Its systemic effect may continue 1–4 weeks after cessation of drug [4].

Conclusion
Preoperative management and evaluation is paramount in creating maximum chance of success of retinal detachment and limiting both ocular and medical complications.

Postoperative Handling

Goals
Optimal postoperative management aims to maximize retinal reattachment result whilst preventing and minimizing complications.

Inpatient versus Outpatient Care
In the past, it was routine to hospitalize patients undergoing retinal detachment surgery. In a 1988 study of 200 patients, 52% required inpatient treatment due to pain, nausea, ocular or medical complications. 79% of these patients indicated that they would have been uncomfortable with outpatient care [10]. Nowadays, there is a shift to outpatient care. A 1992 study of 55 consecutive outpatients showed a satisfaction rate of 88% [11].

Management in the Immediate Postoperative Period
Recovery room management includes monitoring and treating vital signs, blood glucose and urinary retention.

Head Positioning
Optimal positioning promotes retinal reattachment. It is also essential to prevent catarogenic changes due to gas/silicon or corneal touch with the lens. It is most important in eyes with residual subretinal fluid (SRF), where a careful balance of forces has to be maintained. If there is substantial SRF in the presence of a flat retinal break, the patient should be placed so that fluid gravitates away from the break (i.e. the break in a superior position). However, caution must be exercised that this position does not cause fluid to accumulate beneath the macula. Placing the break in the superior position also has the disadvantage of possible vitreoretinal traction, and can prevent a break from settling on a scleral buckle. Inferior positioning of the break has the advantage of reducing traction and obstruction of the break by vitreous gel, thereby promoting SRF absorption. However, it

may cause the SRF to accumulate in the area of the break preventing its closure [12]. Patients undergoing a procedure that includes an intravitreal gas bubble should be placed in a way so that it is in contact with the break. If possible, patients should be placed so that the nasal retina is in the dependent position. This prevents retinal pigment epithelium (RPE) from falling on the macular, reducing the chance of epiretinal membrane formation [12].

Postoperative Activity
This is permitted unless there are open retinal breaks or a giant tear that has not fully flattened. Early ambulation and return to normal activity is essential in preventing medical complications such as thrombophlebitis, pulmonary embolism, constipation and urinary retention. A prospective, masked randomized trial of patients after scleral buckle surgery showed no difference in outcome between restricted and full activity groups, and thus activity should not be restricted [13]. Sleeping with an eye shield is recommended in the first few days, and direct blows to the eye should be avoided. In patients undergoing surgery with insertion of gas into the vitreal cavity, airplane travel, deep sea diving and general anesthesia are dangerous due to gas bubble expansion. At 8,000-ft cabin pressure, intraocular bubble size expands 34% and the increase in pressure outpaces compensatory mechanisms. Some surgeons recommend not flying if the air bubble fills more than 20% of the vitreous cavity [13]. Antiglaucomatous medications are ineffective as they do not lower intraocular volume.

Pain Control
In one series of 200 patients 19% had severe postoperative pain, 50% moderate, 34% mild and 7% no pain [14]. It is important to provide adequate pain relief but also to be aware that severe pain may indicate infection or increased intraocular pressure. Patients with extensive nausea and vomiting should be treated with fluids and electrolyte imbalance corrected.

Management in the Early Postoperative Period
This depends on the type of detachment and treatment received. It also depends on patient factors such as comorbidities and compliance.

Examination
Although examination may be limited by pain or swelling, their presence increases the importance of the examination to rule out infection or elevated intraocular pressure [11].

Visual Acuity
This is important to quantify whether there is a complication that could affect the retina or cause optic nerve ischemia (e.g. secondary to orbital swelling, increased intraocular pressure, IOP, or the needle for retrobulbar injection).

External Examination
Gravity-dependent swelling is common, although severe swelling may be a sign of infection. Scleral buckle infection is rare within the first 6 weeks. Strabismus may appear postoperatively, especially in the presence of scleral buckle surgery with temporal disinsertion of extraocular muscle. Diplopia is usually transient but may require strabismus surgery if it persists for more than 6 months.

Conjunctiva
This should be checked for dehiscence and adhesions.

Cornea
Epithelial defects are often induced intraoperatively to aid visualization and should be treated with topical antibiotics. Topical steroids should be used with caution as they slow the repair of the defect. Topical phenylephrine should be avoided as it penetrates ten times better through an epithelial defect and may cause systemic side effects such as severe hypertension. Edema and Descemet folds are often seen in the presence of an epithelial defect, but increased ocular pressure

and anterior segment ischemia should be ruled out.

Anterior Chamber

Mild flare and cells are common. A severe reaction should alert the physician to the possibility of anterior segment ischemia or endophthalmitis. Reduced chamber depth may indicate pupillary block, choroidal effusion, anterior rotation of the ciliary body or wound leak. Gonioscopy should be performed if the angle is suspicious. Silicon oil or gas may be present and is managed with inferior iridotomy and head positioning.

Lens

Feathery opacities and intraocular lens displacement may occur with gas contact and are initially managed by head positioning.

Intraocular Pressure

Elevated pressure in the presence of open angle should be managed with topical anti-glaucoma medications. If the pressure is greater than 40 mm Hg, systemic treatment should be added. Eyes with gas tamponade should be pressure monitored 4 h after surgery. If the pressure is greater than 50 mm Hg, fluid/gas should be removed from the eye (paracentesis should not be performed it there is a risk of vitreous incarceration in the anterior chamber). Serous choroidal detachment is surgically drained. Mydriatics are administered in the presence of pupillary block with a fibrin membrane, and intraocular tissue plasminogen activator (tPA) can also be considered.

Vitreous

Vitreous should be examined for hemorrhage, fibrin, inflammatory cells and size of gas bubble.

Retina

The retina is examined for evidence of reattachment, presence and dynamics of SRF (failed reabsorption may indicate impaired absorption by RPE or increase fluid due to choroidal exudation). If there is an open break near the surface of a scleral buckle, laser photocoagulation may induce flattening of the retina. In highly elevated breaks, gas injection and head position with subsequent laser may encourage retinal reattachment and closure of the break. Failure of the retina to reattach or inadequate absorption of SRF may indicate a previously undetected break, and reoperation is often required.

Postoperative Medications

Topical medications are administered to prevent infection, suppress inflammation, provide comfort and treat coexisting problems such as elevated intraocular pressure. Routine medication includes a steroid-antibiotic combination (e.g. tobramycin 0.3% + dexamethasone 0.1% [Tobradex]). These are then tapered according the amount of inflammation present. If there is allergy to a component, use separate steroid and antibiotic solutions. A topical mydriatic-cycloplegic is often used to dilate the pupil and prevent posterior synechia, although long-term dilation should be avoided to prevent synechiae between the iris and lens remnants after lensectomy. They are usually discontinued after a month unless more rapid recovery of accommodation is needed. Antiglaucoma medications are tapered when pressure is normal. Carbonic anhydrase inhibitors are discontinued first and pressure is measured 2–7 days after discontinuation of the drug. They are generally not reinitiated if the pressure remains less than 25 mm Hg.

Follow-Up

This is intended to monitor the status of the retina and ensure no complications. Patient education is paramount for prompt treatment and early identification of complications. Routine postoperative follow-up is usually performed at day 1, weeks 1, 3–4 and 6, months 3, 6, and yearly thereafter. Refraction should be performed after the eye has healed as refractive changes may have been induced.

Conclusion

Appropriate postoperative management is important in improving the chance of successful retinal surgery and to detect and treat complications early. Medical complications of surgery must also be managed. Patient education and understanding of their ocular management plan improve compliance and relieve anxiety, ensuring optimal outcome.

References

1 Roysarkar TK, Mitra S, Shanmugam MP, Ravishankar KV, Murugesan R: Effect of flurbiprofen sodium on pupillary dilatation during scleral buckling surgery. Indian J Ophthalmol 1994;42:133–137.

2 Speaker MG, Menikoff JA: Prophylaxis of endophthalmitis with topical povidone-iodine. Ophthalmology 1991; 98:1769–1775.

3 Tani P, Robertson DM, Langworthy A: Prognosis for central vision and anatomic reattachment in rhegmatogenous retinal detachment with macula detached. Am J Ophthalmol 1981;92:611–620.

4 Wilkinson LP, Rice TA: Michels Retinal Detachment, ed 2. St Louis, Mosby, pp 517–536.

5 Roizen MF: Cost-effective preoperative laboratory testing. JAMA 1994:271;319–320.

6 Preoperative tests. The use of routine preoperative tests for elective surgery: evidence, methods and guidance. http://www.nice.org.uk/nicemedia/live/10920/29094/29094.pdf.

7 Richman DC: Ambulatory surgery: how much testing do we need? Anesthesiol Clin 2010;28:185–197.

8 Chung F, Yuan H, Yin L, Vairavanathan S, Wong DT: Elimination of preoperative testing in ambulatory surgery. Anesth Analg 2009;108:467–475.

9 Quigley HA: Mortality associated with ophthalmic surgery. A 20-year experience at the Wilmer Institude. Am J Ophthalmology 1974;77:517–524.

10 Isernhagen RD, Michels RG, Glaser BM, et al: Hospitalization requirements after vitreoretinal surgery. Arch Opthalmol 1988;106:767–770.

11 Cannon CS, Gross JG, Abramson L, et al: Evaluation of outpatient experience with vitreoretinal surgery. Br J Ophthalmol 1992;76:68–71.

12 Wilkinson LP, Rice TA: Michels Retinal Detachment, ed 2. St Louis, Mosby, pp 907–934.

13 Bovino JA, Marcus DF: Physical Activity after retinal detachment surgery. Am J Ophthalmol 1984;98:171–179.

14 Drew FI, Moriarty RW, Shapiro AP: An approach to the measurement of the pain and anxiety responses of surgical patients. Psychosom Med 1968;30:826–836.

Naomi Fischer, MD
Department of Ophthalmology, Tel-Aviv Medical Center
6 Weizman Street
Tel Aviv 64239 (Israel)
Tel. +972 3 9739408, E-Mail naomi797@hotmail.com

Bandello F, Battaglia Parodi M (eds): Surgical Retina.
ESASO Course Series. Basel, Karger, 2012, vol 2, pp 105–108

Making Sense of Prophylaxis for Retinal Detachment

George William Aylward

Moorfields Eye Hospital, London, UK

Abstract

Prophylactic treatment is designed to reduce the risk of retinal detachment, but is a controversial subject, largely due to the poor evidence base. This chapter reviews the principles of prophylaxis, and provides practical advice in a number of common clinical scenarios.

The majority of patients with retinal detachment present with macular involvement [1], resulting in reduced acuity and metamorphopsia even after successful primary surgery. Therefore, there would be significant patient benefit if an effective prophylactic treatment existed. Unfortunately the evidence base of prophylaxis is scant, with no high quality evidence to support treatment. Treatment decisions consequently vary greatly between surgeons in different centres [2].

General Principles

Retinal detachments result from fluid passing through retinal breaks, and can be divided into two distinct groups according to whether a posterior vitreous detachment (PVD) is present. In PVD-related detachments, the vitreous peels away from the retina potentially causing a retinal tear at sites of abnormal vitreoretinal adhesion, such as lattice degeneration (fig. 1). Unfortunately, the vast majority of patients with lattice degeneration do not experience a retinal tear, and in patients who do, the tears are often not related to the lattice. Thus, there is no reliable method of identifying areas of dangerous adhesion prior to the PVD occurring.

Non-PVD-related detachments include those associated with round holes and dialyses. The aetiology of these detachments is poorly understood, but their incidence seems to peak at a relatively young age, with the risk of detachment receding as the patient gets older.

Evidence

The evidence base for prophylactic treatment is poor, but this is largely because of the practical difficulties in addressing the question 'What effect does prophylactic treatment have on the lifetime risk of visual loss'. For example, if a patient receives prophylactic treatment at the age of 20, it might be more than 40 years before a PVD occurs and the value of the treatment can be determined. Given the rarity of retinal detachment, the numbers required in a trial would also be unfeasibly large. Consider for a moment a trial designed to determine whether treatment X was effective in reducing the incidence of retinal detachment by half. Power calculations indicate that 7,263 patients would be required in each arm of the trial. The combination of this large sample size and the long follow-up period means that there will be no randomised controlled prospective trial for the foreseeable future.

In the absence of randomised controlled trials, we have to fall back on observational studies and common sense in making decisions about prophylaxis. We owe a large debt to the painstaking and meticulously documented work of Norman Byer in deriving knowledge of the natural history retinal detachments and predisposing lesions.

A useful way of thinking about prophylaxis is the number needed to treat, defined as the number of patients needing treatment to prevent one bad outcome. Consider for example asymptomatic lattice. A rough estimate of lifetime risk of retinal detachment in the presence of lattice is 0.2%. If we assume that prophylactic treatment were to be successful and reduce the risk to half that (0.1%), then the absolute risk reduction is 0.1. The number needed to treat is the inverse of the absolute risk reduction, so would be 1,000, far higher than anything that is considered reasonable in other fields of medicine.

Risks of Prophylaxis

If we could be sure that prophylactic treatment was completely safe, then it might be reasonable to give some patients the benefit of the doubt, and apply it. However, no treatment is 100% safe, and there are theoretical reasons, as well as emerging evidence of harm. For example, in one study of prophylactic failures (patients who had received treatment but who had developed PVD-associated retinal detachment much later), half the patients had retinal tears on the edge of the treated areas, suggesting that treatment might be simply replacing one abnormal vitreoretinal adhesion with a larger one [3].

Specific Cases

Asymptomatic Lattice

The prevalence of lattice (fig. 2) is estimated at up to 10% of the population, but the incidence of retinal detachment is only 1 in 10,000 adults annually. Simply put, this means that the vast majority of patients with lattice do not develop retinal detachment. Byer followed up 423 eyes for periods up to 25 years, and observed only 3 sub-clinical detachments. As a result, he recommended that 'prophylactic treatment of lattice with or without holes in phakic, non-fellow eyes should be discontinued' [4].

Lattice in the Fellow Eye

The presence of lattice in the fellow eye of a patient with retinal detachment does represent an increased risk of rhegmatogenous retinal detachment in the fellow eye. One non-randomised study suggested that prophylactic treatment to the fellow eye at the time of surgery was associated with a reduced risk of retinal detachment [5]. However, this benefit was not found for eyes with large amounts of lattice, or for eyes with myopia greater than 6 dpt.

Asymptomatic Breaks

The majority of asymptomatic breaks are round holes, since 'U' tears tend to be associated with symptomatic PVD. Byer [6] observed 359 patients with such breaks for up to 18 years. There were 18 subclinical detachments over that period, but no cases requiring treatment.

Traction 'U' Tears

Tears due to vitreous traction occur secondary to a PVD, and have a very high risk of progression to

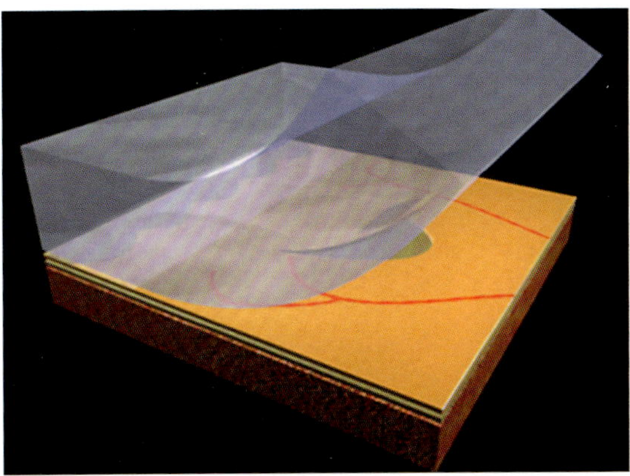

Fig. 1. A 'U' tear occurs as the vitreous, peeling away from the underlying retina, encounters an area of abnormal vitreoretinal adhesion, such as lattice.

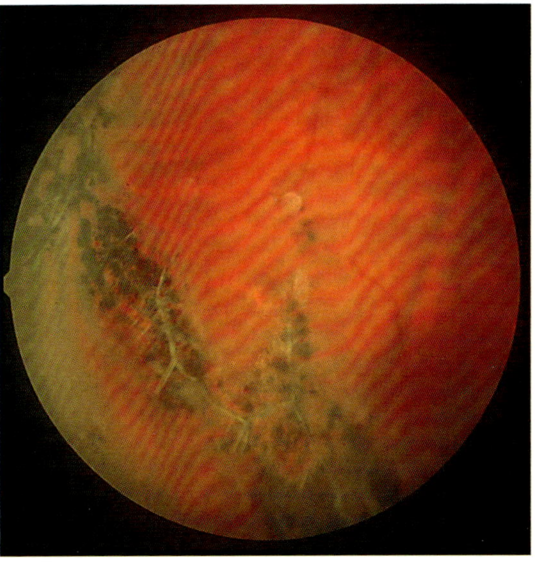

Fig. 2. Lattice degeneration is a common peripheral retinal finding, the presence of which represents an increased risk of retinal detachment.

retinal detachment, at least 30% [6]. While there is no trial evidence to support it, early retinopexy in such cases appears to be effective in preventing detachment in the majority of cases.

Types of Prophylaxis

Laser photocoagulation is the most common form of prophylactic treatment, and is easy and convenient to apply using either slit-lamp lasers or indirect lasers. The aim is to create a continuous chorioretinal adhesion around the break to prevent the passage of fluid. This can be achieved using one or two rows of overlapping spots.

Cryotherapy is less commonly performed because of the associated episcleral inflammation. However, it is useful for tears where the anterior edge is difficult to reach with the slit-lamp laser and an indirect laser is not available.

Whichever method is used, the patient should be reviewed 10 days after retinopexy to ensure that a continuous chorioretinal adhesion has developed.

In summary, the evidence base for prophylactic treatment is poor, and there are reasons to believe it may be harmful in the long-term. In practice, the author recommends that treatment be reserved for traction 'U' tears associated with a PVD, but no other lesions.

References

1 Burton TC: Recovery of visual acuity after retinal detachment involving the macula. Trans Am Ophthalmol Soc 1982;80:475–497.
2 Kreis AJ, Aylward GW, Wolfensberger TJ: Prophylaxis for retinal detachment: evidence or eminence based? Retina 2007;27:468–472.
3 Chauhan DS, Downie JA, Eckstein M, Aylward GW: Failure of prophylactic retinopexy in fellow eyes without a PVD. Arch Ophthalmol 2006;124:968–971.
4 Byer NE: Long-term natural history of lattice degeneration of the retina. Ophthalmol 1989;96:1396–1401.
5 Folk JC, Arrindell EL, Klugman MR: The fellow eye of patients with phakic lattice retinal detachment. Ophthalmol 1989;96:72–79.
6 Byer N: The natural history of asymptomatic retinal breaks. Ophthalmol 1982;89:1033–1039.

George William Aylward, MD
Consultant Vitreoretinal Surgery, Moorfields Eye Hospital
City Road
London EC1V 2PD (UK)
E-Mail bill.aylward@moorfields.nhs.uk

Bandello F, Battaglia Parodi M (eds): Surgical Retina.
ESASO Course Series. Basel, Karger, 2012, vol 2, pp 109–116

Ab externo Surgery of Rhegmatogenous Retinal Detachment: Handling of Intraoperative and Postoperative Complications

Ainat Klein · Anat Loewenstein

Department of Ophthalmology, Tel Aviv Medical Center, Sackler Faculty of Medicine, Tel-Aviv University, Tel-Aviv, Israel

Abstract

Retinal detachment surgery can be associated with multiple complications able to reduce the anatomic success rate and final visual acuity outcomes. Most surgical failures result from inability to detect and treat all retinal breaks, development of proliferative vitreoretinopathy, and errors in surgical judgment or technique. Complications can be divided into pre-, intra- and postoperative conditions. Bad visualization and intraocular inflammation are the main preexisting factors that can complicate the surgery. Intraoperative complications are usually more serious, and can be related to anesthesia, exposure, localization and suturing of the implant, the cryopexy or drainage of subretinal fluids. The important postoperative complications are mainly related to inflammation/infection, ischemia, intraocular pressure, choroidal detachment or hemorrhage and persistent or recurrent retinal detachment. Muscle imbalance and refractive changes are common but easily treated. Buckle intrusion or extrusion can develop even years after the primary procedure.

Retinal detachment surgery can be associated with a various number of complications which can reduce the anatomic success rate and final visual acuity outcomes. Fortunately, serious complications resulting in failure to reattach the retina are infrequent. Most failures are due to inability to detect all retinal breaks, development of proliferative vitreoretinopathy (PVR), and errors in surgical judgment or technique. The aim of this chapter is to review the range and incidence of the complications, emphasize anticipation and prevention of these difficulties and offer possible management options for these complications.

Preexisting Conditions

The main preexisting factors for complications are bad visualization of the retina and intraocular inflammation. Indirect ophthalmoscopy can overcome mild lens opacities, but severe cases require cataract extraction before retinal detachment repair. Nd:YAG laser capsulotomy can be used in cases of significant posterior capsular opacities. Papillary abnormalities that prevent sufficient dilatation can be handled by indirect ophthalmoscopy and by scleral indentation.

Intraoperative Complications

Complications Associated with Anesthesia
In general anesthesia, ocular damage from compression with a gas mask during induction is rare, and can be avoided by taping a shield on the eye. Retreobulbar anesthesia may be complicated by several mechanisms. Retrobulbar hemorrhage can cause physical restriction of the globe and/or elevated intraocular pressure (IOP). The needle can also cause direct damage to the globe or optic nerve (0.1%). This is more frequent in high myopic eyes, and can be avoided by holding the eye at primary position or by the use of peribulbar or subtenon injection. Brain stem anesthesia can be caused if the needle tip penetrates the dural sheath of the optic nerve, so the anesthetic agent is injected actually into the subarachnoid space. This leads to respiratory arrest for 15–30 min.

Complications during Exposure
Complications during exposure are quite rare, and are most likely during reoperations while dissecting abnormal adhesions; tissue planes are indistinct and the sclera is abnormally weak.

Scleral rupture and/or perforation are the most serious complications, and usually occur while dissecting under the rectus muscle. It can be avoided by careful technique, clear operative field, using a blunt muscle hook rather than needle, or holding the needle tangentially. It is also useful to expose the anterior surface of an explant (if it exists) and use it as a plane.

Rectus muscle rupture. If the tendon ruptures near the insertion site, there are usually no serious long-term sequelae. However, rupture of the muscle belly can cause severe postoperative motility disturbances. Therefore, the surgeon should be careful while isolating the muscles, and ensure that the traction sutures are beneath the distal part of the tendon rather than beneath the muscle belly. If anterior rupture of a rectus tendon occurs, it is secured on a 6-0 absorbable suture, and the muscle should be attached to the sclera at the end of surgery. If rupture occurs more posteriorly, both ends of the ruptured muscle belly should be immediately identified and sutured together. This can be aided by elevating Tenon's capsule with forceps to locate the sheath through which muscle passes.

Tear of the vortex veins (VV) is more common in reoperations. The veins are frequently involved in epibulbar scar tissue or may be displaced anteriorly. If they are cut or torn, they should be cauterized to avoid prolonged bleeding that would impair further dissection in that quadrant.

Complications Reducing Visibility
Optimal visualization of the retina is crucial for accurate localization and treatment of all retinal breaks, which is necessary for achieving successful surgery.

Corneal opacities. Punctuate corneal epithelial opacities can result from recurrent topical phenylephrine use, from antiseptic solutions and from direct trauma by lid speculum. The surgeon should avoid drying of the epithelium by intermittent wetting of the cornea. Stromal or epithelial edema can be due to elevated IOP. It is advised to treat the elevated IOP according to its cause and use a cotton tip applicator to remove the epithelium. (Thereafter, wetting is still frequently necessary since the Bowman's membrane is dehydrated rapidly.) Application of 50% sterile glycerin is also useful.

Pupillary constriction usually occurs if the operation is prolonged or when hypotony develops. Using indirect ophthalmoscope may provide adequate visualization even in narrow pupils. In severe cases, it can be treated by subconjunctival injection of a dilating solution. Still, it is sometimes necessary to convert the surgery and use intraoperative techniques as iris hooks.

Hyphema is most likely to occur in cases of hypotony, sometimes during drainage of subretinal fluids (SRF). It is advisable in this case to immediately place cotton-tipped applicators around the eye to indent the sclera and maintain near-normal pressure in order to try and stop the bleeding.

Vitreous hemorrhage. Small hemorrhage is common in acute rhegmatogenic retinal detachment because of tears of blood vessel. Severe hemorrhage is usually associated with other complications and should be treated as discussed above. If the bleeding does not rest and does not allow visualization, vitrectomy must be performed.

Complication of Localization

Improper localization may result in failure to support all edges of the retinal tears leading to persistent leakage. Inadvertent scleral perforation may be caused when the probe is used to localize the breaks, usually when the sclera is thin or necrotic. The sclera should be examined before localization and in areas of thin sclera, diathermy or cautery must not be used, and only slight indentation is applied. Damage to VV may be avoided by identifying the location of the vein before indenting the sclera with the probe.

Complications of Treatment

The main difficulty in applying cryotherapy is the inability to identify the treatment site immediately after the ice ball thaws and difficulty to precisely position the probe tip. This may result in failure to treat some areas, or in inadvertent retreatment. Retreatment can cause excessive necrosis and atrophy of the retina and choroid, additional dispersion of viable retinal pigment epithelium (RPE) cells and prolonged breakdown of blood retinal barrier. Complications may occur from faulty positioning of the cryoprobe tip and treatment of unintended areas. This occurs if the probe is rotated, causing freezing in an adjacent meridian, and is avoided by holding it so that the active surface is always against the sclera. More severe damage can occur if indentation caused by the probe shaft is misinterpreted as being due to the tip, resulting in freezing of the more posterior retina.

The dispersion of RPE cells into the vitreous is common mainly when treating large areas. Those viable cells are capable of causing epiretinal membrane, and/or PVR (further discussed in the section 'Postoperative Complications' below).

Cryotherapy may also cause small intraretinal hemorrhage (with no harmful effect). Choroidal effusion or hemorrhage is more common in highly myopic eyes, intense treatment and retreatment. The bleeding itself is limited because of the tamponade effect of the increased IOP. The VV may be torn while moving the probe, especially if the tip is still frozen to episcleral tissue.

The most severe, but fortunately rare, complication is scleral rupture. It usually occurs during treatment through thin sclera, and if the probe is moved while still frozen to the globe, which causes shearing force that may fracture the sclera and rupture the choroid and retina. The surgeon must therefore wait for the probe to thaw before moving it.

Complications of Scleral Sutures

Complications of scleral sutures are among the most important intraoperative complications as mentioned above. The main concern is inadvertent perforation of the sclera, causing intraocular bleeding, premature SRF drainage with softening of the globe, and additional retinal break. It is more common in myopic eyes with thin sclera. Perforation is indicated by sudden leakage of intraocular fluid or by occurrence of pigment on the suture. As soon as this is noticed, the surgeon must prevent further loss of intraocular fluid by eliminating external pressure and traction on the globe and quickly restoring the integrity of the globe by repairing the wound. Rupture can cause only drainage of SRF, but if the retina is also damaged, or even incarcerated, the area should be treated by diathermy or cryotherapy, and the buckle should be modified to that area. If the perforation is quite anterior and the suture material is not visible by indirect ophthalmoscopy, the suture is left in place and the posterior bite is completed. Visible suture material should always be removed. If perforation occurs during placement of a posterior suture bite, another bite is taken 2 mm posterior to it, and a broader piece of silicone is used.

Choroidal hemorrhage occurs in 15–25% of cases of inadvertent scleral perforation, but the bleeding is usually minimal. If the macula is involved, the eye should be rotated to reduce the risk of SRF migrating beneath the macula. If blood is present under the macula (fig. 1), drainage of all SRF is avoided, so that the blood can be displaced away by postoperative posturing. Extensive hemorrhage beneath the macula can cause severe damage to the photoreceptors in a relatively short time and therefore, surgical removal of the blood should be contemplated.

Insufficient suture depth. Since the explants rely mainly on the scleral sutures to cause the buckling effect, the suture bites must be secure to have a lasting effect until effective chorioretinal scar forms around the retinal break. Later loosening can cause an unsightly external bulge of the explant material, external erosion or extraocular muscle imbalance.

Complications during Drainage of Subretinal Fluids

Partially controlled studies have shown that drainage and non-drainage techniques have similar anatomic success rates. Complications can be minimized by proper selection of the perforation site and careful technique, but cannot be completely avoided. Minor bleeding from the choroid at the sclerotomy site is most common but can be reduced by closely inspecting the choroid before perforation. Bleeding is usually minimal and is visible internally as a small red spot. More extensive subretinal hemorrhage can extend into the macula, and can pass into the vitreous cavity or accumulate as a hemorrhagic choroidal detachment. Active bleeding is treated by elevating IOP by external traction on the rectus muscle sutures or indenting the bleeding site. If the macula is involved by the detachment, the eye is rotated to minimize the chance of blood extending beneath the macula, and drainage should be stopped as mentioned

above. Hemorrhagic choroidal detachment (fig. 1) usually elevates IOP, but if the eye remains soft sutures should be tightened. Usually, this bleeding cannot be drained immediately since blood clots quickly, and sometimes, paracentesis or limited vitrectomy should be performed.

Retinal incarceration can occur at drainage site, usually soon after drainage begins and most commonly if IOP is elevated when choroid is penetrated, and with large opening. Retinal perforation is rare and is avoided by introducing the needle somewhat obliquely and choosing drainage site where which the retina is elevated enough by the SRF. Both incarceration and perforation should be treated by cryopexy and be supported on the buckle.

Drainage of liquid vitreous through a retinal break into the subretinal space and then out through the sclerotomy during drainage occurs especially if the break is large, the retina is immobile or if the drainage site is near a break.

Hypotony. Some degree of softening occurs always during drainage, but significant hypotony is associated with an increased risk of hyphema, choroidal hemorrhage and serous choroidal effusion.

Iatrogenic retinal breaks occur in 1–4% of cases. They may develop during placement of sutures, during drainage of SRF or due to excessive cryotherapy, diathermy or photocoagulation. All breaks should be treated and supported on the buckle.

Complications of the Scleral Buckling

Errors in scleral buckling (SB) size and location. The aim of SB is to close the retinal breaks, offset vitreoretinal traction and alter harmful effects of intraocular fluid currents. Improper localization, size or configuration may result in failure to support all edges of the retinal tears leading to persistent leakage.

Radial retinal folds. Circumferential SB reduces the circumference of the globe and produces radial folds. This can be avoided by limiting the elevation of a circumferential buckle and be treated by adding a radial buckle or by intravitreal gas injection.

Increased IOP. The SB reduces intraocular volume, especially if no drainage procedures are taken. This may result in inadequate perfusion to the optic nerve head or occlusion of the central retinal artery. This is especially dangerous in eyes with glaucoma, systemic vascular disease and elderly patients. Retinal and nerve perfusion is monitored by viewing the central retinal artery and optic nerve by indirect ophthalmoscopy. Elevating systemic blood pressure may be useful.

VV damage. The VV may be compressed by the SB.

Complications of Paracentesis

Paracentesis may be complicated by damage to the lens or incarceration of vitreous so the needle tip must be kept parallel to iris avoiding entering the pupillary space.

Complications of Closure

Conjunctival tissue margins must be differentiated from Tenon's capsule, and this is facilitated by flooding the operative field with saline, which hydrates Tenon's capsule, causing it to swell and turn white. The conjunctiva must be handled with care to avoid tearing, especially in reoperations. Conjunctival incision should be closed with a small-diameter absorbable sutures.

Early Postoperative Complications (within 6 Weeks after Operation)

Lid swelling (fig. 2) usually resolves after 48–72 h and if not improving, cellulitis should be considered.

Conjunctival adhesions between bulbar and palpebral surfaces may occur, and should be interrupted with cotton-tipped applicator.

Corneal injuries. Mild corneal epithelial damage is common, especially in diabetic patients, but reepithelization usually occurs in 2–4 days. Erosions are treated by topical medications and patching. Dellen (fig. 3) is treated by ointment and patching to minimize drying until conjunctival swelling subsides and the cornea returns to normal.

Mild extraocular muscle imbalance is common and may lead to transient diplopia that resolves by 4–6 weeks (see also 'Late Postoperative Complications').

Mild intraocular inflammation in the anterior or posterior segment is common, and treatment with topical steroid is usually sufficient.

Periocular infection is rare and more common in sponge than solid silicone. The risk can be reduced by soaking the buckle material in antibiotic solution before use, although the source is usually periocular surfaces contaminated by *Staphylococcus aureus*, *Proteus* or *Pseudomonas aeruginosa*. Injection, chemosis, mucopurulent discharge, localized atypical pain or massive subconjunctival hemorrhage should raise the suspicion of infection, which should be differentiated from acute scleral necrosis, anterior segment ischemia, and endophthalmitis (which is very rare). Bacterial cultures should be taken, and prompt broad spectrum systemic antibiotics are begun. Sometimes SB removal is needed.

Anterior segment ischemia is caused by interruption of blood flow in the anterior ciliary arteries by disinsertion of rectus muscles, cryodamage to the long posterior ciliary arteries or compression of the VV reducing uveal blood flow. Ischemia is more common in old age, systemic vascular problems, hemoglobin diseases, and in cases of increased IOP. Treatment is aimed to improve blood flow to the anterior segment (sometimes by cutting or loosening the encircling band) and treating complications by topical steroids, cycloplegia and antibiotics. Some eyes recover with minimal residual damage, but others progress to phthisis bulbi.

Posterior segment ischemia may not be recognized early, and should be suspected by poor postoperative vision despite good anatomic outcome. It may result from reduced blood flow in the retinal, choroidal or optic nerve circulation.

Increased IOP. Preexisting primary open angle glaucoma or postoperative secondary open angle glaucoma resulting from obstruction of the trabecular meshwork by cells and extracellular debris can be usually be treated by medications. Some cases will require surgical intervention. Primary angle closure glaucoma, in cases of predisposed shallow anterior chamber, should be treated with laser iridotomy. Secondary angle closure glaucoma is most commonly caused by serous choroidal detachment causing anterior rotation of ciliary body, which displaces the peripheral iris into the anterior chamber angle. This usually resolves spontaneously, though it can be treated by topical steroids and cycloplegia. Sometimes, laser iridotomy is required.

Serous choroidal detachment (fig. 4) is the most common postoperative complication, more frequent in older patients, after drainage of SRF, and long circumferential and/or posterior located buckle (fig. 4). It is caused by vascular damage to the VV combined with increased transmural pressure and increased choroidal vascular pressure due to the buckle. It is typically evident 24–48 h after surgery, increases until 72 h, and remains unchanged for 10 days and then resolves. Treatment by systemic or periocular steroids can help. Kissing choroidal detachment, secondary angle closure glaucoma with IOP above 30 mm Hg, marked generalized shallowing of the anterior chamber or corneal decompensation are all indications for drainage.

Hemorrhagic choroidal detachment is less common and usually related to accidental scleral perforation. Drainage should be deferred to 7–14 days.

Failure to attach the retina. Residual SRF results from ineffective removal of SRF by the RPE, and usually occurs in elderly patients, in cases of choroidal detachment or increased protein content in the SRF. Recurrent/persistent detachment is caused by open retinal breaks (that were not closed properly, that were not detected at the initial procedure or iatrogenic tears caused during the operation). Ineffective closure of breaks can be caused by inaccurate placement of SB, failure to bring break into contact with RPE, radial fold, or progressive VR traction. Open breaks are treated either by laser photocoagulation (if located on the buckle), by pneumatic retinopexy or by additional surgery.

Late Postoperative Complications

Eyelids. Mild ptosis is common (13%) due to dehiscence of levator muscle aponeurosis and usually improves after 4–8 weeks. Other complications are upper lid retraction from excessive stimulation of the levator, and inferior lid ectropion from severing of the inferolateral canthal ligament and faulty closure of conjunctival incision.

Conjunctival scarring and symblepharon may result. Epithelial cyst may result from improper edge to edge closure of the conjunctiva. Large cyst may be excised, or treated with cryotherapy.

Muscle imbalance is a common (50%), usually temporary, complication, more frequent in reoperations, and often involves the inferior rectus muscle. It can be prevented by avoiding temporary disinsertion of the extraocular muscles and by avoiding the use of a bulky scleral buckle material beneath the rectus muscle insertion.

Corneal complications comprise reduced sensitivity with neurotrophic keratitis (when encircling buckle is used or from damage to the ciliary nerve causing neurotrophic changes), recurrent erosions (if epithelium was removed and more common in DM and after extensive cryosurgery or broad SB), and astigmatic changes (more common in radial buckle and silicone sponge and usually improve gradually).

Modification to the eyeball and refractive error changes. An encircling buckle usually causes an increase in axial length causing myopic shift, so as increased scleral rigidity (which can render applanation tonometry less accurate). Marked indentation and tightening of sutures usually cause

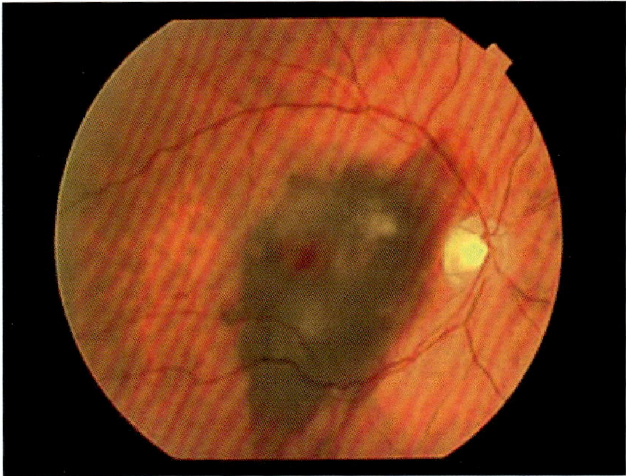

Fig. 1. Color picture of right eye fundus presenting submacular accumulation of blood secondary to choroidal hemorrhage.

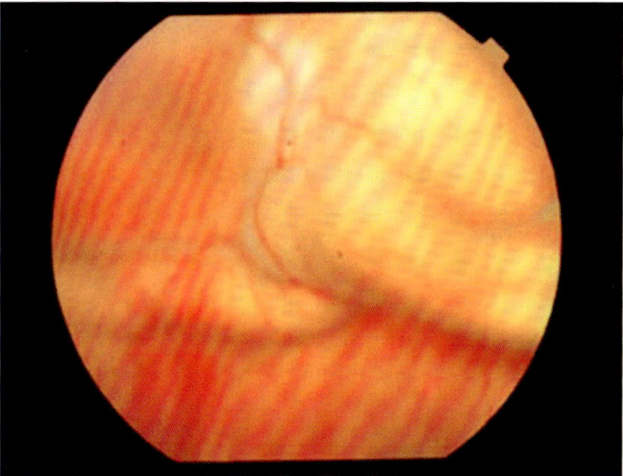

Fig. 4. Serous choroidal detachment, the most common complication during the first 2 weeks after retinal reattachment.

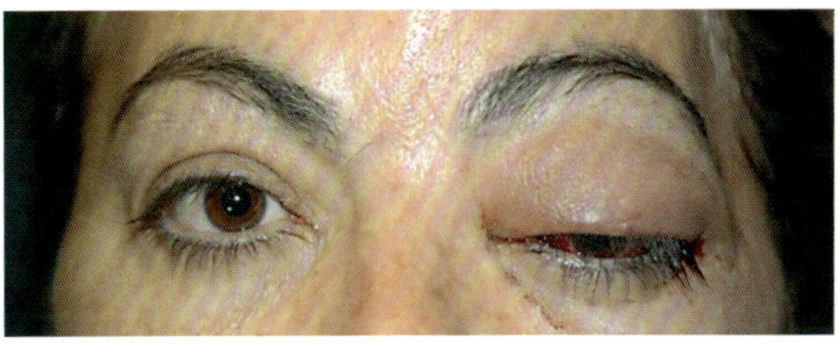

Fig. 2. Marked swelling of left eyelids on first postoperative day. More common after circular scleral buckle, extensive cryosurgery, or reoperations. Swelling resolved gradually through 3–4 days. Left hypotropia is also present.

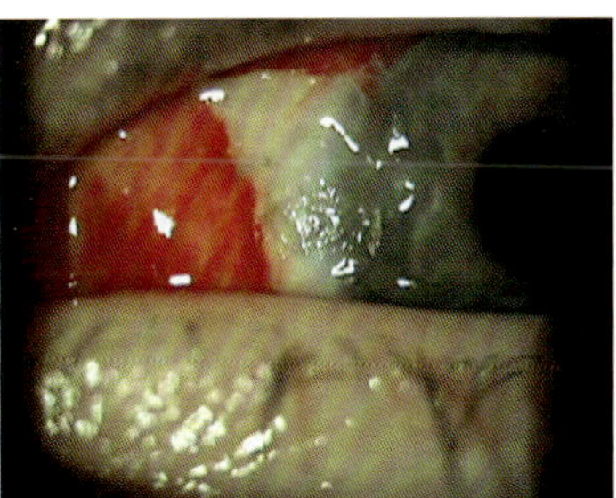

Fig. 3. Subconjunctival hemorrhage and elevated edematous conjunctiva adjacent to the limbus disturbing the tear film resulting in dellen.

reduction in axial length and induce hyperopic shift. An encircling buckle also causes anterior displacement of the lens, increasing any myopic change and decreasing hyperopic change.

Late infection and/or exposure of the buckle is probably due to contamination by relatively non-virulent organisms at time of surgery. In those cases, the buckle should be removed. It is recommended to apply laser treatment to reinforce the chorioretinal scars in areas with residual traction, 2 weeks before the removal. Transscleral intrusion is rare (fig. 5), more common in eyes with thin sclera, high and narrow encircling buckle, improperly shaped and trimmed silicone element or cases of scleral necrosis. In these cases, the implant must be removed.

Anterior segment complications. Most occur during immediate postoperative period (discussed above). Cataract develops especially in longstanding detachment, hypotony or marked preoperative intraocular inflammation.

Macular changes. Postoperative cystoid macular edema, macular hole, epiretinal membrane with macular pucker and subretinal neovascularization are rare but possible complications that reduce visual acuity.

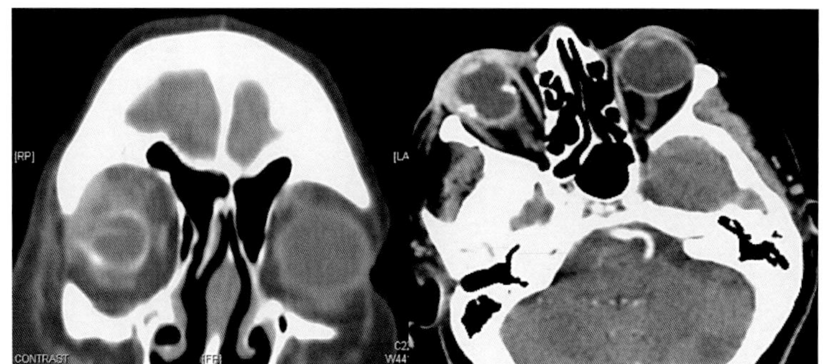

Fig. 5. Sagittal CT scan demonstrating hyperechogenic structure surrounding right eye globe, causing a typical buckling effect. Coronal section of the same patient demonstrating the intrusion of the implant through the sclera and retina.

PVR is the most important complication, causing recurrent retinal detachment and complicating surgeries. It is a cell-mediated process that correlates with conditions that predispose to RPE cell release into the vitreous (as large tears and cryotherapy), and/or breakdown of the blood-aqueous barrier. The cellular membranes contract causing distortion and decreased mobility of the detached retina. Pigment cell release can be minimized by limiting the intensity of each cryotherapy application, avoiding re-treatment, applications only around the break (and not within it) and minimize indentation of the sclera after applying cryotherapy.

Late recurrent retinal detachment is the most significant complication, and occurs in 10% of cases. It usually develops later than 6 weeks after the initial surgery. It can be due to the presence of recurrent tears (rhegmatogenous detachment) or vitreoretinal or epiretinal membrane traction alone (tractional detachment). It is treated by modification of the buckle and/or vitreous surgery according to the cause.

References

1 Guyer DR, Yannuzzi LA, Chang S, et al: Retina, Vitreous, Macula, ed 1. Philadelphia, Saunders, 1999, chapter 110, pp 1248–1270.

2 Schepens CL: Schepen's Retinal Detachment and Allied Diseases, ed 2. Oxford, Butterworth-Heinemann, 2000, chapter 37, pp 721–738.

3 Ryan SJ: Retina, ed 4. St. Louis, Mosby, 2006, chapter 118, pp 2056–2067.

4 Schepens CL: Management of retinal retachment. Ophthalmic Surg 1994;25:427–431.

5 American Academy of Ophthalmology: The repair of rhegmatogenous retinal detachments. Ophthalmology 1990;97:1562–1572.

6 Michels RG: Scleral buckling methods for rhegmatogenous retinal detachment. Retina 1986;6(1):1–49.

Ainat Klein, MD
Department of Ophthalmology, Tel-Aviv Sourasky Medical Center
6 Weizman Street
Tel Aviv 64239 (Israel)
Tel. +972 3 9739408, E-Mail euriya@gmail.com

Bandello F, Battaglia Parodi M (eds): Surgical Retina.
ESASO Course Series. Basel, Karger, 2012, vol 2, pp 117–120

Vitrectomy for Rhegmatogenous Retinal Detachment

George William Aylward

Moorfields Eye Hospital, London, UK

Abstract

This chapter is a guide to the use of vitrectomy in the management of rhegmatogenous retinal detachment. It contains practical advice on each component of the procedure, including the vitrectomy itself, searching for retinal breaks, choice of retinopexy, and the fluid-gas exchange. It also provides hints and tips on how to avoid common problems and complications.

This chapter describes the use of vitrectomy in the primary management of rhegmatogenous retinal detachment. The first successful surgical intervention for rhegmatogenous retinal detachment was thermocautery introduced by Jules Gonin in 1922 [1]. Since then, surgery for retinal detachment has become increasingly successful, and a routine component of the ophthalmological armamentarium. However, controversy continues to surround the choice of optimal technique, particularly for the initial operation. A recent survey conducted by the American Society of Retinal Specialists asked which technique respondents would use to repair a straightforward retinal detachment associated with a single retinal tear. The results are summarised in table 1, and show that surgeons were almost equally divided between four very different techniques [2].

Case Selection

There is little difference of opinion in the use of vitrectomy in complex retinal detachments such as those associated with giant retinal tears, or in cases with vitreous haemorrhage. However, in many centres, vitrectomy is becoming common as the initial choice of procedure for straightforward retinal detachments [3]. This shift is associated more with local circumstances and training, rather than being evidence based. The SpR study was a very important contribution to the literature on this subject, and was a large-scale, multicentre, randomised controlled trial comparing scleral buckling and vitrectomy in the primary management of retinal detachments of medium complexity [4]. It showed that scleral buckling was superior to vitrectomy in phakic eyes, but that vitrectomy was superior to scleral buckling in pseudophakic eyes.

Table 1. Results of the PAT survey [2]

Technique	Choice, %
Scleral buckle	27
Vitrectomy	31
Vitrectomy with supplementary buckle	15
Pneumatic retinopexy	27

Vitrectomy

A vitrectomy is carried out in the normal way using the system and gauge of your choice. In the vast majority of eyes, there is already a posterior vitreous detachment (PVD), as this was the likely cause of the retinal tears which led to the detachment in the first place. While the PVD makes the vitrectomy easier, the presence of detached, mobile retina means that care has to be taken to avoid iatrogenic breaks and incarceration. Breaks are more likely when trimming the vitreous base adjacent to detached retina, as it can easily 'jump' into the jaws of the cutter. The risk can be reduced by using low suction, and higher cutting speed. In cases of bullous detachment, removal of the instruments, particularly at an early stage of the vitrectomy (before there is free flow of fluid), can result in incarceration of vitreous and retina in the sclerostomy. The risk can be reduced by switching off the infusion prior to removing the instruments. In very bullous detachments, the cutter can be used to aspirate subretinal fluid to reduce the size of detachment. The aim of the vitrectomy is to remove as much vitreous as possible, particularly around the areas of the breaks, including removal of the operculum (fig. 1). Some surgeons like to trim the vitreous base using indentation, but the author does not consider this necessary.

Search
Once the vitrectomy is complete, the peripheral retinal can be searched thoroughly for any retinal breaks that were not detected pre-operatively. An effective method of doing this is to plug one port, and use a flat-bladed squint hook to indent the periphery. The combination of a light pipe and a wide-angle viewing system provides a very good view which should be sufficient to detect the majority of breaks. Effective indentation requires that fluid refluxes up the infusion, and this will only happen if the vitreous has been cleared from the tip of the infusion in the previous step. If the eye hardens on indentation, or if the scleral plug tends to 'pop out', then it is worth carrying out more vitrectomy around the infusion port. In rare cases, very small retinal breaks are not visible, even on deep indentation. In cases were no breaks are found, the use of subretinal trypan blue can be a valuable aid for detecting them [5]. Breaks that are visible in a fluid-filled eye can sometimes be very difficult to see after the fluid is exchanged for air. This problem can be solved by marking the break with a small spot of diathermy. An intraocular diathermy, set on low power, is positioned on the apex of the retinal break and turned on briefly (fig. 2).

Fluid Air Exchange

The goal is to replace the subretinal and preretinal fluid with air. An airline is attached to the three-way tap and the other end attached to a source of air set to 30 mm Hg. It is important that the air supply is switched on at the machine, since otherwise turning the three-way tap results in hypotony. A flute needle is then inserted and positioned, the ideal location being through the most posterior break, and the air supply switched on. During the early phase of the fluid-air exchange, a clear view of the break and the tip of the flute is not possible, and this can be alarming. However, it returns once the fluid bubble is larger than about 50%. The subretinal fluid is then drained until the edges of the break are apposed

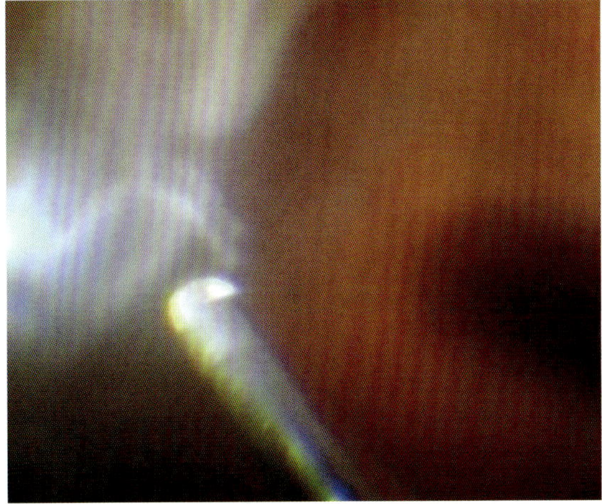

Fig. 1. The cutter should be used to trim the vitreous attachments to the retina around the tear, and to remove the operculum.

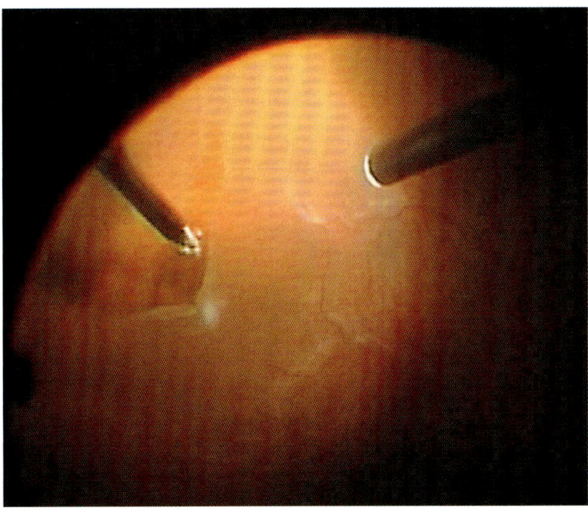

Fig. 2. The breaks should be marked using a small spot of diathermy. This makes them much easier to find later on the case when applying retinopexy.

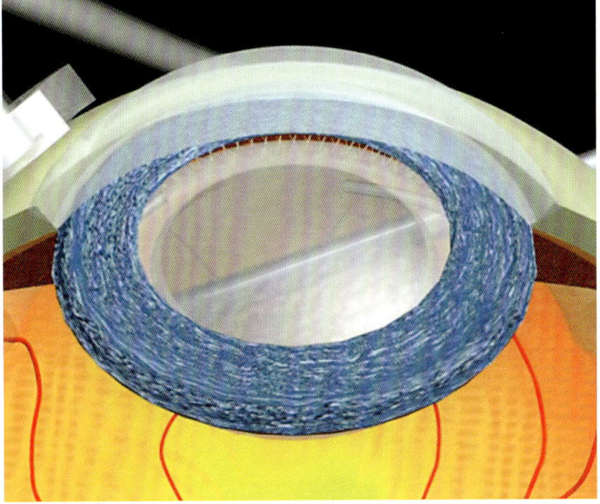

Fig. 3. Removing condensation from the posterior surface of an IOL by wiping with the edge of the flute needle.

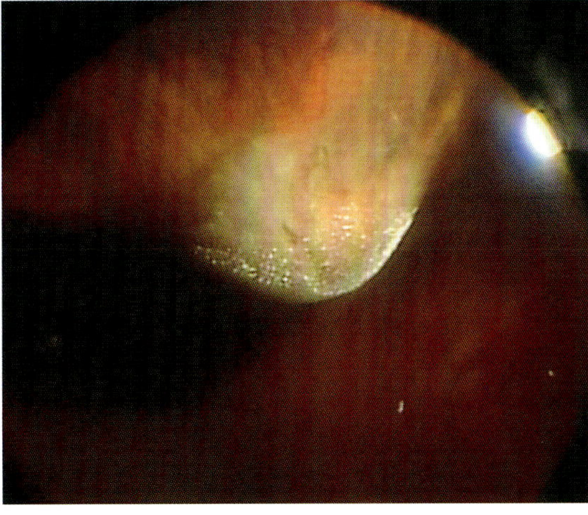

Fig. 4. Thawing of the frozen retina in an air filled eye takes some time because of the insulating effect of the gas.

to the pigment epithelium. At this point, the flute is moved to the most dependent part of the globe, usually the optic disk, in order to remove the preretinal fluid.

In some pseudophakic eyes, condensation on the posterior surface of the IOL can cloud the view. This can be dealt with temporarily by wiping the lens with the edge of the flute needle (fig. 3). If the condensation returns rapidly, then a small blob of viscoelastic placed on the posterior surface of the IOL is an effective method of preserving the view for the remainder of the case.

Retinopexy

Once the retina around the breaks is attached, retinopexy can be applied. Either laser or cryotherapy can be applied to seal the break. Cryotherapy is easier to apply in an air-filled eye, but there are theoretical concerns about increasing the risk of proliferative vitreoretinopathy. However, for a small number of tears, cryotherapy is acceptable. Air acts as an insulator, so take care not to apply the cryotherapy for too long. The foot pedal should be released as soon as retinal whitening appears, and the probe must be kept still until thawing is complete (fig. 4).

Gas Injection

The decision of which gas to use depends on a number of factors, but in practice 20% SF6 is suitable for the majority of cases. A 50-ml syringe is prepared containing the gas mixture, and then attached to the three-way tap in place of the airline (the tap is switched off for the changeover). A scleral plug is then removed, and the gas slowly injected, aiming to pass 40 ml through the eye. The ports can then be closed, and the case is complete.

References

1 Gonin J: Le traitement de décollement retinien. Ann Oculist 1921;158:175–178.
2 PAT Survey. American Society of Retinal Specialists. 2006.
3 Minihan M, Tanner V, Williamson TH: Primary rhegmatogenous retinal detachment: 20 years of change. Br J Ophthalmol 2001;85:546–548.
4 Heimann H, et al: Scleral buckling versus primary vitrectomy in rhegmatogenous retinal detachment. A prospective randomised multicentre clinical study. Ophthalmology 2007;114:2142–2154.
5 Wong R, Gupta B, Aylward GW, Laidlaw DA: Dye extrusion technique (DE-TECH): occult retinal break detection with subretinal dye extrusion during vitrectomy for retinal detachment repair. Retina 2009;29:492–496.

George William Aylward, MD
Consultant Vitreoretinal Surgery, Moorfields Eye Hospital
City Road
London EC1V 2PD (UK)
E-Mail bill.aylward@moorfields.nhs.uk

Bandello F, Battaglia Parodi M (eds): Surgical Retina.
ESASO Course Series. Basel, Karger, 2012, vol 2, pp 121–126

Scleral Buckling Materials

S. Rizzo · F. Genovesi-Ebert · L. Allegrini

U.O. Chirurgia Oftalmica, Azienda Ospedaliera Universitaria Pisana, Pisa, Italy

Abstract

Currently, scleral buckling (SB) surgery is considered the gold standard for uncomplicated rhegmatogenous retinal detachment. In SB, the eye wall is indented toward the vitreous in order to support or close retinal breaks and to relieve the forces of vitreous tractions. A scleral buckle is a piece of silicone sponge, rubber, or semi-hard plastic that is placed on the sclera, and sewn to keep it in place. The buckle effect may cover only the area behind the detachment, or it may encircle the globe like a ring. There are different types of SB, e.g. encircling versus segmental or radial versus circumferential, absorbable versus non-absorbable. The height of a scleral buckle has to be greater if substantial vitreous tractions are associated with the tears, and lower if there are minimal tractions. The height is affected by the choice of the buckle: radial wedge or radial sponge may create a very high buckling effect; moreover, mattress suture can be placed to increase the indent. The minimal buckle height necessary to achieve closure of the break is preferred, because it leads to less manipulation and distortion of the globe.

In scleral buckling (SB) surgery, the wall of the eye is indented toward the vitreous in order to support or close retinal breaks and to relieve the forces of vitreous tractions that would otherwise keep them open. A scleral buckle is a piece of silicone sponge, rubber, or semi-hard plastic that is placed on the sclera, and sewn to keep it in place. It is usually left permanently in order to push in, or 'buckle', the sclera toward the middle of the eye. The buckle effect may cover only the area behind the detachment, or it may encircle the eyeball like a ring.

The degree of indentation required varies, but it should reduce the vitreous traction and indent the break to close it by apposing the RPE to the break or the break to solid vitreous gel, thus decreasing the communication of liquid vitreous with the subretinal space.

There are different types of SB, e.g. encircling versus segmental or radial versus circumferential, absorbable versus non-absorbable.

The choice of the indentation depends on several factors such as size of the retinal detachment, size, number and localization of the tears. If the tears show a radial orientation, also the buckle will be radially placed; if they are localized circumferentially, a circumferential indentation will be chosen. Different SB procedures may have different success rates and are associated with some common or specific complications [1, 2].

Absorbable buckling components include native fascia lata, human donor sclera and gelatin. Gelatin (hydrolyzed collagen) is the most popular form of absorbable material: it is available as dehydrated sheets that when rehydrated swell. However, if placed before being fully hydrated, gelatine may increase the buckling effects as it swells, and sometimes can minimize the needs for drainage of subretinal fluid. It may also be placed under a permanent buckling material to increase the initial buckling effect. As the gelatine is absorbed over 2–4 months, the buckling effect decreases. The choice of the indentation depends on several factors such as: size of the retinal detachment, size, number and localization of the tears. If the tears show a radial orientation, also the buckle will be radially placed, if they are localized circumferentially, a circumferential indentation will be chosen. It is essential that all components inserted for SB be trimmed of sharp edges to prevent postoperative erosion into adjacent tissues [3, 4].

Non-absorbable buckling components include solid silicone buckles and bands, silicone sponges and hydrogel implants. In 1960, Dr. Charles Schepens introduced silicone and sponge as a material to be used as an implant in treating retinal detachment.

The solid silicone is designed to provide the appropriate softness and tensile strength. The solid silicone implants are produced from a soft, resilient silicone elastomer formulated from medical grade silicone that is firm, non-allergenic and resistant to bacteria. It can be easily cut into desired shapes. It provides a smooth buckling effect without the risk of erosion that is present with polyethylene tubing, and it does not become softer or lose its buckling effect as do absorbable materials [4, 5]. The most used are silicone encircling bands, usually fixed into a sleeve (fig. 1), strips, tires (fig. 2, 3) and radial wedges (fig. 4).

The silicone sponge implants are produced from a small-cell medical grade elastomer sponge. Silicone sponges have numerous air cells, and are therefore more easily moldable than solid silicone. However, in modeling the sponge, the air cells can be damaged and become a nidus for infection.

Therefore, sponges are often soaked preoperatively in broad-spectrum antibiotics to reduce the risk of infection. A sponge placed intraoperatively may initially cause only a small indentation. As the globe decompresses and subretinal fluid is reabsorbed after surgery, the buckling effect becomes more pronounced (fig. 5).

Hydrogel implants made from soft and moldable hydrophilic acrylate can be cut into shapes. They do not contain air cells, and may absorb and release antibiotics; however, over time they become brittle, cause irritation and possible erosion, and must be removed.

Many sizes and shapes of buckling element exist, some with grooves for encircling bands and other without. The height of a scleral buckle has to be greater if substantial vitreous tractions are associated with the tears, and lower if there are minimal tractions. The height is affected by the choice of the buckle: radial wedge or radial sponge may create a very high buckling effect; moreover, mattress suture can be placed to increase the indent.

Although a tight encircling element may increase buckle height, it also impairs the circulation of the eye, so encircling band has to be not so tight to cause IOP increase. The minimal buckle height necessary to achieve closure of the break is preferred, because it leads to less manipulation and distortion of the globe [4, 5].

It is essential that all components inserted for SB be trimmed of sharp edges to prevent postoperative erosion into adjacent tissues.

Choice of the Scleral Buckling Element and Procedure

Currently, SB surgery is considered the gold standard for uncomplicated rhegmatogenous retinal detachment (RRD). It is the treatment of choice for many retinal detachment cases, particularly those with peripheral retinal breaks, and may be used successfully in some cases of

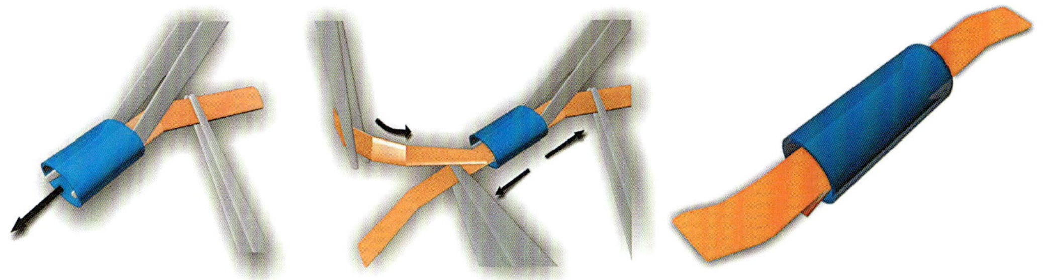

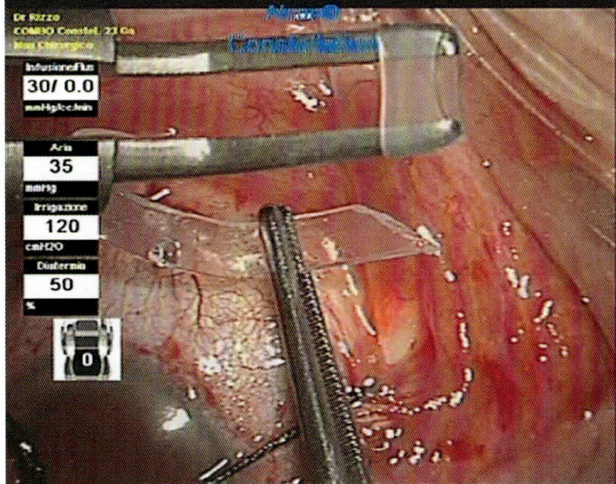

Fig 1. Positioning of silicone sleeve for fixing an encircling band.

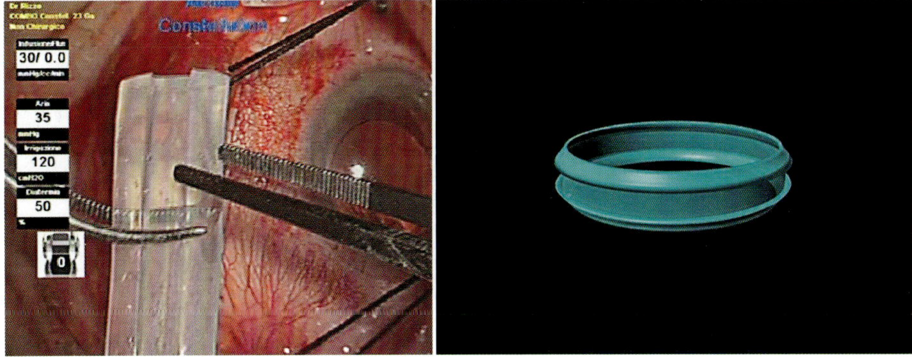

Fig. 2. Hard grooved silicone rubber tire.

proliferative vitreoretinopathy (PVR). However, RRD is not homogeneous: it may be caused by a flap tear due to acute posterior vitreous detachment or by several atrophic holes with extensive lattice degeneration. Different types of retinal detachments behave differently, and may need special considerations in the selection of SB procedures rather than a 'routine method' [6]. For instance, in eyes with PVR, broad and high encircling SB may be preferred since it provides

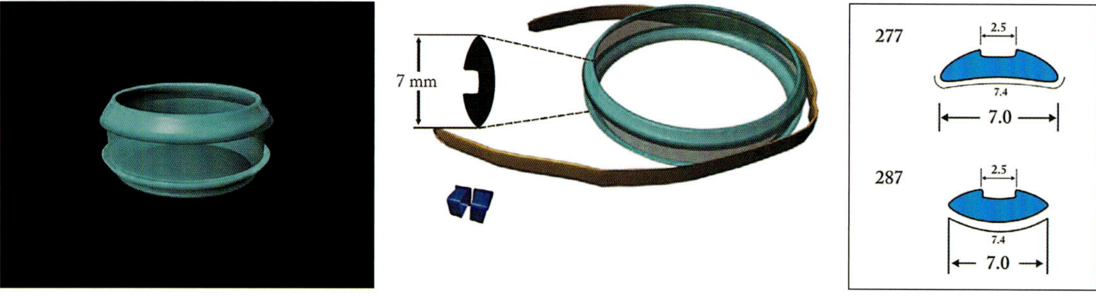

Fig. 3. Hard grooved silicone rubber tire.

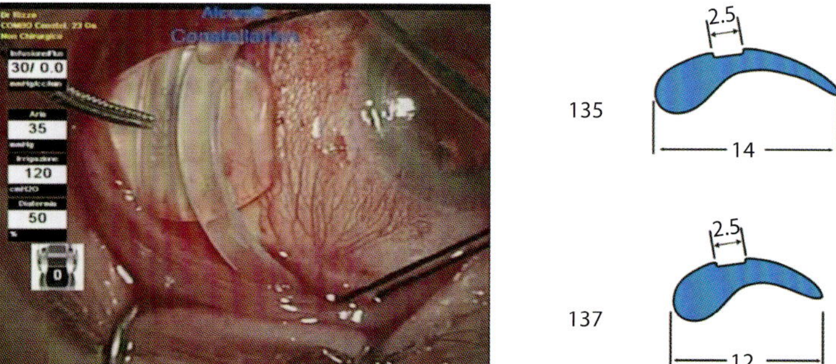

Fig. 4. Hard silicone grooved radial wedge positioned under the encircling band.

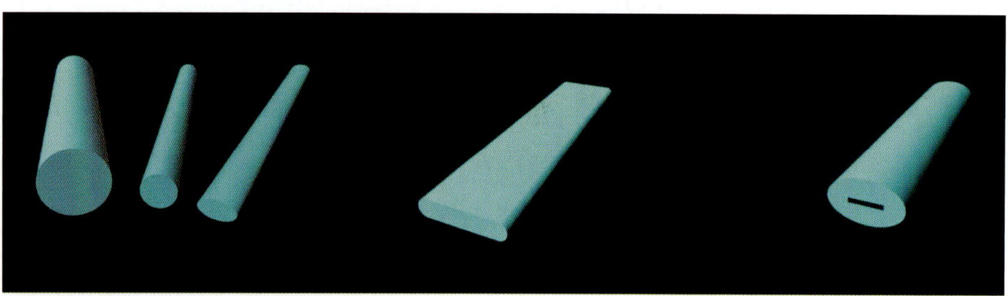

Fig. 5. Silicone sponges.

a wider retinal support and may have a higher success rate. In horseshoe-shaped tears, segmental buckling, especially a radial sponge, can be successfully used because it avoids radial retinal folds (fishmouthing).

Therefore, guidelines have been suggested for the selection of an SB procedure, and they are presented below [1, 3, 6].

Guidelines for the Selection of Scleral Buckling Procedure

1 Radial segmental buckling: Single retinal break, an atrophic hole, or a flap tear, a large horseshoe tear, two retinal breaks located in different quadrants (fig. 6), posterior retinal breaks with or without lattice degeneration.

Rizzo · Genovesi-Ebert · Allegrini

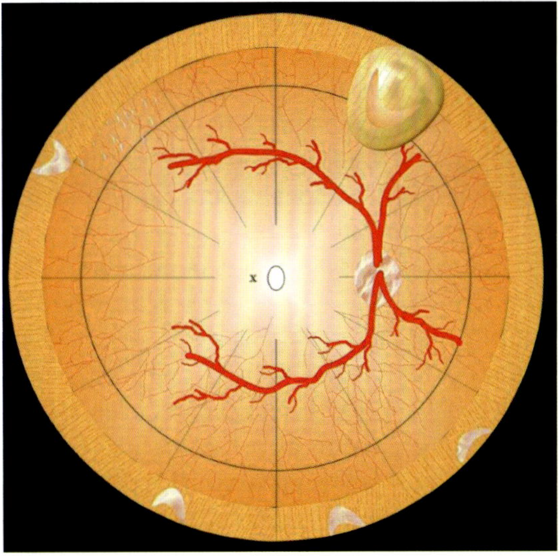

Fig. 6. Radial + encircling band.

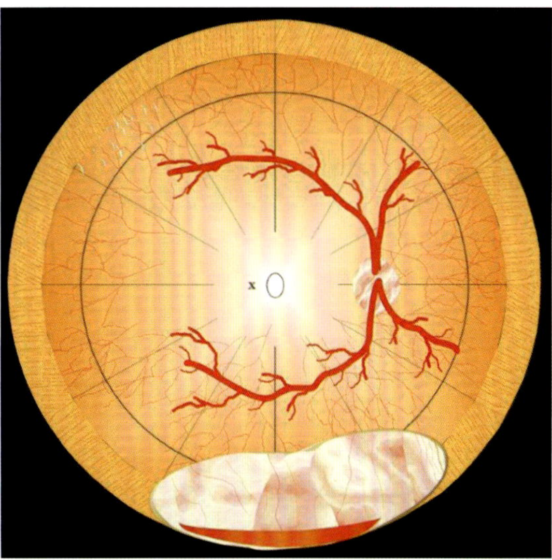

Fig. 7. Circumferential sponge

2 Circumferential segmental buckling: Multiple adjacent retinal breaks, retinal breaks with limited lattice degeneration, anterior retinal breaks or retinal dialysis (fig. 7).
3 Encircling buckling: Multiple retinal breaks in multiple quadrants (fig. 8), multiple retinal breaks with extensive lattice degeneration, absence of recognized breaks, total, chronic detachment with preretinal proliferative changes or extensive subretinal fibrosis.

Final anatomic success rates of greater than 94% after SB surgery have consistently been reported, and a recent retrospective follow-up study by Schwartz et al. [6] demonstrated the stability and longevity of the procedure, with 95% reattachment at 20 years. Vision is preserved, with postoperative visual acuity in uncomplicated RRD of 20/50 or better.

The most common reported cause of failure in surgery for retinal detachment is PVR. If PVR develops, patients typically require further surgical intervention, including vitrectomy. Detachment of the choroid is a frequently reported complication

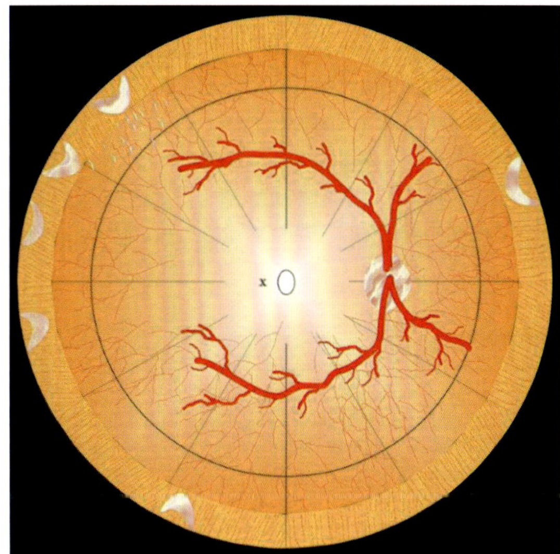

Fig. 8. Encircling band.

following SB surgery. However, recent evidence suggests that the frequency of choroidal detachments after SB (2.4%) may be similar to that following PPV (2.1%). Choroidal detachments usually develop one or two days after surgery and may increase in size for 2 or 3 days. However, they usually heal within 2 weeks without further treatment.

Commonly cited disadvantages of SB surgery include intraoperative hemorrhage or retinal incarceration during drainage procedure (that sometimes can be avoided when dealing with segmental elements). Additionally, small or multiple breaks may not be identified in the SB procedure, although definitive data on the prevalence of missed breaks are lacking.

Postoperatively, disadvantages include prolonged recovery time, pain, induced refractive error with increased myopia, floaters, and ocular motility disturbances. Unusual risks include vitreous or subretinal hemorrhage, infection, swelling or inflammation of the macula, cataracts, increased intraocular pressure.

Complications due to the buckle include distortion of the shape of the eye (causing a refractive error and affecting vision) and interference with extraocular muscles (leading to strabismus or diplopia). The most frequent reported complication after SB was ocular motility disturbance although usually temporary. Long-term diplopia, however, is seen in 5–25% of patients. Deokule et al. [7] report that the most common reasons for scleral explant removal after RRD repair are extrusion, pain, infection, and scleritis/redness.

Some of these complications might be prevented with the use of a segmental buckle instead of an encircling band, without a significant difference in reattachment rates.

Factors associated with anatomic failure of SB include the presence of multiple retinal breaks, breaks larger than three quadrants or three disc diameters, and detachments lasting longer than one week. Poor visual outcome has been associated with these factors as well as macular detachment and poor preoperative visual acuity.

In conclusion, taking in account the suggested guidelines, an appropriate buckling procedure and a suitable indenting element can be selected.

Segmental buckling is as effective as encircling buckling, but without the subsequent complications of significant myopic changes, longer operation times, and higher frequencies of subretinal fluid drainage. The suspicious degenerative areas per se do not necessarily require buckling [8].

Perhaps the guidelines can be of help for retinal surgeons to achieve optimal surgical results when operating on this heterogeneous group of patients.

References

1   Williams GA, Aaberg TM: Techniques of scleral buckling; in Ryan SJ, Glaser BM (eds): Retina. St Louis, Mosby, 1994, vol 3, pp 1979–2017.
2   Michels RG: Scleral buckling methods for rhegmatogenous retinal detachment. Retina 1986;6:1–49.
3   Robertson DM: Scleral buckling choices for primary retinal detachment: vitreoretinal update. American Academy of Ophthalmology, subspecialty day, 1997, pp 147–150.
4   Hartnett ME: Primary rhegmatogenous retinal detachment; in Schepens CL, Hartnett ME, Hirose T (eds): Schepens' Retinal Detachment and Allied Diseases, ed 2. Woburn, Butterworth-Heinemann, 2000, pp 303–305.
5   Ho CL, Chen KJ, See LC: Selection of scleral buckling for primary retinal detachment. Ophthalmologica 2002;216: 33–39.
6   Schwartz SG, Kuhl DP, McPherson AR, et al: Twenty-year follow-up for scleral buckling. Arch Ophthalmol 2002;120: 325–329.
7   Deokule S, Reginald A, Callear A: Scleral explant removal: the last decade. Eye 2002;17:697–700.
8   Sodhi A, Leung SH, Do DV, et al: Recent trends in the management of rhegmatogenous retinal detachment. Surv Ophthalmol 2002;53:50–67.

Stanislao Rizzo, MD
Ospedale Cisanello, Via Paradisa, Edificio 30A
Azienda Ospedaliera Universitaria Pisana
IT–56100 Pisa (Italy)
Tel. +39 3357076057, E-Mail stanislao.rizzo@gmail.com

Bandello F, Battaglia Parodi M (eds): Surgical Retina.
ESASO Course Series. Basel, Karger, 2012, vol 2, pp 127–131

Pneumatic Retinopexy

S. Rizzo · F. Genovesi-Ebert · L. Allegrini

U.O. Chirurgia Oftalmica, Azienda Ospedaliera Universitaria Pisana, Pisa, Italy

Abstract

Pneumatic retinopexy is indicated for uncomplicated rhegmatogenous retinal detachments, including superior retinal breaks smaller than one clock hour, or multiple breaks not extending for more than one clock hour. It is especially effective in eyes with superior breaks and cooperative patients, but requires extraordinary examination of retina pre- and postoperatively. Pneumatic retinopexy is successful 80% of the time with a single operation and an appropriate case selection. The patient must also understand the need for posttreatment head positioning.

The principle of pneumatic retinopexy (PR) is that an intravitreous bubble of an inert gas can be used to seal a retinal break from overlying liquid vitreous, thus allowing the RPE pump to reabsorb subretinal fluid without continued ingress of liquid vitreous into the subretinal space (fig. 1). The gas injection is performed in combination with photocoagulation or cryotherapy to create a permanent chorioretinal adhesion around the break. Rarely, gas is used to drive fluid from under the detached retina through the open break and into the vitreous cavity to reattach the retina.

PR has traditionally been indicated for uncomplicated rhegmatogenous retinal detachments (RRDs), including superior retinal breaks smaller than one clock hour, or multiple breaks not extending for more than one clock hour. It is especially effective in eyes with superior breaks and cooperative patients. However, PR requires extraordinary examination of retina pre- and postoperatively: if you cannot see 360° of the periphery, do not try PR. Additional indications are macular hole, salvage for failing sclera buckle, giant retinal tears, inverted positioning for inferior retinal breaks or creation of posterior vitreous detachment.

Contraindications to PR include inferior breaks, PVR, lattice degeneration, media opacities, uncontrolled glaucoma, and pseudophakia or aphakia, and young patients with trauma. You must be careful if general anesthesia is performed by using N_2O. Tissue nitrogen enters gas bubble in response to partial-pressure gradient.

Frequently cited advantages of the minimally invasive procedure include reduced postoperative morbidity and recovery time as non-buckling operations are less traumatic and will likely result in better vision than buckling operations.

Disadvantages of the procedure include the necessity for correct postoperative positioning and close follow-up, as well as avoidance of air travel in the immediate postoperative period.

The most frequent problems from PR include misplaced gas injection, PVR, and persistent subretinal fluid or trapped gas. More rarely, patients may experience endophthalmitis, macular folds, an increase in intraocular pressure, choroidal detachment, and vitreous or subretinal hemorrhage.

The most serious complication of PR reflects the nature of the procedure. Because PR does not relieve vitreoretinal traction (as opposed to scleral buckling, SB, or pars plana vitrectomy, PPV), new breaks may form, previously unidentified breaks may be recognized, or the original break may reopen. These issues are manifest by a more common need for more than one surgery to reattach the retina after PR than with either SB or PPV [1].

In a retrospective study by Eter et al. [2], 19.4% of reattached retinas redetached during the first 3 months after procedure, with an additional 4.5% redetached after 6 months. Although a failed attempt at PR does not appear to disadvantage the eye for reoperation with SB, suitable criteria for selection of candidates for primary PR are warranted.

Additionally, the appropriate secondary surgical approach (PR vs. SB or PPV) for RRDs that fail (or re-detach after) PR remains to be addressed.

The use of inverted PR for treating RRD associated with inferior retinal breaks was recently reported by Chang et al. [3]. Initially suggested by Friberg and Eller in 1988 [4], this procedure requires inverted positioning of the patient after placement of the gas bubble. Chang et al. [3] demonstrated that positioning of the patient for 8 h was sufficient for retinal reattachment, suggesting that long-acting gas bubbles (and prolonged positioning up to 16–21 h a day for 1–3 weeks after the surgery) may not be necessary for successful RRD repair by PR.

Surgical Technique

Retrobulbar anesthesia is commonly used. The IOP is reduced by topical iopidine (1% drop administered 30 min before). The eye is prepared with several drops of povidone-iodine. An eyelid speculum is placed in the eye. Some gas (100%) is bled, and then drawn up into a tuberculin syringe through a 22-nm Millipore filter by allowing the pressure of the gas to push the plunger of the syringe back. The correct technique for air or gas preparation follows 4 steps: (1) draw through Millipore filter; (2) flush line with gas; (3) draw pure (100%) gas into tuberculin syringe; (4) connect 30-gauge needle.

Gas is ejected from the syringe until the exact volume of the gas to be injected into the vitreous is left in the syringe: 0.5–0.6 ml SF6, 0.3–0.4 ml C3F8 or C2F6.

If a large break exists, the injection should not be done over the retinal break in order to avoid air bubbles entering the subretinal space. To avoid multiple air bubbles, the injection site should be uppermost in the globe and the needle perpendicular to the floor. A limbal paracentesis of approximately 0.2–0.4 ml of aqueous is performed.

Where to inject? The needle is placed into the vitreous cavity in temporal pars plana 3/3.5 mm (in aphakic or pseudophakic eyes) to 4 mm (phakic eyes) posterior to the limbus and is visualized in the pupil. The needle is withdrawn until 2–3 mm remains in the vitreous. Avoid the crystalline lens and the retina. Rotate head/eye so that at the highest point gas is injected smoothly to produce a single gas bubble in the vitreous gel rather than multiple small bubbles or fish eggs (fig. 2, 3). Perform a brisk, steady injection by adding gas into the bubble. The patient's head is turned to allow the bubble to move away from the injection site, the needle is withdrawn completely and a cotton-tipped applicator is applied over the site to prevent release of fluid or gas.

How much gas to inject? Remember the gas basics: the amount of 0.3 ml of gas has an arc of contact of 90°, 1.0 ml of 120°, 3.0 ml of 180°. The gas expansion is shown in table 1.

At the end of the procedure, first check the central retinal artery, then check the IOP: if the IOP is very high or the central retinal artery is not patent, be prepared to perform a paracentesis by aspirating 1–2 ml (or by passive flow) with a tuberculin syringe 27/30 gauge needle. Try to

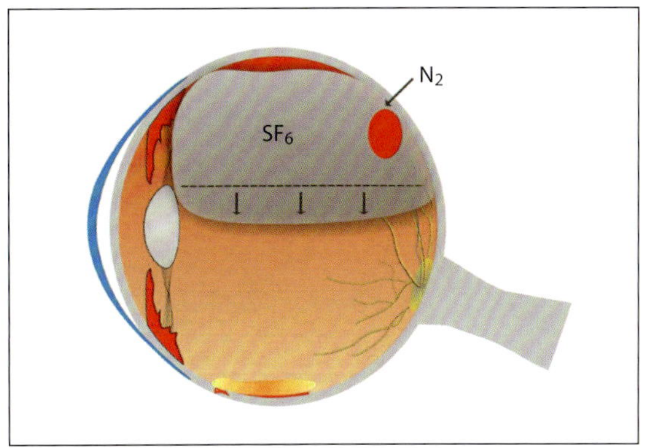

Fig. 1. An intravitreous bubble of an inert gas can be used to seal a retinal break.

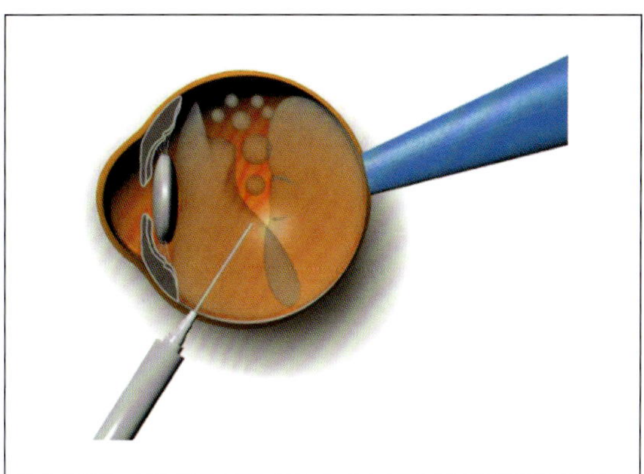

Fig. 3. Multiple small bubbles or fish eggs.

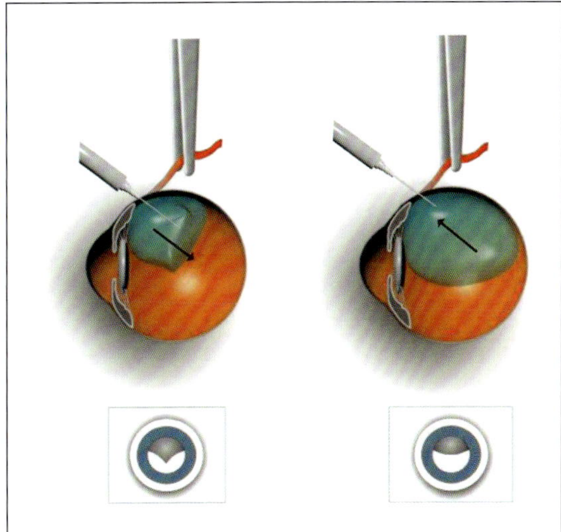

Fig. 2. Rotate the head/eye, so that at the highest point gas is injected smoothly to produce a single gas bubble in the vitreous gel.

Table 1. Gas basics

Expansion	Days	Concentration, %	Amount, ml
Air 0	1	100	0.5–1.0
SF$_6$ 2.0–2.5×	2.5	18	0.5
C$_3$F$_8$ 4×	4	14	0.3

retina, steam roller maneuver is indicated. The technique is as follows. After gas injection, place the patient in the prone position, then rotate slowly the head in 10 min so that the bubble rolls toward the biggest and more elevated tear. Be careful because if the tear is small the maneuver may be ineffective (fig. 4).

If the retina is adherent, cryopexy is immediately performed, if not photocoagulation is applied after 24 h. The retinal breaks must be completely surrounded with cryotherapy spots.

achieve a small wound to avoid the lens and to mark the pathway.

If retinal detachment is too bullous and CRA pulsation cannot be visualized, if there is a risk of macular shift of retinal fluid or a risk that subretinal fluid migrates under inferior tears on flat

Postoperative Care

The patient is positioned so that the bubble adequately covers the open break, and the position is explained to the patient and to his relatives. Air

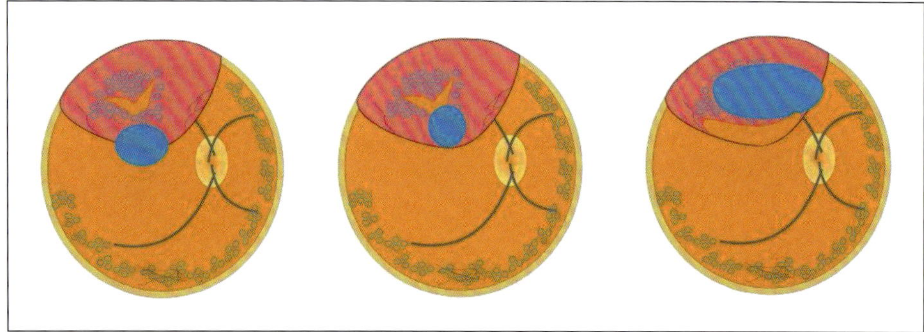

Fig. 4. After gas injection, place the patient in the prone position, then rotate slowly the head in 10 min, so that the bubble rolls toward the biggest and more elevated tear.

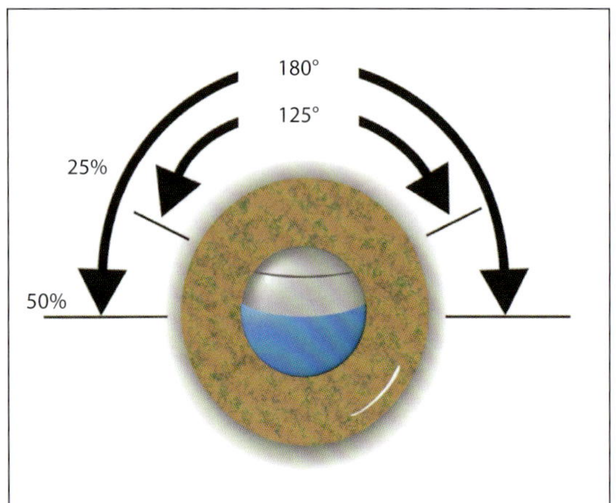

Fig. 5. The bubble has to adequately cover the open break; 0.25 ml covers 90° at the equator, 2.50 ml covers 180° at the equator.

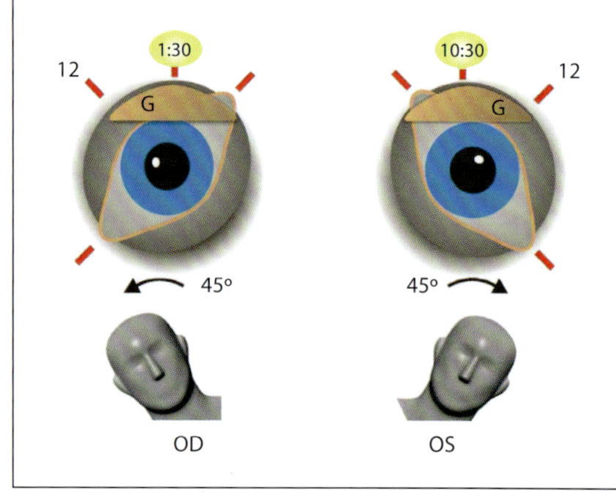

Fig. 6. The position is explained to the patient and to his relatives.

travel must be avoided. Continue topical antibiotic for 3 or 4 days, keep the position for 5–7 days (fig. 5, 6).

Tricks

Tornambe [5] suggests that especially for pseudophakic eyes, 360 retinopexy between the insertion of the vitreous base and ora will improve the success rate by 5–10%. He also recommends using the shortest acting gas bubble which gets the job done (therefore C3F8 should be reserved for large eyes, with large and/or posterior breaks, about 5% of cases).

Conclusions

Success with PR, as with other surgical procedures, depends on proper case selection and surgical technique. Ideal case selection and peripheral 360° retinopexy can increase the success rate to 97%. Even with reoperations, PR is more cost-effective than SB [5].

References

1 Sodhi A, Leung SH, Do DV, et al: Recent trends in the management of rhegmatogenous retinal detachment. Surv Ophthalmol 2008;53:50–67.

2 Eter N, Böker T, Spitznas M: Long-term results of pneumatic retinopexy. Graefes Arch Clin Exp Ophthalmol 2000;238: 677–681.

3 Chang TS, Pelzek CD, Nguyen RL, et al: Inverted pneumatic retinopexy: a method of treating retinal detachments associated with inferior retinal breaks. Ophthalmology 2003;110:589–594.

4 Friberg TR, Eller AW: Pneumatic repair of primary and secondary retinal detachments using a binocular indirect ophthalmoscope laser delivery system. Ophthalmology 1988;95:187–193.

5 Tornambe PE: Pneumatic retinopexy: the evolution of case selection and surgical technique. A twelve-year study of 302 eyes. Trans Am Ophthalmol Soc 1997; 95:551–578.

Stanislao Rizzo, MD
Ospedale Cisanello, Via Paradisa, Edificio 30A
Azienda Ospedaliera Universitaria Pisana
IT–56100 Pisa (Italy)
Tel. +39 3357076057, E-Mail stanislao.rizzo@gmail.com

Bandello F, Battaglia Parodi M (eds): Surgical Retina.
ESASO Course Series. Basel, Karger, 2012, vol 2, pp 132–135

Retinal Detachment by Giant Tear or Dialysis

Elad Moisseiev · Anat Loewenstein

Department of Ophthalmology, Tel Aviv Medical Center, Sackler Faculty of Medicine, Tel Aviv University, Tel Aviv, Israel

Abstract

This chapter deals with retinal detachments secondary to giant retinal tears or dialyses. The etiology, epidemiology and pathogenesis are thoroughly reviewed. Management options are discussed, with an emphasis on surgical techniques and considerations.

Retinal Dialysis

Definition

A retinal dialysis is a tear of the retina from its insertion at the ora serrata [1]. It consists of circumferential, linear breaks that occur along the anterior and posterior vitreous base [2]. Retinal dialyses are most commonly seen in the inferotemporal quadrant. The majority of retinal dialyses are secondary to blunt ocular trauma, but may also be idiopathic. Idiopathic cases tend to be bilateral [1].

It has been estimated that about 4.4% of retinal detachments are secondary to dialyses [3]. They occur in younger patients (mean age of 30 years), and with a slight male preponderance [1].

Natural History

There is often a long time delay between the creation of a retinal dialysis and the development of a symptomatic retinal detachment [1]. This time delay may extend for years, but most cases occur within 2 years [4]. This means that previous blunt ocular trauma should be suspected as a cause even in patients who deny it.

Usually, the vitreous is not liquefied and remains attached to the retina. This causes the slow progression of the detachment, which typically becomes symptomatic only when the macula is involved [1].

Management

Patients who have retinal dialysis with signs of chronicity, such as tidemarks and retinal cysts, are usually stable and have a low risk of progression [1]. However, most cases are usually treated by laser demarcation or surgically [2, 5].

Limited detachments may be demarcated by laser to prevent their progression. As most dialyses are inferotemporal, this results in a superonasal visual field defect, which is usually well tolerated by these patients [1].

The surgical procedure of choice for the treatment of retinal detachment secondary to dialysis is segmental sclera buckling. Reported success rates of this form of treatment are very high, ranging from 94 to 100% [3, 6–8].

Giant Retinal Tear

Definition
A giant retinal tear (GRT) extends circumferentially for 90° (3 clock hours) or more [2]. It usually occurs at the posterior edge of the vitreous base, and may also include a radial component. The incidence of GRTs is estimated to be 0.05 per 100,000 of the general population per year, and it accounts for about 0.5% of rhegmatogenous retinal detachments [9].

Etiology
The most common type of GRTs is idiopathic, which constitutes 70% of cases. They are associated with high myopia and have a male preponderance [10]. It has been postulated that myopic expansion of the globe or traction at the vitreous base initiate the creation of a GRT.

GRTs are associated with trauma, intraocular surgery, acute retinal necrosis, large areas of chorioretinal scarring or lattice degeneration, lenticular colobomas and hereditary conditions such as retinitis pigmentosa, Marfan's syndrome and Stickler's syndrome [9, 10].

Pathogenesis
Vitreous syneresis and liquefaction occur early in cases of GRT [9]. Circumferential vitreoretinal traction at the vitreous base can lead to the formation of a retinal ridge and significant tension on the retina. Tangential traction caused by myopic or traumatic globe expansion causes the retina to tear along the posterior edge of the vitreous base. The vitreous base pulls away the anterior retinal flap and the free posterior flap fold over. In GRT secondary to trauma, the posterior vitreous may not be liquefied and can prevent the posterior retinal flap from slipping back.

GRTs may also result from coalescence of multiple retinal tears at the vitreous base.

Proliferative vitreoretinopathy (PVR) develops in about 50–78% of GRT patients [9–11]. The high incidence of PVR is attributed to the large area of exposed retinal pigment epithelium (RPE) and the release of a high number of RPE cells into the vitreous [9, 11]. Vitreous hemorrhage and increased cytokine production may also contribute to PVR formation [9]. PVR causes the posterior edge of GRTs to contract and stiffen, which complicates their treatment.

Clinical Presentation
GRTs may present with floaters and flashes, similar to other cases of rhegmatogenous retinal detachment. Visual acuity may be as good as 20/20 until the macula is involved.

Some cases present as a large floater that intermittently blurs the vision. This symptom may result from a mobile retinal flap or bellowing of the detached retina.

Inferior GRTs may be asymptomatic or cause blurred vision.

Fellow Eyes
Fellow eyes in patients with GRT have an increased risk of developing a GRT. Bilateral GRTs occur in 12.8–16.5% of cases, but the incidence may rise to 90% in cases with predisposing factors such as large areas of lattice degeneration or Stickler's syndrome. Fellow eyes are also at risk for non-GRT retinal detachment, which may occur in up to 36% of them [9].

Management
Careful preoperative examination is helpful in planning the surgical approach to each case. It is important to know the size, location and morphology of the GRT, as well as the extent of the retinal detachment and whether additional tears are present. It is also important to be aware of the nature of vitreous traction, the presence of vitreous hemorrhage and PVR. The lens status should also be taken into consideration [11]. Patients should not be subjected to extensive manipulation or physical activity prior to surgery, as that may cause extension of the GRT.

Scleral buckling may be useful for GRTs smaller than 2 quadrants in circumference. The goal of the buckle is to reduce circumferential and tangential traction on the GRT. It is not placed at the posterior border of the tear but along the vitreous base, which it is supposed to support [11]. In cases with mild retinal folding, intravitreal injection of expanding C3F8 gas may be used.

The placement of the buckle is critical. It is recommended to place a broad, low scleral buckle, which prevents fish-mouthing by extending support well posterior to the posterior flap. The buckle should extend 360° to ensure that the entire circumference of the vitreous base is supported. New tears often develop in unsupported parts of the retina. Creating strong chorioretinal adhesions anteriorly toward the ora serrata and beyond both ends of the tear prevents posterior seepage of fluid. This is usually achieved by cryopexy. Subretinal fluid (SRF) should be drained posteriorly to the posterior flap, where it accumulates the most.

Cases of GRT complicated by PVR, posterior slippage of the retinal flap, cataract, vitreous hemorrhage or a radial component are usually managed by pars plana vitrectomy. Panoramic viewing systems and perfluorocarbon (PFC) liquids have facilitated this surgical procedure [11]. A sclera buckle should be placed prior to pars plana vitrectomy, if the final posterior flap position can be accurately estimated before reattachment. This also enables better control of the buckle contour and the intraocular pressure. In cases of folded over flaps or 180° or greater breaks, the lens should be removed in order to facilitate removal of anterior vitreous cortex and anterior PVR. Anterior vitrectomy should precede the lensectomy. Endocapsular lensectomy is performed by a 20-gauge fragmenter, or by the vitrectome in soft lenses.

It is important to perform meticulous vitrectomy over the vitreous base in order to release all anterior traction, especially in cases with PVR. Prudent use of low suction force and high cutting rate is advocated to avoid more traction on the tear and damaging the retina. In cases where release of the anterior flap is not possible, the vitreous and anterior retinal flap can be excised together. Peeling of epiretinal membranes is necessary to enable retinal flattening and reattachment. In cases with advanced anterior PVR, circumferential relaxing retinotomy may be required.

In smaller GRTs with little retinal folding, it is possible to drain SRF and attach the retina by fluid-air exchange. PFC liquids are very useful in cases with extensive GRTs and PVR [11] as they stabilize the retina and aid in peeling of residual membranes and reattachment of the retina. The PFC liquids are denser than the infusion fluid and the retina. They migrate to the lower part of the eye and cause the retina to roll back into its original position. The PFC is injected on the anterior side of the retina near the optic nerve with a 25- or 27-gauge cannula, and the BSS is allowed to leak around it.

After retinal reattachment, continuous laser endophotocoagulation is along the posterior and anterior flaps to prevent seepage of fluid from the edges of the GRT [11]. It is possible to perform circumferential cryopexy as well, but it is thought to cause more PVR and retinal slippage [12]. Since PFC cannot remain in the eye, it is removed. Postoperative tamponade may be achieved by C3F8 gas or silicone oil [10, 11]. Silicone oil may be directly exchanged with PFC, and enables earlier visual rehabilitation [13]. C3F8 gas is associated with less postoperative PVR, but has several significant disadvantages such as short-term efficacy due to its absorption, limited view of the retina and inability to travel by air. Silicone oil is preferred in cases that require internal tamponade for over one month and in recurrent retinal detachments.

Prognosis

Anatomical retinal reattachment is achieved in 56–95% of cases of GRT [11]. Visual recovery occurs in 80–90% of cases. Factors associated with poorer prognosis include young age, high myopia,

PVR, large GRT, an elevated anterior flap, residual SRF, Marfan's syndrome and Stickler's syndrome.

Complications

The leading complication after surgery for GRT repair is PVR, which leads to recurrent retinal detachment. Postoperative hypotony may be associated with choroidal detachment or hemorrhage. Additional complications include slippage of the posterior edge of the GRT flap and accumulation of SRF.

Management of Fellow Eye

Although no prospective randomized controlled trial on prophylactic treatment of fellow eyes of patients with GRT has been performed, a review of the literature concluded it is an effective and safe option [9]. Most clinicians perform 360° prophylactic laser photocoagulation or cryotherapy in fellow eyes. Previous studies have shown that prophylactic treatment reduces that risk of GRT in fellow eyes to 2.1%, and that of non-GRT retinal detachment to 16.7%. No procedure has been proven more effective than the other [9]. It is especially prudent to offer prophylactic treatment in fellow eyes with predisposing factors, and some clinicians recommend prophylactic encircling sclera buckling in such eyes.

References

1 Aylward GW: Optimal procedures for retinal detachments; in Ryan SJ, Schachat AP, Wilkinson P, Hinton DR (eds): Retina, ed 4. St Louis, Mosby, 2004.

2 Peripheral retinal abnormalities; in Retina and Vitreous. American Academy of Ophthalmology Basic and Clinical Science Course. San Francisco, American Academy of Ophthalmology.

3 Kennedy CJ, Parker CE, McAllister IL: Retinal detachment caused by retinal dialysis. Aust NZ J Ophthalmol 1997;25:25–30.

4 Cox MS, Schepens CL, Freeman HM: Retinal detachment due to ocular contusion. Arch Ophthalmol 1966;76:678–685.

5 Preferred Practice Patterns Committee, Retina Panel: Management of Posterior Vitreous Detachment, Retinal Breaks and Lattice Degeneration. San Francisco, American Academy of Ophthalmology, 1998, p 13.

6 Bonnet M, Moyenin P, Pecoldowa C, et al: Retinal detachment caused by a tear at the ora serrata. J Fr Ophthalmol 1986;9:231–242.

7 Ross WH: Traumatic retinal dialyses. Arch Ophthalmol 1981;99:1371–1374.

8 Johnston PB: Traumatic retinal detachment. Br J Ophthalmol 1991;75:18–21.

9 Ang GS, Townend J, Lois N: Interventions for prevention of giant retinal tear in the fellow eye. Cochrane Database Syst Rev 2009;CD006909.

10 Ghosh YK, Banerjee S, Savant V, et al: Surgical treatment and outcome of patients with giant retinal tears. Eye 2004;18:996–1000.

11 Chang S, Lopez JM: Giant retinal tears with proliferative vitreoretinopathy; in Ryan SJ, Schachat AP, Wilkinson P, Hinton DR (eds): Retina, ed 4. St Louis, Mosby, 2004.

12 Campochiaro PA, Kaden IH, Vidaurri-Leal J, et al: Cryotherapy enhances intravitreal dispersion of viable retinal pigment epithelial cells. Arch Ophthalmol 1985;103:434–436.

13 Kertes PJ, Wafapoor H, Peyman GA, et al: The management of giant retinal tears using perfluoroperhydrophenanthrene. Ophthalmology 2001;108:1179–1183.

Elad Moisseiev, MD
Department of Ophthalmology, Tel Aviv Sourasky Medical Center
Weitzman 6 St.
Tel Aviv, 64239 (Israel)
Tel. +972 3 6973408, E-Mail elad_moi@netvision.net.il

Bandello F, Battaglia Parodi M (eds): Surgical Retina.
ESASO Course Series. Basel, Karger, 2012, vol 2, pp 136–145

Macular Hole Surgery

Jose Garcia-Arumi · Carme Macia Badia

Hospital Vall Hebrón, Barcelona, Spain

Abstract

Idiopathic macular hole is a relatively frequent condition which can be effectively managed with surgery in most of the cases. This review describes pathogenesis, clinical aspects, and therapeutic perspectives of macular hole.

Idiopathic full-thickness macular hole (MH) is a relatively frequent retinal condition and a known cause of poor central visual acuity in patients older than 50 years. MHs occur most commonly in the seventh decade of life, although patients can present at a younger age. There is a predominance in women, with a reported incidence of 67–91% [1]. A theory attributing vitreous traction in the pathogenesis of MH was proposed by Gass [2]. Observations in subjects before formation of a hole have shown a shallow elevation of the central fovea [2, 3]. Tangential traction of the posterior hyaloid face has been hypothesized as the cause of impending MH. Continued traction can lead to the development of a full-thickness hole, although spontaneous resolution may occur in some cases [2]. Treatment can result in a satisfactory anatomic and visual outcome [4, 5]. Vitrectomy has become one of the most common procedures for this condition in many vitreoretinal departments. The development of new surgical techniques such as internal limiting membrane (ILM) peeling and the use of various stains have generated considerable interest in recent years [6–12].

Histopathology

MH formation typically evolves over a period of weeks to months through a series of stages that were first described by Gass [13, 14]. In his classification, stage 1A and 1B lesions represent impending MHs with foveolar and foveal detachment, respectively. Approximately 60% of eyes undergo spontaneous vitreofoveal separation with relief of the retinal traction and show no further progression. Recent ocular coherence tomography (OCT) data suggest that perifoveal posterior hyaloid separation with persistent adherence of the posterior hyaloid to the foveal center is the first event in MH formation [15–18]. This results in an intraretinal split that progresses into intraretinal cystic changes corresponding to the clinical features of stage 1 MH. In stage 2, there is a small retinal defect (hole) inside the yellow ring. OCT demonstrates stage 2 to be a complete, full-thickness retinal defect. Stage 3 is characterized by a larger (>400 μm) hole with a rim of elevated retina and complete separation of the posterior hyaloid from the macula. An operculum on the posterior hyaloid may or may not be clinically apparent, but is usually seen on OCT. In 20–40% of eyes, vitreous detachment with complete separation of the vitreous from the macular retina and optic nerve occurs, and the hole is classified as stage 4 [19].

Vision in patients with stage 1 and stage 2 MH is typically between 20/25 and 20/80. In eyes with stage 3 and stage 4 holes, vision is usually 20/100 to 20/400. The vision in stage 3 and stage 4 eyes rarely improves spontaneously.

Indications for Treatment

Most retina specialists agree that symptomatic patients with MH who have reduced visual acuity and metamorphopsia are likely to obtain some degree of visual improvement after surgery. Surgery is contemplated in most eyes with moderate to large stage 3 or 4 holes that cause symptoms and reduced visual acuity in the range of 20/60 to 20/400. Surgical treatment may also be indicated in small, but definite, full-thickness stage 2 or 3 MHs causing symptoms in a patient with visual acuity in the range of 20/40 to 20/60. MH formation is aborted in 60% of stage 1 lesions, and posterior vitreous detachment is generally believed to confer protection from progression of MH. Eyes with the poorest preoperative acuity experience the greatest improvement following surgery. Eyes with MHs and visual acuity of less than 20/400 should alert the clinician to possible coexisting ocular conditions that may contribute to vision loss and prevent postoperative visual improvement (fig. 1a–f) [1].

Differential Diagnosis and Diagnostic Testing

Clinically, full-thickness MH can be confused with pseudo-cyst, pseudo-holes, and lamellar holes. OCT can differentiate and help to confirm the relationships between these conditions. By improving our understanding of the role of vitreoretinal adhesions in the pathogenesis of these entities, OCT has become invaluable in the pre- and postoperative management of affected patients [20].

Advances in retinal imaging have helped to demonstrate possible causes of delayed or incomplete visual recovery after anatomically successful surgical repair. Several studies have reported a possible association between the integrity of the photoreceptor inner and outer segment (IS/OS) junction and postoperative visual acuity after successful MH repair [21–23]. The structural integrity of the IS/OS line may simply enhance the status of the photoreceptor OS at the time of examination, but not fully reflect the photoreceptor cell survival, which seems to be more critical for predicting postoperative visual prognosis. Wakabayashi et al. [24] suggested that early postoperative reconstruction of the external limiting membrane (ELM) line is important for morphologic and functional recovery of the foveal photoreceptor layer in surgically closed MHs. Whether the initial closure of the hole (foveal defect) is achieved by the bridging of the ELM or by proliferating glial cells seems to be crucial for early visual recovery in patients after MH repair. In closed MHs, the pattern of foveal reconstruction may depend on a balance between the proliferating glial cells filling the foveal defect and the centripetal bridging of the ELM with subsequent reapproximation of the normal photoreceptors to the central fovea. Because there are currently no surgical techniques that can ensure perfect restoration of the photoreceptor IS/OS and ELM in surgically closed MHs, the current SD-OCT findings only provide a better understanding of the foveal microstructural changes and a possible reason for the differences in visual recovery after successful MH repair (fig. 1g–j) [24, 25].

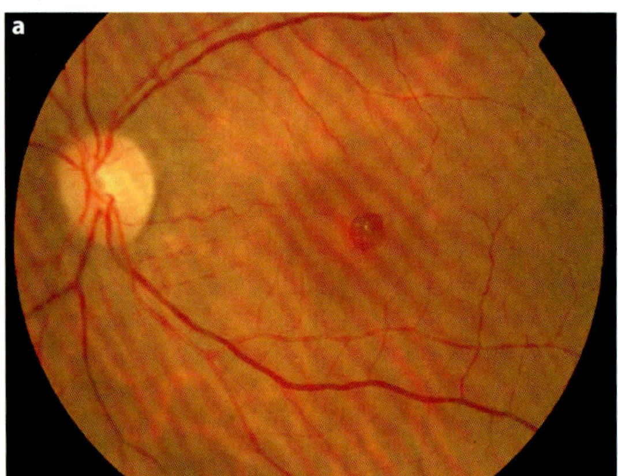

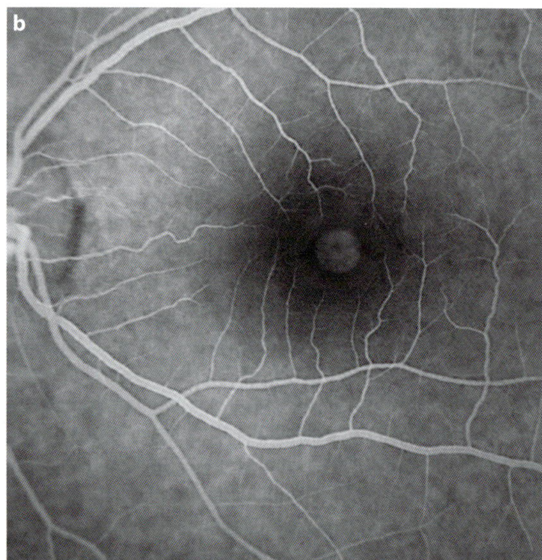

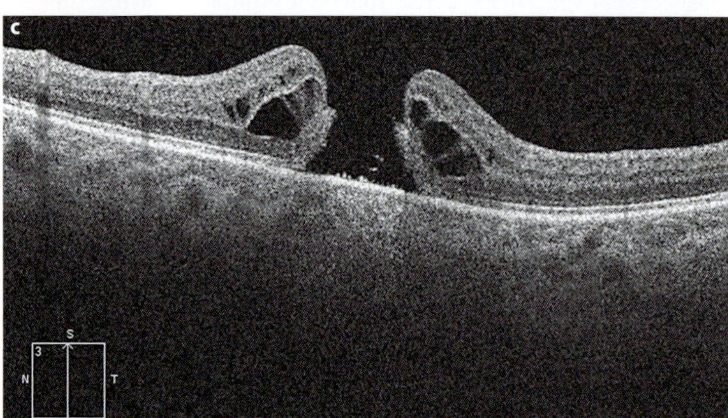

Fig. 1. a, b Fundus photograph before surgery. Stage 4 MH with a surrounding macular detachment. The VA is 20/200 in the left eye. **c** SD-OCT showing stage 4 MH. **d** Color fundus photograph obtained 2 months after the operation. **e, f** An SD-OCT image obtained 2 months after successful MH repair. Despite a focal disruption of the photoreceptor IS/OS line, the foveal ELM line is well reconstructed. The visual acuity is 20/60. Eyes with reconstruction of the ELM have a higher chance of achieving concomitant or subsequent restoration of a normal IS/OS.

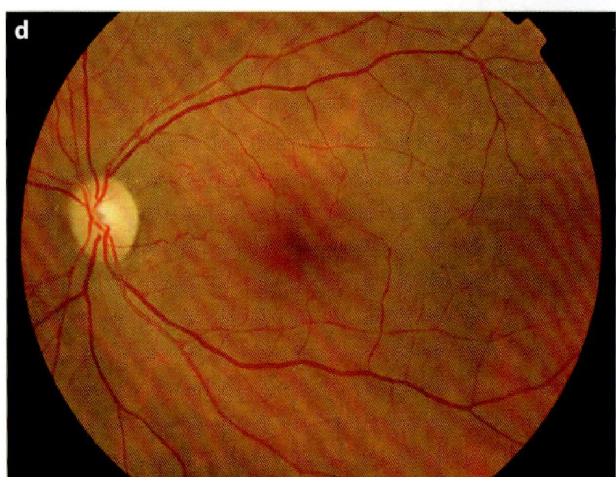

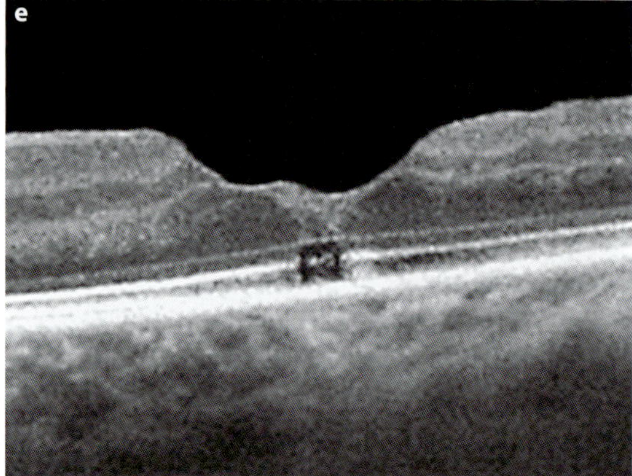

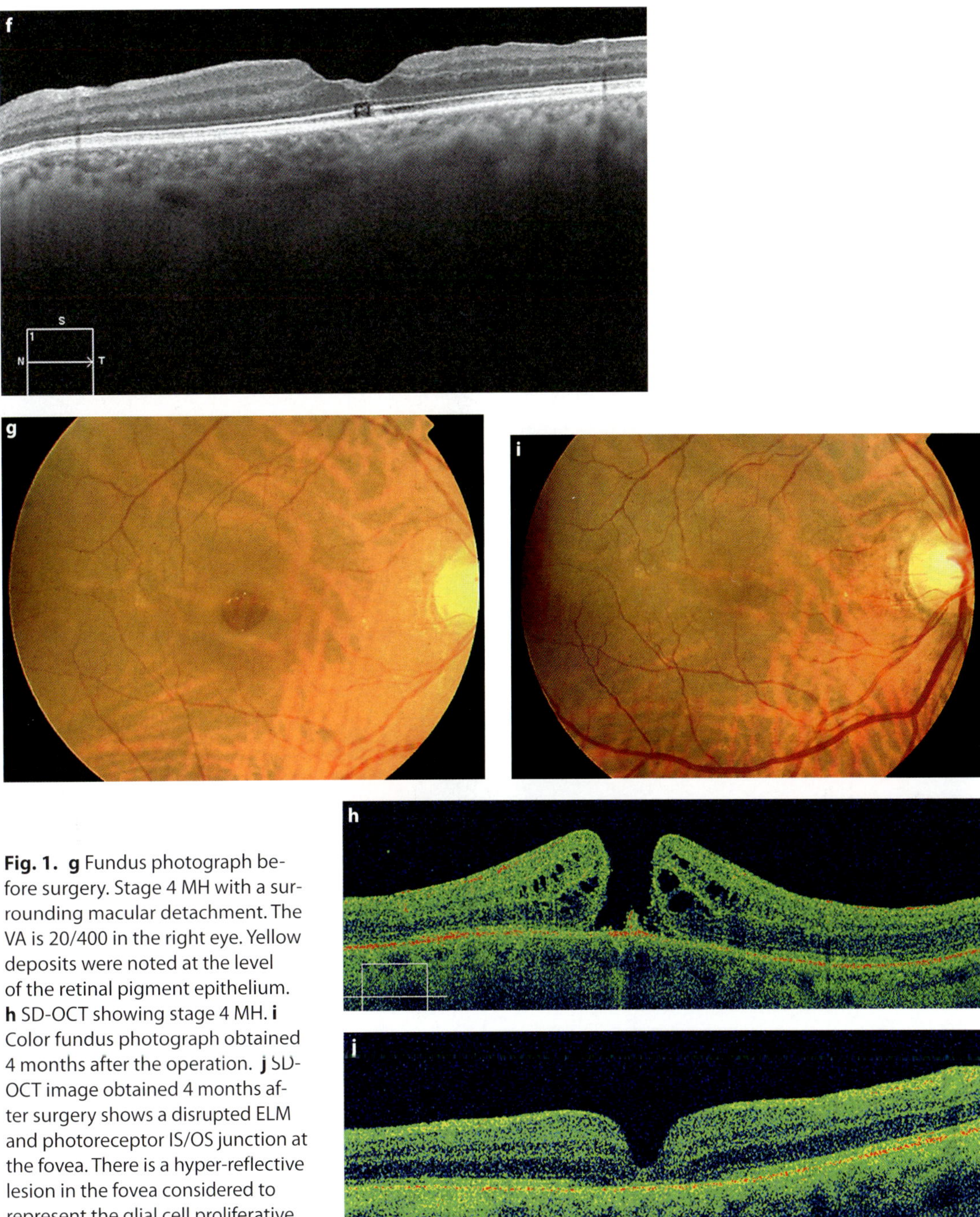

Fig. 1. g Fundus photograph before surgery. Stage 4 MH with a surrounding macular detachment. The VA is 20/400 in the right eye. Yellow deposits were noted at the level of the retinal pigment epithelium. **h** SD-OCT showing stage 4 MH. **i** Color fundus photograph obtained 4 months after the operation. **j** SD-OCT image obtained 4 months after surgery shows a disrupted ELM and photoreceptor IS/OS junction at the fovea. There is a hyper-reflective lesion in the fovea considered to represent the glial cell proliferative events at the foveal defect. The foveal hyper-reflective lesion replaces all intraretinal layers. The VA is 20/40.

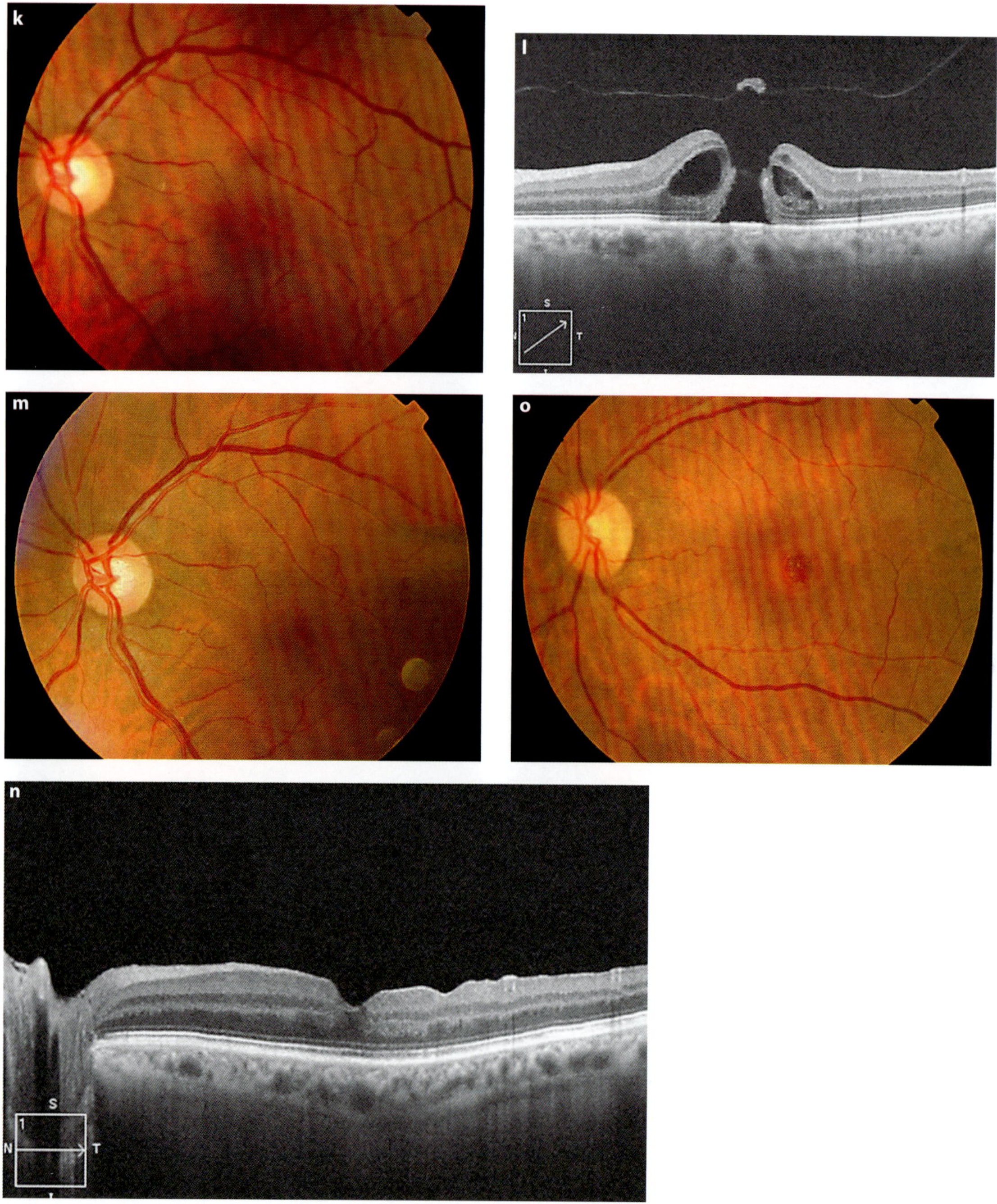

Fig. 1. **k** Preoperatively, there is submacular fluid and elevation of the edges of the MH. **l** An SD-OCT image obtained before surgery shows a stage 3 MH. **m** Postoperative appearance after pars plana vitrectomy and intraocular gas tamponade. Postoperatively, the lesion is flat and the borders of the lesion are imperceptible. **n** The patterns of the photoreceptor IS/OS junction and ELM at the fovea obtained by SD-OCT after MH repair. The restoration of both the ELM and the photoreceptor IS/OS junction 3 weeks after MH repair. The VA is 20/20 in the left eye. **o** Fundus photograph before surgery. Stage 4 MH with a surrounding macular detachment. Yellow deposits were noted at the level of the retinal pigment epithelium.

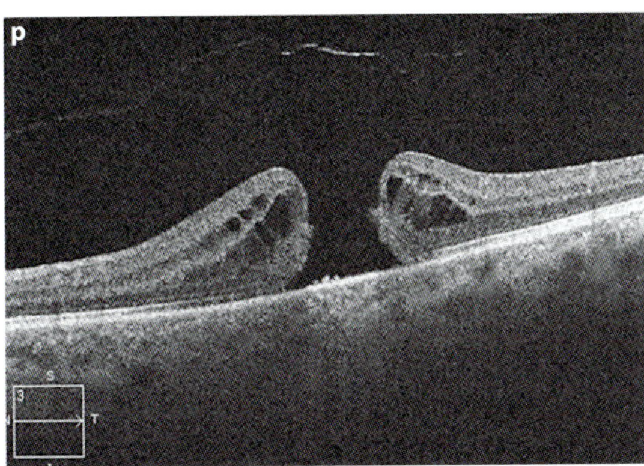
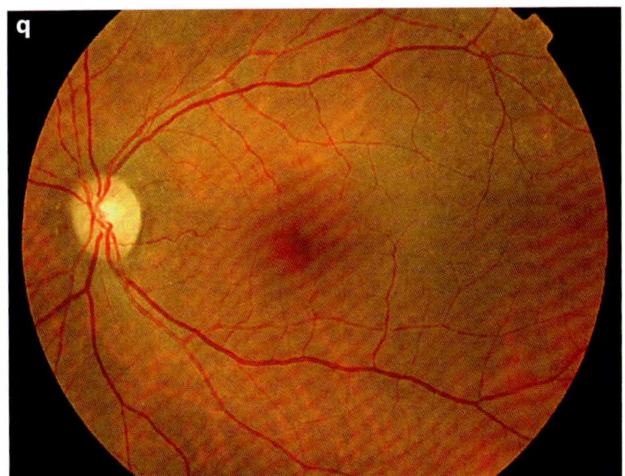
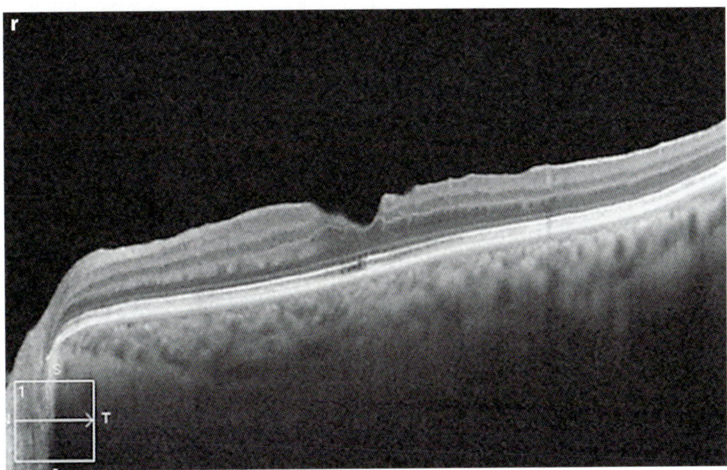

Fig. 1. p An SD-OCT image obtained before surgery shows a full-thickness stage 4 MH. **q** Color fundus photograph obtained 3 weeks after the operation. **r** The patterns of the photoreceptor IS/OS junction and ELM at the fovea obtained by SD-OCT after MH repair. The restoration of both the ELM and the photoreceptor IS/OS junction 3 weeks after MH repair. The VA is 20/25 in the left eye.

Management of Macular Hole Lesions

In 1991, Kelly and Wendel [26] reported on vitrectomy, removal of cortical vitreous and epiretinal membranes, and strict face-down gas tamponade to stabilize or improve vision in full-thickness age-related MHs. Their hypothesis was that by removing tangential vitreous and membrane forces, they could flatten the MH and possibly reduce the adjacent cystic retinal changes and neurosensory macular detachment. The overall results of their initial report were a 58% anatomic success rate and visual improvement of two or more lines in 42% of eyes (73% of anatomically successful eyes) [1].

Nowadays, the most commonly indicated procedure is a standard three-port vitrectomy with 23-G/25-G sutureless surgery. A critical surgical step is the induction of a posterior vitreous detachment with an actively aspirated soft-tipped silicone suction cannula, which is swept over the retinal surface near the major retinal vascular arcades and temporal to the macular or adjacent to the optic nerve: engagement of the often invisible cortical vitreous with active suction results in the 'fish strike' sign or bending of the soft silicone cannula. Epiretinal membranes, when clinically significant, may be removed using intraocular picks and forceps, as is performed in macular pucker surgery. Often, the surface of the retina has an abnormal refractile sheen that surrounds the retinal hole, but there is no apparent surface traction as evidenced by retinal striae or retinovascular distortion. This sheen may represent a minimal epiretinal membrane such as the ILM seen in cellophane maculopathy. However, this sheen also may represent the ILM, which is often seen in patients with retinal thickening or retinal vascular disorders [27]. In our experience, removal of the residual cortical vitreous and epimacular membranes seems to provide the greatest chance for anatomic success. Intentional ILM peeling was started in an effort to completely remove all contractile cells from the edge of the MH. Although the ILM has no inherent contractile properties, it does act as a scaffold for contractile tissue to exert tangential traction on the umbo. Subsequently, ultrastructural features of tissue removed during MH surgery showed cells with myofibroblastic differentiation on the ILM [1]. ILM peeling may also help by ensuring complete removal of any epiretinal tissues above the ILM that could cause foveal traction, and by stimulating gliosis [28].

ILM peeling has given the best anatomic and visual results in the literature to date for recent and chronic MHs, and reopened and failed MHs, and was statistically superior to eyes without ILM peeling [12]. Visual function of the successful eyes without ILM peeling was equivalent to eyes with ILM peeling. ILM peeling should be performed in all MHs greater than 300 μm in size, including reopened and/or primarily failed MHs. Recently, reports of more than 90%

primary closure have appeared in the literature, and ILM removal was considered the most important variable [29, 30]. There is a higher failure and/or reopening rate in eyes without ILM peeling compared with eyes with ILM peeling [12].

The peripheral retina is inspected carefully for iatrogenic retinal tears, which are often not associated with sclerotomy sites and are likely related to the process of vitreous separation [31]. Total air-fluid gas exchange is performed to desiccate the vitreous cavity, and accumulated posterior retinal fluid is followed by a non-expansible concentration of long-acting gas. Strict face-down positioning to position the gas bubble against the MH for at least 24 h and as long as 3 or 4 weeks is as important as the technical components of the procedure.

In an effort to increase the anatomic and visual success rates of MH surgery, several surgical adjunctive agents have been used with varying degrees of reported success. Autologous blood products [32–35], such as platelets, serum [32] and plasma, and commercial thrombin, and other biologic modifiers have been used, although their role in MH surgery remains investigational at present. Future studies will most probably evaluate the safety and efficacy of these and other agents more thoroughly (fig. 1k–n).

Surgical Results

Surgery for primary MHs is successful in closing the hole in about 69–94% of eyes, according to several relatively large published series [36–39]. Late reopening of the hole after initial successful closure occurred in 4.8% of eyes in two reports [40, 41] and 6.9% of eyes in a third report [42]. Prior studies have demonstrated that repeat surgery can close recurrent MHs and improve visual acuity in most eyes with one recurrence. Patients with multiple recurrent MHs need to be advised whether to consider a third operation to try to close an MH that has failed two prior surgeries [43]. Eyes in which one of the prior surgeries temporarily closed the MH have a much better prognosis for MH closure and improvement in visual acuity. Successful closure of the MH with a third MH surgery does improve the visual acuity. Patients with multiple recurrent MHs and prior successful closure of the MH should be encouraged to consider additional surgery on the basis of the patients' symptoms and visual needs [43]. OCT demonstrates closure of the hole as soon as 24 h postoperatively (fig. 1o–r) [44].

Complications

The immediate complication for the surgical patient is the strict, 1-week, face-down positioning requested by most surgeons [45]. Potential surgical candidates also need to be informed about possible surgical complications, including the high rate of subsequent nuclear cataract progression (up to 81% after 2 years) [46]; at least 25% of patients will require postoperative cataract surgery [26]. Simultaneous cataract and MH surgery is an option. Other surgical complications of intraocular surgery for MH have been reported, including retinal tears (3%), rhegmatogenous retinal detachment (14%), enlargement of the hole (2%), late reopening (2–7%) [47], photic toxicity or retinal pigment epithelial alterations (1%) [47], exudative retinal detachment, glaucoma, and proliferative vitreoretinopathy [1].

Secondary Macular Holes

Ocular trauma accounts for up to 9% of eyes that develop full-thickness MH [48]. Although the initiating factors of traumatic holes are quite different from idiopathic MHs, the results of vitrectomy surgery indicate that the prognosis is good [2]. If we combine previous reports of traumatic MHs, successful closure of the hole after one vitrectomy surgery occurred in 83% of cases [48–52].

Secondary MH can occur in eyes with high myopia, and the characteristics and demographics of these MH differ from most idiopathic holes. These MH tend to develop in younger subjects and may be associated with a rhegmatogenous retinal detachment surrounding the hole [53]. The exact relationship between retinoschisis and MH formation is not known; it has been suggested that retinoschisis develops prior to the MH [54]. MH surgery can provide substantial visual acuity improvement in myopic eyes, but the results do not seem to be as favorable as those reported for typical idiopathic MH in recent series. The one-operation success of MH surgery in myopes seems to be lower than that of typical idiopathic MH. The visual results with one or more surgeries are good, with similar mean final visual acuity and improvement of three or more Snellen lines compared with series of idiopathic MH [55]. We believe that MH surgery should be considered in subjects who have myopic MH [56, 57].

MH can also develop after retinal detachment repair. In our experience, this occurs most commonly after macula-off repair with vitrectomy procedures. Surgical treatment is effective in achieving anatomic closure and good visual outcome. The prior macular-off retinal detachment and macular edema probably limit the functional outcome.

References

1 Ho AC, Guyer DR, Fine SL: Macular hole. Surv Ophthalmol 1998;42:393–416.
2 Gass JD: Idiopathic senile macular hole. Its early stages and pathogenesis. Arch Ophthalmol 1988;106:629–639.
3 Johnson RN, Gass JD: Idiopathic macular holes. Observations, stages of formation, and implications for surgical intervention. Ophthalmology 1988;95: 917–924.
4 Ezra E, Gregor ZJ: Surgery for idiopathic full-thickness macular hole: two-year results of a randomized clinical trial comparing natural history, vitrectomy, and vitrectomy plus autologous serum: Morfields Macular Hole Study Group Report No. 1. Arch Ophthalmol 2004;122:224–236.
5 la Cour M, Friis J: Macular holes: classification, epidemiology, natural history and treatment. Acta Ophthalmol Scand 2002;80:579–587.
6 Casuso LA, Scott IU, Flynn HW Jr, et al: Long-term follow-up of unoperated macular holes. Ophthalmology 2001;108:1150–1155.
7 Cheung CM, Munshi V, Mughal S, et al: Anatomical success rate of macular hole surgery with autologous platelet without internal-limiting membrane peeling. Eye (Lond) 2005;19:1191–1193.
8 Burk SE, Da Mata AP, Snyder ME, et al: Indocyanine green-assisted peeling of the retinal internal limiting membrane. Ophthalmology 2000;107:2010–2014.
9 Da Mata AP, Riemann CD, Nehemy MB, et al: Indocyanine green-assisted internal limiting membrane peeling for macular holes to stain or not to stain? Retina 2005;25:1119.
10 Ho JD, Tsai RJ, Chen SN, et al: Cytotoxicity of indocyanine green on retinal pigment epithelium: implications for macular hole surgery. Arch Ophthalmol 2003;121:1423–1429.
11 Kimura T, Takahashi M, Takagi H, et al: Is removal of internal limiting membrane always necessary during stage 3 idiopathic macular hole surgery? Retina 2005;25:54–58.
12 Brooks HL Jr: Macular hole surgery with and without internal limiting membrane peeling. Ophthalmology 2000;107:1939–1948, discussion 1948–1949.

13 Gass JD: Macular hole opercula: ultrastructural features and clinicopathologic correlation. Arch Ophthalmol 1998;116:965–966.
14 Gass JD: Reappraisal of biomicroscopic classification of stages of development of a macular hole. Am J Ophthalmol 1995;119:752–759.
15 Hee MR, Puliafito CA, Wong C, et al: Optical coherence tomography of macular holes. Ophthalmology 1995;102:748–756.
16 Gaudric A, Haouchine B, Massin P, et al: Macular hole formation: new data provided by optical coherence tomography. Arch Ophthalmol 1999;117:744–751.
17 Haouchine B, Massin P, Gaudric A: Foveal pseudocyst as the first step in macular hole formation: a prospective study by optical coherence tomography. Ophthalmology 2001;108:15–22.
18 Mori K, Abe T, Yoneya S: Dome-shaped detachment of premacular vitreous cortex in macular hole development. Ophthalmic Surg Lasers 2000;31:203–209.
19 Benson WE, Cruickshanks KC, Fong DS, et al: Surgical management of macular holes: a report by the American Academy of Ophthalmology. Ophthalmology 2001;108:1328–1335.
20 Mirza RG, Johnson MW, Jampol LM: Optical coherence tomography use in evaluation of the vitreoretinal interface: a review. Surv Ophthalmol 2007;52:397–421.
21 Sano M, Shimoda Y, Hashimoto H, et al: Restored photoreceptor outer segment and visual recovery after macular hole closure. Am J Ophthalmol 2009; 147:313–318 e1.
22 Oh J, Smiddy WE, Flynn HW Jr, et al: Photoreceptor inner/outer segment defect imaging by spectral domain OCT and visual prognosis after macular hole surgery. Invest Ophthalmol Vis Sci 2010;51:1651–1658.
23 Inoue M, Watanabe Y, Arakawa A, et al: Spectral-domain optical coherence tomography images of inner/outer segment junctions and macular hole surgery outcomes. Graefes Arch Clin Exp Ophthalmol 2009;247:325–330.
24 Wakabayashi T, Oshima Y: Restoration of ELM reflection line crucial for visual recovery in surgically closed MH. Retina Today 2010;1:48–51.

25 Wakabayashi T, Fujiwara M, Sakaguchi H, et al: Foveal microstructure and visual acuity in surgically closed macular holes: spectral-domain optical coherence tomographic analysis. Ophthalmology 2010;117:1815–1824.
26 Kelly NE, Wendel RT: Vitreous surgery for idiopathic macular holes. Results of a pilot study. Arch Ophthalmol 1991;109:654–659.
27 Sjaarda RN: Macular hole. Int Ophthalmol Clin 1995;35:105–122.
28 Abdelkader E, Lois N: Internal limiting membrane peeling in vitreo-retinal surgery. Surv Ophthalmol 2008;53:368–396.
29 Olsen TW, Sternberg P Jr, Capone A Jr, et al: Macular hole surgery using thrombin-activated fibrinogen and selective removal of the internal limiting membrane. Retina 1998;18:322–329.
30 Park DW, Sipperley JO, Sneed SR, et al: Macular hole surgery with internal-limiting membrane peeling and intravitreous air. Ophthalmology 1999;106:1392–1397, discussion 1397–1398.
31 Sjaarda RN, Glaser BM, Thompson JT, et al: Distribution of iatrogenic retinal breaks in macular hole surgery. Ophthalmology 1995;102:1387–1392.
32 Liggett PE, Skolik DS, Horio B, et al: Human autologous serum for the treatment of full-thickness macular holes. A preliminary study. Ophthalmology 1995;102:1071–1076.
33 Bresgen M, Heimann K: Idiopathic macular foramen: new aspects of staging and possible therapeutic concepts (in German). Klin Monbl Augenheilkd 1995;206:2–12.
34 Gaudric A, Massin P, Paques M, et al: Autologous platelet concentrate for the treatment of full-thickness macular holes. Graefes Arch Clin Exp Ophthalmol 1995;233:549–554.
35 Korobelnik JF, Hannouche D, Belayachi N, et al: Autologous platelet concentrate as an adjunct in macular hole healing: a pilot study. Ophthalmology 1996; 103:590–594.
36 Freeman WR, Azen SP, Kim JW, et al: Vitrectomy for the treatment of full-thickness stage 3 or 4 macular holes. Results of a multicentered randomized clinical trial. The Vitrectomy for Treatment of Macular Hole Study Group. Arch Ophthalmol 1997;115:11–21.

37 Wendel RT, Patel AC, Kelly NE, et al: Vitreous surgery for macular holes. Ophthalmology 1993;100:1671–1676.

38 Thompson JT, Smiddy WE, Williams GA, et al: Comparison of recombinant transforming growth factor-beta-2 and placebo as an adjunctive agent for macular hole surgery. Ophthalmology 1998; 105:700–706.

39 Thompson JT, Glaser BM, Sjaarda RN, et al: Effects of intraocular bubble duration in the treatment of macular holes by vitrectomy and transforming growth factor-beta 2. Ophthalmology 1994; 101:1195–1200.

40 Christmas NJ, Smiddy WE, Flynn HW Jr: Reopening of macular holes after initially successful repair. Ophthalmology 1998;105:1835–1838.

41 Duker JS, Wendel R, Patel A, et al: Late re-opening of macular holes after initially successful treatment with vitreous surgery. Ophthalmology 1994;101:1373–1378.

42 Paques M, Massin P, Santiago PY, et al: Late reopening of successfully treated macular holes. Br J Ophthalmol 1997;81:658–662.

43 Thompson JT, Sjaarda RN: Surgical treatment of macular holes with multiple recurrences. Ophthalmology 2000;107:1073–1077.

44 Kasuga Y, Arai J, Akimoto M, Yoshimura N: Optical coherence tomography to confirm early closure of macular holes. Am J Ophthalmol 2000;130:675–676.

45 Tornambe PE, Poliner LS, Grote K: Macular hole surgery without face-down positioning. A pilot study. Retina 1997;17:179–185.

46 Thompson JT, Glaser BM, Sjaarda RN, et al: Progression of nuclear sclerosis and long-term visual results of vitrectomy with transforming growth factor beta-2 for macular holes. Am J Ophthalmol 1995;119:48–54.

47 Park SS, Marcus DM, Duker JS, et al: Posterior segment complications after vitrectomy for macular hole. Ophthalmology 1995;102:775–781.

48 Rubin JS, Glaser BM, Thompson JT, et al: Vitrectomy, fluid-gas exchange and transforming growth factor-beta-2 for the treatment of traumatic macular holes. Ophthalmology 1995;102:1840–1845.

49 Garcia-Arumi J, Corcostegui B, Cavero L, et al: The role of vitreoretinal surgery in the treatment of posttraumatic macular hole. Retina 1997;17:372–377.

50 Margherio AR, Margherio RR, Hartzer M, et al: Plasmin enzyme-assisted vitrectomy in traumatic pediatric macular holes. Ophthalmology 1998;105:1617–1620.

51 Madreperla SA, Benetz BA: Formation and treatment of a traumatic macular hole. Arch Ophthalmol 1997;115:1210–1211.

52 Chow DR, Williams GA, Trese MT, et al: Successful closure of traumatic macular holes. Retina 1999;19:405–409.

53 Morita H, Ideta H, Ito K, et al: Causative factors of retinal detachment in macular holes. Retina 1991;11:281–284.

54 Tano Y: Pathologic myopia: where are we now? Am J Ophthalmol 2002;134:645–660.

55 Patel SC, Loo RH, Thompson JT, et al: Macular hole surgery in high myopia. Ophthalmology 2001;108:377–380.

56 Sulkes DJ, Smiddy WE, Flynn HW, et al: Outcomes of macular hole surgery in severely myopic eyes: a case-control study. Am J Ophthalmol 2000;130:335–339.

57 Garcia-Arumi J, Martinez V, Puig J, et al: The role of vitreoretinal surgery in the management of myopic macular hole without retinal detachment. Retina 2001;21:332–338.

Jose Garcia-Arumi, MD
Hospital Vall Hebrón, 119–129
Passeig de la Vall d'Hebron
ES–08035 Barcelona (Spain)
Tel. +34 932746000, E-Mail jgarcia.arumi@gmail.com

Bandello F, Battaglia Parodi M (eds): Surgical Retina.
ESASO Course Series. Basel, Karger, 2012, vol 2, pp 146–152

Vitrectomy for Epiretinal Membrane

Alain Gaudric · Ramin Tadayoni

Hôpital Lariboisière, AP-HP, Université Paris 7 Diderot, Paris, France

Abstract

Macular epiretinal membranes (ERM) are formed by glial cell proliferation that covers the macular surface, and result in retinal thickening and distortion when they contract. These membranes are in most cases idiopathic, i.e. exclusively due to posterior vitreous detachment, even if it is incomplete. Idiopathic ERM usually occurs in the elderly. In some cases, the macular profile presents as a macular pseudohole. In others, the persistent adherence of the posterior hyaloid to the ERM results in a vitreomacular traction syndrome. The indication for surgery mainly depends on the degree of vision loss and of the impairment of binocular vision due to metamorphopsia. Surgery is usually indicated when vision drops to 0.4 or 0.5. Vitrectomy by sutureless transconjunctival incisions has become the standard procedure for this surgery, and if necessary, may easily be combined with cataract surgery. Visual results are fairly good, with significant improvement of vision in more than 70% of cases once the cataract has been operated on. Vision may improve for up to one year after surgery, although the macular profile rarely returns to normal.

Macular epiretinal membranes (ERM) are formed by the self-limiting proliferation of cells of retinal origin, mainly glial cells [1]. These membranes cover the macular area and posterior pole, and result in retinal folding when they contract [2]. In 80% of cases, ERM are idiopathic, i.e. exclusively due to the occurrence of a posterior vitreous detachment; in most of the remaining cases, ERM are secondary to other diseases, including diabetic retinopathy, posterior and intermediate uveitis, and retinal detachment, of which they complicate the course. ERM mostly occur in the elderly, but in rare cases may affect young adults or even children, and are probably congenital [4].

Idiopathic Macular Epiretinal Membranes

Optical coherence tomography (OCT) shows the anomalies in the macular profile caused by the contraction of the membrane. Spectral domain (SD) OCT is able to show even very thin membranes adhering firmly to the retinal surface. They are more clearly visible when they bridge inner retinal folds.

In some cases, the posterior hyaloid remains partially adherent to the ERM, and it may be difficult to differentiate between them. The posterior hyaloid is usually less reflective than the ERM and tends to move away from the retinal surface at the periphery of the macula.

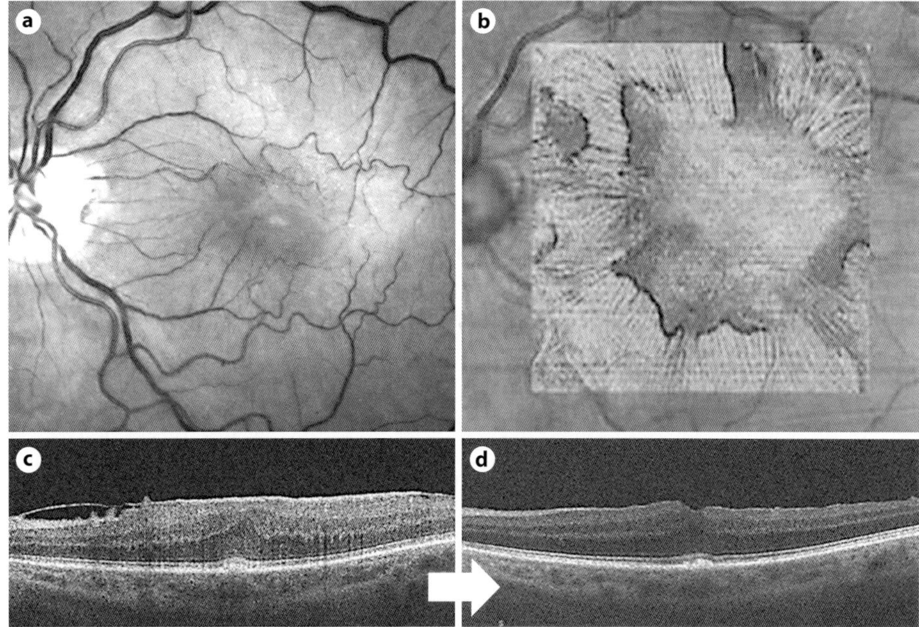

Fig. 1. ERM resulting in contraction of the posterior pole. **a** Red-free fundus photo showing the distortion of retinal vessels. **b** En face OCT image showing a contracted ERM with a smooth surface causing radial retinal folds. **c** OCT scan, showing the ERM on the surface of the thickened retina. **d** Six months after surgery, improvement of the macular profile on OCT scan but the macula did not return to normal.

ERM contraction results in the formation of retinal folds. These folds may only be superficial and include the internal limiting membrane (ILM) and optic nerve fiber layer, or they may affect the entire thickness of the retina. The severity of the changes in the inner nuclear layer might account for the presence of metamorphopsia [5]. The outer limiting membrane and inner segment/outer segment line are seldom distorted.

ERM contraction also results in macular thickening. Flattening of the foveal pit is the first effect of ERM contraction on the retinal macular architecture. Macular thickening is maximal under the epicenter(s) of ERM contraction and corresponds to the compression of the retina due to its great plasticity (fig. 1). The disappearance of the usual landmarks of the macular profile may make it difficult to locate the foveal center. However, in most cases it is still possible to recognize the center of the compressed and closed foveal pit. In some cases, cystoid cavities are present and may be combined with dye pooling on fluorescein angiography.

In almost 20% of ERM cases, fundus examination shows the presence of a subfoveal yellow dot. On OCT, this dot corresponds to a hyperreflective subretinal deposit, which tends to disappear slowly after membrane peeling [6].

Macular Pseudoholes

The term macular pseudohole refers to an ophthalmoscopic image on which the center of the fovea has a round reddish appearance. OCT clearly shows that this image is due to the verticalization of the edge of the foveal pit. As Allen and Gass already suggested 30 years ago [7], this verticalization is caused by the centripetal contraction of an ERM. The thickness of the outer retina at the umbo is normal or slightly thicker, foveal thickness has increased, and on the OCT scans profile, the foveal edge is clearly thicker [8] (fig. 2). Sometimes, the ERM bridges the opening of the fovea, and may be difficult to distinguish from a central foveal cyst. The visual prognosis of macular pseudoholes after surgery is the same as for ERM in general [9]. SD OCT has now shown that the edge of the pseudohole may exhibit various degrees of dissociation of the Henle fibers, due to foveal stretching by the asymmetric contraction of the ERM.

Vitreomacular Traction Syndrome
Vitreomacular traction syndrome (VMTS) is an anomaly of the vitreoretinal junction at the macula, in which the posterior hyaloid is partially detached from the retina but still adheres to the foveal center, the optic disc and often the temporal vessels, and exerts traction on the fovea, resulting in microcystic foveal thickening. OCT gives meaningful images of VMTS.

The posterior hyaloid is thicker and more reflective than normally, probably due to the lining of the posterior surface of the hyaloid by the proliferation of a fibroglial membrane coming from the retina [10, 11]. The membrane then tends to seal off the vitreous even more firmly from the retina, thus preventing its subsequent detachment and increasing the effect of the traction exerted by the vitreous on the retina. This traction may create major deformation of the inner boundary of the fovea, which assumes the characteristic shape of a truncated cone, and is often combined with foveal cystic cavities (fig. 3).

Secondary Epiretinal Membranes

Epiretinal membranes may also be secondary to other retinal diseases such as retinal detachment (macular pucker) [12], posterior or intermediate uveitis, vascular retinal diseases or retinal dystrophies. On OCT, they do not look very different from idiopathic ERM. Macular pucker usually consists of thick and very contractile membranes. In posterior uveitis, ERM are often combined with cystoid macular edema, which is also the case in diabetic retinopathy, retinal vein occlusion sequelae or Coats' disease.

Epiretinal Membrane in the Young

Epiretinal membrane is extremely rare in young people. When present, it is often fortuitously disclosed and does not result in loss of vision. However, there are rare cases in which the ERM contracts and causes visual loss requiring surgery [4]. In young people, ERM are usually white and opaque, and have an extrafoveal epicenter. In rare cases, they may be associated with combined hamartoma of the retina and retinal pigment epithelium [13].

Surgery is indicated when vision drops, and visual results are usually good. Complete ERM dissection may sometimes be difficult when the membrane is firmly attached to a retinal vessel.

Foveal Thickness, Visual Acuity and the Decision to Operate

Foveal thickness (i.e. the mean retinal thickness of the central area 1 mm in diameter) is inversely correlated with visual acuity, but this correlation is relatively weak, and includes extremely variable individual values, making it quite impossible to predict visual acuity from foveal thickness in any particular case. Foveal thickening on OCT is therefore not a sufficient criterion for surgical decision-making. On the other hand, it is unlikely that an ERM which has not resulted in foveal thickening of at least 340 μm on SD OCT would cause significant loss of vision. Thus, in

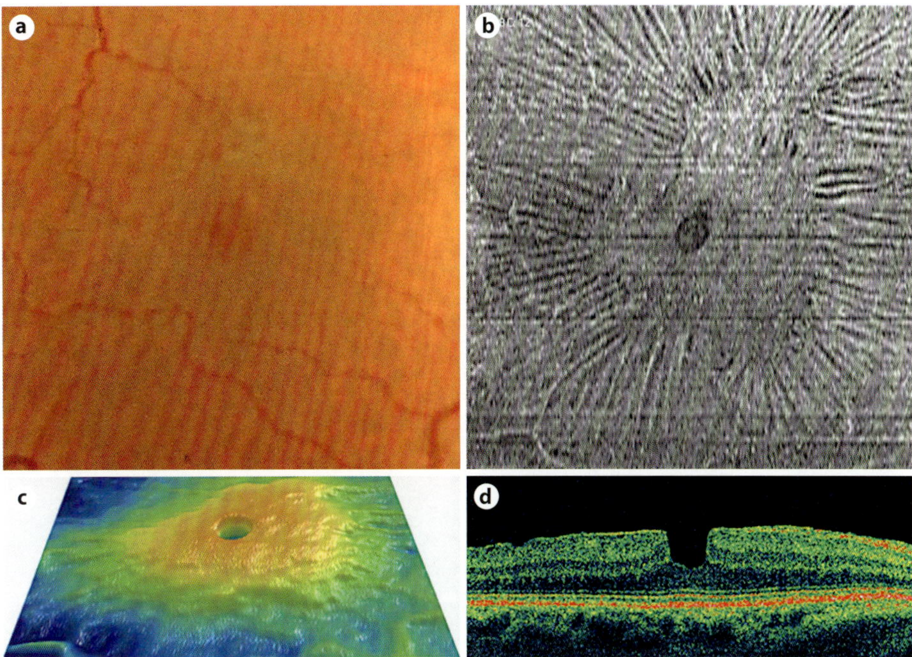

Fig. 2. Epiretinal membrane contraction inducing a macular pseudohole. **a** Color fundus photograph exhibiting the typical feature of a reddish rounded fovea known as a pseudohole. **b** En face OCT image showing a contracted ERM causing radial retinal folds. **c** OCT volume of the macula showing the pseudohole. **d** OCT scan illustrating the verticalization of the foveal pit edge.

such cases, OCT is useful in encouraging the search for another cause of visual loss associated with ERM. The decision to operate is then mainly based on the objective decrease in vision and the complaint expressed by the patient. The visual threshold for deciding on surgery has gradually moved from 0.3 to 0.5 or more, depending on the degree of metamorphopsia and binocular vision impairment [15].

Surgery for Epiretinal Membranes and Vitreomacular Traction Syndrome

Surgery is mostly performed by small sutureless transconjunctivoscleral 23- or 25-gauge incisions. Only core vitrectomy is needed. However, in VMTS, the posterior hyaloid has to be opened around the area of its adherence to the fovea, in order to obtain access to the membrane. It is usually necessary to peel off an ERM to allow complete removal of the cone of vitreous cortex attached to the fovea.

The epiretinal membrane is usually grasped with an end-gripping forceps and progressively peeled off the macular surface in one or several pieces (fig. 4). When one observes the whitening of the peeled retinal surface and the occurrence of small petechiae, this indicates that the ILM has been peeled off together with the ERM, a circumstance which occurs in at least 70% of cases. However, at this point in the surgical procedure, vital dyes (trypan blue or brilliant blue G) can be used to stain any ILM or ERM remnants and achieve the epiretinal dissection. There is no proof that complete ablation of the ILM improves

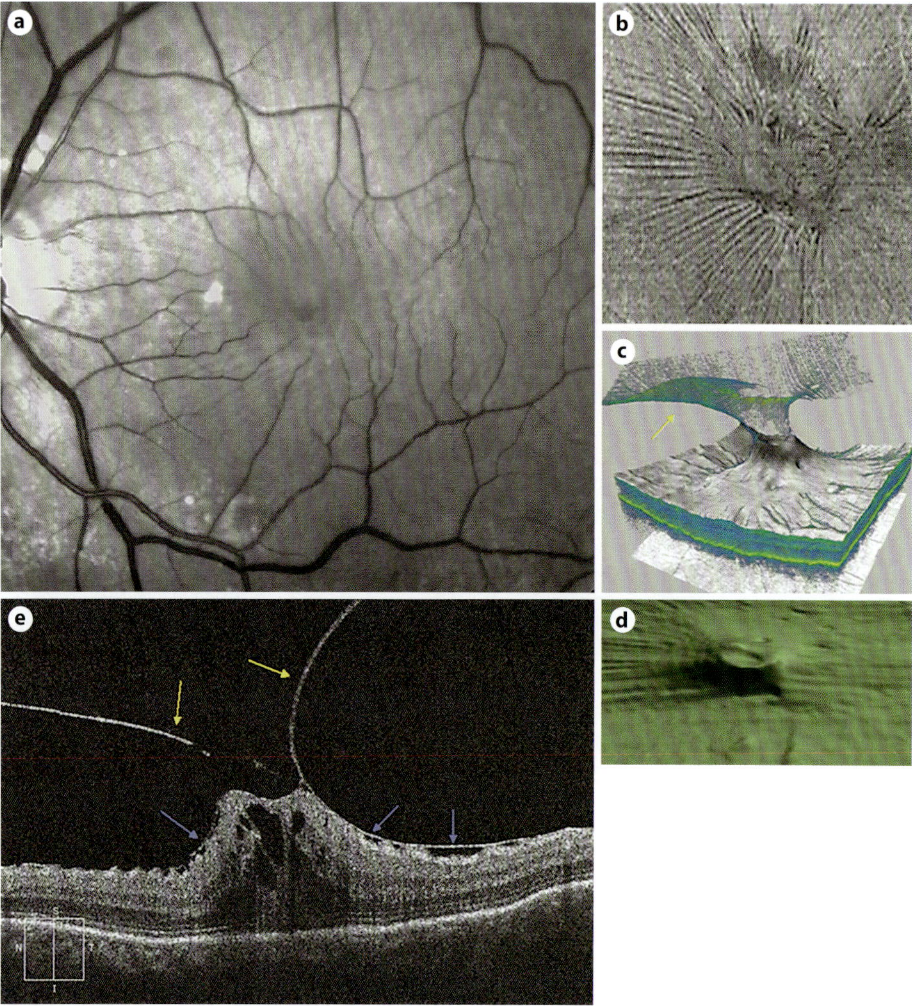

Fig. 3. VMTS. **a** Red-free fundus photograph showing only moderate distortion of retinal vessels in the macula. **b** En face OCT image showing a contracted ERM causing complex retinal folds. **c** Three-dimensional OCT showing traction of the posterior hyaloid on the elevated surface of the fovea. Note the hyperreflectivity of the posterior hyaloid (arrow) corresponding to the proliferation of an ERM at the posterior hyaloid surface. **d** OCT retinal surface showing elevation of the fovea. **e** OCT scan showing foveal elevation due to traction exerted by the posterior hyaloid; an ERM covers the retinal surface (blue arrows) and lines the posterior hyaloid (yellow arrows).

visual results, but it ensures that all ERM have been removed [16]. On the other hand, ILM ablation may reduce the recurrence rate, which is in general less than 10%. Before surgery is completed, the retinal periphery must be carefully examined for treatment of any accidental breaks.

Surgical Results

After epiretinal membrane dissection, foveal thickness usually decreases, but the macular profile rarely returns to normal, and some degree of retinal thickening persists.

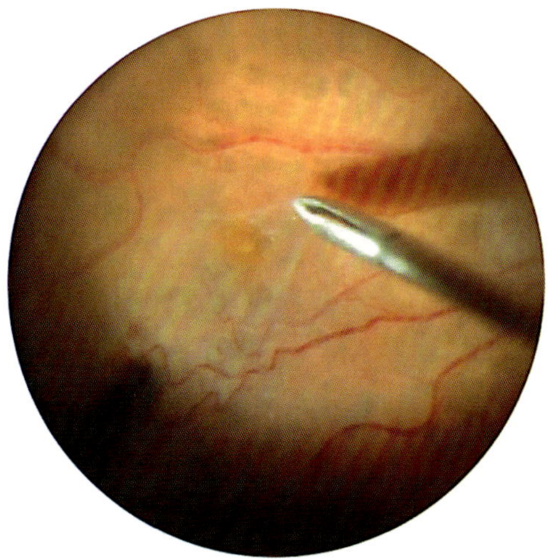

Fig. 4. Peroperative photo of ERM peeling. The ERM is peeled off with a 23-gauge forceps, and detached from the retina. Note the whitening of the denuded retina and presence of petechiae characteristic of the ablation of the ILM together with the ERM.

The foveal surface often remains slightly convex on the scan profile, and on SD OCT, foveal thickness remains at 320–340 μm, whether or not the ILM has been peeled off. Sometimes, however, a faint image of a foveal pit reappears. The macular profile may gradually improve for up to one year after surgery [18]. There is no clear correlation between the persistence of some degree of foveal thickening and the improvement of visual acuity. If the patient is phakic, nuclear sclerosis will occur soon after surgery, thus preventing significant visual improvement at 3 months. Maximum vision recovery will only be possible after cataract surgery [15]. In cases of combined cataract and ERM surgery, visual improvement may only be maximal after 1 year.

References

1 Bringmann A, Wiedemann P: Involvement of Müller glial cells in epiretinal membrane formation. Graefes Arch Clin Exp Ophthalmol 2009;247:865–883.

2 Foos RY: Vitreoretinal juncture over retinal vessels. Albrecht Von Graefes Arch Klin Exp Ophthalmol 1977;204:223–234.

3 Klein R, Klein B, Wang Q, Moss SE: The epidemiology of epiretinal membranes. Trans Am Ophthalmol Soc 1994;92:403–425, discussion 425–430.

4 Benhamou N, Massin P, Spolaore R, Paques M, Gaudric A: Surgical management of epiretinal membrane in young patients. Am J Ophthalmol 2002;133:358–364.

5 Watanabe A, Arimoto S, Nishi O: Correlation between metamorphopsia and epiretinal membrane optical coherence tomography findings. Ophthalmology 2009;116:1788–1793.

6 Dupas B, Tadayoni R, Erginay A, Massin P, Gaudric A: Subfoveal deposits secondary to idiopathic epiretinal membranes. Ophthalmology 2009;116:1794–1798.

7 Allen AWJ, Gass JMD: Contraction of perifoveal epiretinal membrane simulating a macular hole. Am J Ophthalmol 1976;82:684–691.

8 Haouchine B, Massin P, Tadayoni R, Erginay A, Gaudric A: Diagnosis of macular pseudoholes and lamellar macular holes by optical coherence tomography. Am J Ophthalmol 2004;138:732–739.

9 Massin P, Paques M, Masri H, et al: Visual outcome of surgery for epiretinal membranes with macular pseudoholes. Ophthalmology 1999;106:580–585.

10 Koizumi H, Spaide RF, Fisher YL, Freund KB, Klancnik JM Jr, Yannuzzi LA: Three-dimensional evaluation of vitreomacular traction and epiretinal membrane using spectral-domain optical coherence tomography. Am J Ophthalmol 2008;145:509–517.

11 Chang LK, Fine HF, Spaide RF, Koizumi H, Grossniklaus HE: Ultrastructural correlation of spectral-domain optical coherence tomographic findings in vitreomacular traction syndrome. Am J Ophthalmol 2008;146:121–127.

12 Machemer R: The surgical removal of epiretinal macular membranes (macular puckers) (in German). Klin Monbl Augenheilkd 1978;173:36–42.

13 Zhang X, Dong F, Dai R, Yu W: Surgical management of epiretinal membrane in combined hamartomas of the retina and retinal pigment epithelium. Retina 2010;30:305–309.

14 Massin P, Allouch C, Haouchine B, et al: Optical coherence tomography of idiopathic macular epiretinal membranes before and after surgery. Am J Ophthalmol 2000;130:732–739.

15 Thompson JT: Epiretinal membrane removal in eyes with good visual acuities. Retina 2005;25:875–882.

16 Schumann RG, Gandorfer A, Eibl KH, Henrich PB, Kampik A, Haritoglou C: Sequential epiretinal membrane removal with internal limiting membrane peeling in brilliant blue G-assisted macular surgery. Br J Ophthalmol 2010;94:1369–1372.

17 Treumer F, Wacker N, Junge O, Hedderich J, Roider J, Hillenkamp J: Foveal structure and thickness of retinal layers long-term after surgical peeling of idiopathic epiretinal membrane. Invest Ophthalmol Vis Sci 2011;52:744–750.

18 Kim J, Rhee KM, Woo SJ, Yu YS, Chung H, Park KH: Long-term temporal changes of macular thickness and visual outcome after vitrectomy for idiopathic epiretinal membrane. Am J Ophthalmol 2010;150:701–709.e1.

Prof. Alain Gaudric
Service d'Ophtalmologie, Hôpital Lariboisière, AP-HP, Université Paris 7 Diderot
2 rue Ambroise Paré
FR–75010 Paris (France)
E-Mail alain.gaudric@lrb.aphp.fr

Bandello F, Battaglia Parodi M (eds): Surgical Retina.
ESASO Course Series. Basel, Karger, 2012, vol 2, pp 153–158

Irvine-Gass Syndrome

Anselm Kampik

Augenklinik der LMU, Klinikum der Universität München, München, Germany

Abstract

Cystoid macular edema developing following cataract surgery is also called Irvine-Gass syndrome. The frequency is described as being between 7 and 70% depending on the definition of the syndrome, and occurs usually 2–3 months after surgery. Etiology is thought to be from an inflammatory reaction or a vitreous traction leading to inflammation resulting in cystoid macular edema, sometimes with visual disturbances. The disease is thought to be self-limiting in most cases. Pharmacologic therapy as well as surgical vitreoretinal therapy are discussed for the more severe cases of Irvine-Gass syndrome. The published data on the different therapeutic approaches are also discussed.

Cystoid macular edema (CME) developing following cataract surgery, if it is thought to be directly related to the surgery, is referred to as Irvine-Gass syndrome. It is the leading cause of unfavorable visual outcomes after cataract surgery in the absence of other retinal diseases. The greatest incidence is observed 1–3 months after surgery.

The visual acuity is affected initially but recovers in the majority of cases. Therapy of this condition is controversial and usually involves anti-inflammatory drugs to restore visual acuity.

The initial description was presented by Irvine in 1953 [1]. Thirteen years later, following fluorescein-angiographic studies, a further description was given by Gass [2]. Fluorescein

studies demonstrate that the pathogenesis of the macular and optic nerve lesions involves leakage of fluid from the retinal and optic nerve head capillaries.

The incidence of the Irvine-Gass syndrome has allegedly dramatically decreased with the introduction of extracapsular techniques and phakoemulsification. However, hard data confirming this assumption are not available.

According to different observational studies, the angiographic frequency of CME after cataract surgery is in the range between 3 and 70%. In contrast, a clinically relevant Irvine-Gass syndrome is clinically observed in the range between 0.1 and 12%. This variation of incidence between different clinical studies is due to the ill definition of the disease, surgical techniques, and follow-up criteria. According to a cohort study, a clinical CME resulting in a visual acuity below 20/40 had a prevalence of 0.4% [3]. In an older prospective study, the incidence of clinical CME resulting in a visual acuity below 20/40 after 6 months was 1.7% [4].

Risk Factors for Irvine-Gass Syndrome

The reason for the occurrence of CME in Irvine-Gass syndrome is unclear. Therefore, many factors are accused of being causative factors. One is the type of surgery with intracapsular cataract surgery having a higher risk than extracapsular or phako-surgery of the lens. The placement of the lens in the posterior chamber seems to have a lower risk than a lens placed in contact with the iris either in the sulcus ciliaris or in the anterior chamber. A defect of the posterior lens capsule appears to be a risk factor. Also, the operating microscope light and even the environmental light are blamed for potentially fostering the occurrence of CME after cataract surgery. Sometimes, it is associated with complicated cataract surgery and may occur after (1) intraoperative vitreous loss or (2) vitreous adhesion to the iris or to the corneoscleral wound. Alteration of the iris, such as iris incarceration in the wound is another risk factor. Even the use of epinephrine during cataract surgery for dilating the pupil is under discussion as a risk factor.

Additional influencing factors include the occurrence of contralateral CME, older age, systemic vascular disease, race (white > black), ocular inflammatory disease, and the use of topical latanoprost for glaucoma therapy.

Pathophysiology

Pathophysiology of Irvine-Gass syndrome is not completely understood. Principally, the macular area is predisposed for edema development due to anatomic peculiarities. The avascularity of the foveolar zone restricts fluid absorption. The anatomic structure of the outer plexiform layer has a horizontal course in the macular area and extends transversely from cone nuclei to bipolar cells giving space for accumulation of intracellular transudation. CME in general is a nonspecific intraretinal reaction, often associated with intraocular inflammatory or vascular diseases.

Inflammation is thought to be the major etiologic factor for CME following cataract surgery. CME following cataract surgery is most likely caused by cytokines released by activated inflammatory cells (prostaglandins, other vasopermeability factors). These molecules lead to breakdown of the blood-retinal barrier, a hyperpermeability of macular capillaries resulting in macular edema. Cysts result either from edematous, degenerating Müller cells or from expansion of extracellular spaces in the inner plexiform and inner nuclear layers caused by serous exudates.

Histopathology

Findings from clinicopathologic correlations revealed retinal capillary dilatation, serous fluids in the outer plexiform and inner nuclear layers, and inflammatory cells around blood vessels in the iris and ciliary body. Transudation can involve most of the retinal layers, displacing rod and cone nuclei and receptor cell axons. Perifoveal cysts, sometimes confluent were seen from expansion of extracellular spaces.

Clinical Findings and Diagnosis

CME in Irvine-Gass syndrome is suspected if visual function is deteriorating or not recovering after cataract surgery. Some patients notice besides a decreased visual acuity a positive central scotoma or even metamorphopsia.

On biomicroscopic slit lamp examination, an absence of the foveal light reflex is suggestive of Irvine-Gass syndrome. Intraretinal cystoid spaces in a concentric fashion around the fovea are visible in more pronounced cases. A complete posterior vitreous detachment is usually present. Rarely, there is a vitreomacular attachment accompanying the wet macula. The diagnosis is confirmed by fluorescein angiography demonstrating a typical flower-like appearance of the leakage in the macular area. Thickening of the macular area correlates more with visual impairment than the angiogram grading. Of importance is the wide variety of differential diagnoses. Thus, other causes of macular edema have to be ruled out before making the diagnosis of Irvine-Gass syndrome.

Monitoring is best performed by high-resolution optical coherence tomography of the macular area, where cystoid spaces are found typically in the inner aspect of the retina, mostly not involving the deeper retinal structures or the RPE.

Clinical Course and Therapy

Acute Irvine-Gass syndrome may resolve spontaneously, but chronic forms (>6 months duration) remain difficult to treat. 50–75% resolve spontaneously, achieving improved vision within 6 months [5].

Targets of treatment in Irvine-Gass syndrome are (1) the inflammatory component of the disease, and (2) potential vitreous traction or adhesion.

Therapeutic attempts so far include the following: (1) topical steroids/NSAIDs; (2) grid laser photocoagulation; (3) intravitreal anti-VEGF; (4) intravitreal steroids; (5) vitrectomy.

Available data on these therapeutic options will be given and evaluated for their clinical usefulness.

Topical Steroids/Nonsteroidal Anti-Inflammatory Drugs as Prophylactic Measure
A meta-analysis on this form of treatment found medical prophylaxis/medical treatment with nonsteroidal anti-inflammatory drugs (NSAIDs) are significantly beneficial [6]. In another study, diclofenac 0.1% eye drops were compared with steroids (fluorometholone 0.1% eye drops) as a prophylaxis of CME after small-incision phako. In this study, an angiographic CME was found postoperatively in 5.7% in the diclofenac group and in 54.7% in the fluorometholone group [7].

Clinical practice probably is not really affected by these findings since the incidence of Irvine-Gass syndrome is so variable that results like those presented above are not sufficient to treat prophylactically all patients for cataract surgery. Studies giving data on the numbers needed to treat to cure or avoid postoperative pseudophakic clinically relevant macular edema are missing so far.

Grid Laser Photocoagulation
One study reports on 20 patients with CME due to uveitis (n = 14) or Irvine-Gass (n = 6) in which a modified macular grid with a yellow dye laser (wavelength 577 nm) using a pattern of 20–40 spots in the central edematous area (500 μm) was applied. The mean visual acuity before treatment was 0.16. The mean visual acuity after 2 months was 0.3, which persisted during 12 months of follow-up. Fluorescein leakage was reduced. The results were reported to be similar in uveitis/Irvine-Gass syndrome. When the duration of the edema was >2 years, the prognosis was worse [8].

Due to the very small numbers of patients in this series, laser treatment most probably is not the choice of treatment any longer.

Intravitreal Anti-VEGF
In a multicenter study during the years 2005–2006, 28 eyes of 25 consecutive patients with pseudophakic CME received a minimum of 1 injection with 1.25 mg (16 eyes) or 2.5 mg (12 eyes) bevacizumab. After 6 months, 20 patients (71.4%) improved >2 ETDRS lines, 8 patients (28.6%) were stable. Eight eyes had a second injection, 4 eyes a third injection. No significant differences between the two doses of bevacizumab were observed. The edema resolved completely in only one patient [9]. Another study examined 16 eyes of 16 patients refractory to current standard therapy (topical NSAIDs or topic steroids) in which intravitreal anti-VEGF injections were applied [10]. The mean duration of the CME was 7 months (3 weeks to 19 months); the mean visual acuity before injection was 20/100. 1.25 mg of bevacizumab was injected. As a result, the visual acuity was the same in 13 patients, worse in 2 patients, and better in 1 patient. Repeated injections

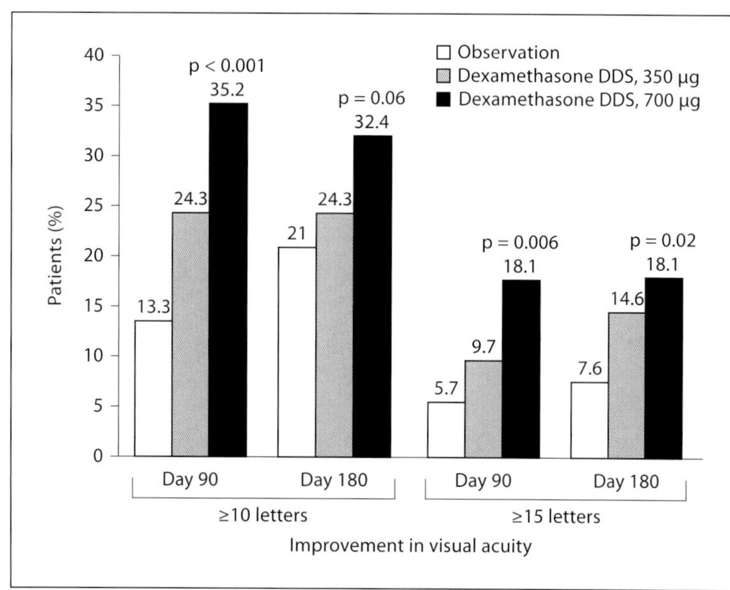

Fig. 1. Influence of dexamethason implant to treat Irvine-Gass syndrome.

gave no better visual outcome. However, the retinal thickness decreased >10% in 9 patients (81%), was unchanged in 4 patients, and increased >10% in 3 patients. Thus, the studies demonstrated only a very limited improvement with the use of intravitreal anti-VEGF treatment.

Intravitreal Steroids

In a recent study, 315 patients with persistent CME were randomized (41 with Irvine-Gass) to intravitreal steroid. This latter subgroup received a posterior segment drug delivery system. As a result, a >2 lines ETDRS improvement after 3 months was seen in 41.7% of the patients receiving 350 µg dexamethasone, and in 53.8% in those receiving 700 µg dexamethasone. A significant reduction of leakage was observed in fluorescein angiographic examinations. The increase in intraocular pressure of 10 mm Hg or more was seen in 5 of 13 patients in the 700 µg group, 1 of 12 patients in the 350 µg group (fig. 1) [11].

Although these results are promising, they are not really specific for the Irvine-Gass syndrome. Future experience with intravitreal slow-release steroid application still has to demonstrate its value for the treatment of postsurgical pseudophakic CME.

Vitrectomy

In a retrospective analysis of 23 consecutive eyes of 23 patients with pseudophakic CME unresponsive to medical treatment after mostly complicated cataract surgery, the result of vitrectomy was analyzed [12]. The mean interval between cataract surgery and vitrectomy was 32.4 months. The complex situation is evidenced by the vitreous adherent to the iris or IOL in 52.2% and the vitreous present in the anterior chamber in 30.4%. The median preoperative visual acuity was 20/200. The median postoperative visual acuity improved to 20/60 with a mean follow-up of 30.2 months (table 1).

In a similar case series of complicated cataract surgery with subsequent Irvine-Gass syndrome, 24 consecutive patients with pseudophakic macula edema resistant to conservative treatment were treated with vitrectomy. Twenty-three eyes had preoperative evidence of vitreous adhesions

Table 1. Effect of vitrectomy in the treatment of Irvine-Gass syndrome

Median best-corrected preoperative VA	20/200
Median best-corrected final postoperative VA	20/60*
Number of lines of improvement	
Mean ± SD	3.3 ± 2.6
Range	0–11
Percent change in best-corrected final VA	
Median	70
Range	0–99
CME status	
Resolved	23 (100%)
Persistent	0
Final best-corrected VA distribution	
≥20/50	9 (39.1%)
20/60–20/100	12 (52.2%)
20/200	2 (8.7%)
Time for resolution of CME, months	
Mean	3.3
Range	1–12
Follow-up, months	
Mean ± SD	30.2 ± 31.2
Range	2–109

VA = Visual acuity. * p < 0.0001, Wilcoxon signed rank test.

at the anterior chamber, 1 eye had iris capture. The mean preoperative visual acuity was 20/190 (range 20/50–20/300). Postoperatively, the visual acuity improved by 4.7 Snellen lines (mean) in all

patients. A longer time interval between cataract surgery and vitrectomy did not influence visual outcome [13].

Peyman et al. [14] reported on 2 patients who had received vitrectomy with additional internal limiting membrane peeling. The two eyes had pseudophakic CME of 11–22 months. Case 1 had prior treatment with oral and topical steroids, topical diclofenac, 4 injections of sub-Tenon's steroids, and 5 intravitreal triamcinolone injections. Visual acuity was 20/70 before vitrectomy and 20/40 at 3.5 and 11 months after vitrectomy (on 1% topical prednisolone twice a day). Case 2 had prior treatment with acetazolamide in addition to oral and topical NSAIDs. Because of a reported corticosteroid allergy, no steroids were administered. Preoperative visual acuity of 20/400 remained unchanged for 4 weeks postoperatively, but improved to 20/80 during 5- to 9-month follow-up.

Thus, these case series demonstrate a useful effect of vitrectomy, especially in those patients who have had complicated cataract surgery.

In summary, Irvine-Gass syndrome in most cases is probably an inflammatory disease, as originally stated by Gass. Thus, the time course or – in more severe cases – pharmacologic anti-inflammatory treatment or anti-VEGF treatment may play an important role. However, in some instances vitreoretinal microsurgery, eventually even including internal limiting membrane peeling, may be a helpful adjunct for treating the most recalcitrant cases.

References

1 Irvine SR: A newly defined vitreous syndrome following cataract surgery. Am J Ophthalmol 1953;36:599–619.
2 Gass JD, Norton EW: Cystoid macular edema and papilledema following cataract extraction. A fluorescein fundoscopic and angiographic study. Arch Ophthalmol 1966;76:646–661.
3 Norregaard JC, Bernth-Petersen P, Bellan L, et al: Intraoperative clinical practice and risk of early complications after cataract extraction in the United States, Canada, Denmark, and Spain. Ophthalmology 1999;106:42–48.
4 Wright PL, Wilkinson CP, Balyeat HD, et al: Angiographic cystoid macular edema after posterior chamber lens implantation. Arch Ophthalmol 1988;106:740–744.
5 Levin DS, Lim JI: Update on pseudophakic cystoid macular edema treatment options. Ophthalmol Clin North Am 2002;15: 467–472.

6 Rosetti L, Chaudhwi J, Dickersin K: Medical prophylaxis and treatment of cystoid macular edema after cataract surgery. The results of a meta-analysis. Ophthalmology 1998;105:397–405.

7 Miyake K, Ibaraki N: Prostaglandins and cystoid macular edema. Surv Ophthalmol 2002:47(suppl 1):S203–S218.

8 Lardenoye CWTA, van Schooneveld MJ, Treffers WF, Rothova A: Grid laser photocoagulation for macular oedema in uveitis or the Irvine-Gass syndrome. Br J Ophthalmol 1998;82:1013–1016.

9 Arevalo JF, Garcia-Amaris RA, Roca JA, Sanchez JG, Wu L, Berrocal MH, Maia M, Pan-American Collaborative Retina Study Group: Primary intravitreal bevacizumab for the management of pseudophakic cystoid macular edema: pilot study of the Pan-American Collaborative Retina Study Group. J Cataract Refract Surg 2007;33:2098–2105.

10 Spitzer MS, Ziemssen F, Yoeruek E, Petermeier K, Aisenbrey S, Szurman P: Efficacy of intravitreal bevacizumab in treating postoperative pseudophakic cystoid macular edema. J Cataract Refract Surg 2008;34:70–75.

11 Wiiliams G, Haller JA, Kuppermann BD, Blumenkranz MS, Weinberg DV, Chou C, Withcup SM, on behalf of the dexamethasone DDS phase II Study group: Dexamethasone posterior-segment drug delivery system in the treatment of macular edema resulting from uveitis or Irvine-Gass syndrome. Am J Ophthalmol 2009;147:1048–1054.

12 Pendergast SD, Marherio RR, Williams GA, Cox MS: Vitrectomy for chronic pseudophakic cystoid macular edema. Am J Ophthalmol 1999;128:317–323.

13 Harbour JW, Smiddy WE, Rubsamen PE, Murray TG, Davis JL, Flynn HW Jr: Pars plana vitrectomy for chronic pseudophakic cystoid macular edema. Am J Ophthalmol 1995;120:302–307.

14 Peyman GA, Canakis C, Livir-Rallatos C, Conway MD: The effect of internal limiting membrane peeling on chronic recalcitrant pseudophakic cystoid macular edema: a report of two cases. Am J Ophthalmol 2002;133:571–572.

Prof. Dr. Anselm Kampik, FEBO
Augenklinik der LMU, Klinikum der Universität München, Campus Innenstadt
Mathildenstrasse 8
DE–80336 München (Germany)
Tel. +49 89 5160 3800, E-Mail akampik@med.uni-muenchen.de

Bandello F, Battaglia Parodi M (eds): Surgical Retina.
ESASO Course Series. Basel, Karger, 2012, vol 2, pp 159–173

Endophthalmitis

Marco A. Zarbin

Institute of Ophthalmology and Visual Science-New Jersey Medical School, Newark, N.J., USA

Abstract

Effective treatment of infectious endophthalmitis depends on early recognition of infection, proper biopsy and culture of material, and proper selection of antibiotics. When, what, and how to biopsy and treat endophthalmitis depends on the clinical setting and findings. The prognosis depends heavily on the culture result (better prognosis if culture negative), the time at onset (better prognosis if late onset, unless associated with trabeculectomy), and the virulence of the pathogen (worst outcomes typically are associated with *Streptococcus* species, Gram-negative species, and *Bacillus* species). The classification, physical findings, risk factors, and treatment of endophthalmitis in various clinical settings are considered in detail.

Endophthalmitis can be classified as infectious vs. non-infectious (table 1) [1]. In this chapter, features of each class of inflammation are reviewed and suggested treatment paradigms are described.

Infectious Endophthalmitis

Acute Postoperative Endophthalmitis

Acute postoperative endophthalmitis can have variable clinical findings including: decreased visual acuity, pain, hypopyon, corneal edema (or infiltrate), fibrinoid anterior chamber reaction, vitritis, retinitis, retinal vasculitis, afferent pupillary defect, chemosis/lid edema, and, in cases of panophthalmitis, restriction of extraocular motility and proptosis. To ensure that one does not miss a small hypopyon, one should be sure to retract gently the lower lid during slit lamp examination to visualize directly the inferior anterior chamber. The incidence of retinal detachment after acute postoperative endophthalmitis ranges from 10 to 16%, and the prognosis with concurrent retinal detachment depends on the virulence of the associated pathogen(s).

The incidence of acute (i.e. within 6 weeks of surgery) postoperative endophthalmitis ranges from 0.05 to 0.4%, depending on the type of surgical intervention (table 2). The incidence tends to be highest after secondary intraocular lens (IOL) placement and lower after pars plana vitrectomy. In a report of 28,622 intraocular surgical procedures in which all patients were prepped with povidone iodine on the lid margins and conjunctiva (pHisoHex if allergic), the median visual acuity after treatment was 20/200 [2]. The visual outcome was significantly better for secondary IOLs (20/40; often caused by *Staphylococcus epidermidis*) and significantly worse after vitrectomy (no light perception).

Table 1. Classification of endophthalmitis

Infectious endophthalmitis
  Postoperative endophthalmitis
  • Acute
  • Delayed onset (onset ≥6 weeks after surgery)
  • Conjunctival filtering bleb associated
  Endogenous endophthalmitis
  Posttraumatic endophthalmitis
Noninfectious endophthalmitis
  Sterile uveitis
  Phacoanaphylactic endophthalmitis
  Sympathetic ophthalmia

Table 2. Incidence of acute postoperative endophthalmitis [2]

Intervention	Incidence of endophthalmitis, %
Phacoemulsification/ extracapsular cataract extraction + IOL	0.07–0.12
Secondary IOL	0.366
Penetrating keratoplasty (PK)	0.11–0.18
PK + cataract extraction	0.194
Glaucoma filtering procedures	0.06–1.8
Glaucoma filtering + cataract extraction	0.114
Pars plana vitrectomy	0.046–0.07

Table 3. Risk factors for acute postoperative infectious endophthalmitis

Risk factor
Blepharitis
Conjunctivitis
Canaliculitis
Dacryocystitis
Lacrimal duct obstruction
Contact lens wear
Ocular prosthesis in fellow orbit
Host immune suppression (including diabetes mellitus)
Upper respiratory tract infection (especially children)
Atopic dermatitis and keratoconjunctivitis sicca (high rate of *Staphylococcus* colonization)

Micro-organisms that have colonized the eyelids, lacrimal sac, and conjunctiva are the usual source of infection [3]. Gram-positive organisms cause ~90% of cases. Gram-negative species cause ~7% of cases, and fungi cause ~3% of cases. In the Endophthalmitis Vitrectomy Study (EVS), of the 69% of patients with confirmed microbiologic growth, 70% grew coagulase-negative micrococci (mostly *S. epidermidis*), 9.9% grew *Staphylococcus aureus*, 9.0% grew *Streptococcus* species, 2.2% grew *Enterococcus* species, 3.1% grew other Gram-positive species, and 5.9% grew Gram-negative species [4]. Gram-negative organisms did not grow from any eye in which retinal vessels could be visualized with indirect ophthalmoscopy; 61.9% of such eyes had equivocal or no growth. Factors predictive of a ≥50% chance of infection by either Gram-negative or 'other' Gram-positive organisms include: corneal infiltrate, wound abnormalities, afferent pupillary reflex, loss of the red reflex, and symptom onset within 2 days of surgery [5]. A positive Gram stain or infection with species other than Gram-positive, coagulase-negative micrococci was associated with a significantly worse visual outcome in the EVS [6]. Initial visual acuity was a more powerful predictor of visual outcome and favorable response to vitrectomy than were microbiological data. The ocular surface and adnexa are the primary sources of bacteria in culture-positive cases (table 3) [7].

Intraoperative risk factors for acute postoperative endophthalmitis include inadequate eyelid/conjunctival disinfection (5% povidone iodine in the conjunctival sac reduces the incidence of endophthalmitis [8]), prolonged (>60 min) surgery, use of prolene haptic IOL (bacteria adhere to prolene and are protected by extracellular biofilm), unapparent/unplanned ocular penetration during ocular surgery (e.g. radial keratotomy, strabismus, retro-/peribulbar anesthesia), and contamination of donor cornea.

Postoperative risk factors for endophthalmitis include suture removal, vitreous incarceration in the wound, inadequately buried sutures, and wound leak/dehiscence/filtering bleb. Sutureless clear corneal incisions may also be a risk factor [9, 10].

Although preclinical data indicate that subconjunctival antibiotics (e.g. ceftazidime, gentamicin, ciprofloxacin) prevent endophthalmitis after cataract extraction, clinical data are not conclusive. While it seems reasonable to consider using subconjunctival cefazolin (or vancomycin in penicillin-allergic patients) or ceftazidime after cataract surgery, one probably should not use gentamicin due to the risk of macular infarction [for a more detailed discussion of this issue, see Kresslof et al. 1]. The European Society of Cataract and Refractive Surgeons Endophthalmitis Study Group assessed the value of intraoperative intraocular antibiotic infusion in endophthalmitis prophylaxis [11]. In this study, all patients received topical 5% povidone iodine. Use of intracameral cefuroxime was associated with a 5-fold decreased risk of endophthalmitis. However, the rate of endophthalmitis in the control group was much higher than the rate in other studies, and the rate of endophthalmitis was comparable to the rates in the United States when pre- and postoperative topical antibiotics are used. Thus, the value of intracameral antibiotic use is debated.

Chronic Postoperative Endophthalmitis

Factors influencing the time of onset of chronic postoperative endophthalmitis (i.e. occurring ≥6 weeks after surgery) include the virulence of the pathogen, the use of antibiotics and/or anti-inflammatory agents, and host characteristics. The most frequent causative organisms include: coagulase-negative *Staphylococcus* species, *Propionibacterium acnes*, fungi (especially *Candida* species), anaerobic *Streptococcus* species, *Actinomyces* species, and *Nocardia asteroides*.

Patients can present with any of the signs or symptoms characteristic of acute postoperative endophthalmitis, but typically, they present with low grade, persistent, granulomatous uveitis that responds initially to topical corticosteroids. The inflammation may appear to be related to retained lens cortex or may follow Nd:YAG capsulotomy (which can release sequestered organisms). Sometimes, beaded fibrin strands are present in the anterior chamber. Mutton-fat keratic precipitates can be present on the corneal endothelium and/or IOL. White plaque can be present on the posterior capsule or associated with retained lens material (both in bacterial and fungal infection) and represents a sequestrum (fig. 1). Finally, small hypopyon may be present that sometimes is visible only with gonioscopy.

Post-Trabeculectomy Endophthalmitis

Infection can develop acutely or years after filtering surgery. Infection after filtering surgery has several possible manifestations including blebitis and bleb-associated endophthalmitis (table 4; fig. 2). The microbiological spectrum of late-onset bleb-associated endophthalmitis differs from acute-onset postoperative infectious endophthalmitis [12, 13]. The greater virulence of organisms in the former case probably reflects the different mechanism of bacterial entry into the eye (i.e. penetration of conjunctiva vs. entry via an open wound). Risk factors for post-trabeculectomy endophthalmitis are numerous (table 5). It is important to treat conjunctivitis and blebitis promptly and aggressively in order to prevent endophthalmitis.

Endogenous Endophthalmitis

Endogenous infectious endophthalmitis tends to occur in debilitated/immune-compromised hosts. Endophthalmitis occurs in of 5/10,000 hospitalized patients, and 2–15% of cases are endogenous. If a source is not apparent, systemic workup should include evaluation of the heart (e.g. transesophageal echocardiogram to identify valvular vegetations), skin (e.g. Osler nodes and Janeway lesions), genitourinary tract (e.g. abdominal CT/MRI to identify perinephric/prostatic abscess) [14], gastrointestinal tract (e.g. colon

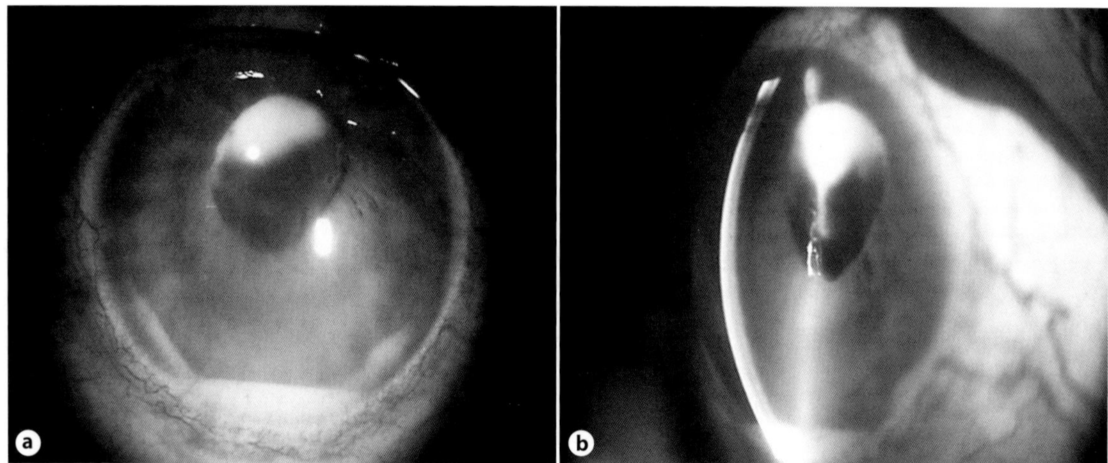

Fig. 1. *S. epidermidis* chronic endophthalmitis in a 78-year-old man. Note the white plaque posterior to the posterior chamber IOL and hypopyon. **a** Frontal view. **b** Tangential view. Reproduced with permission from Kresloff et al. [1].

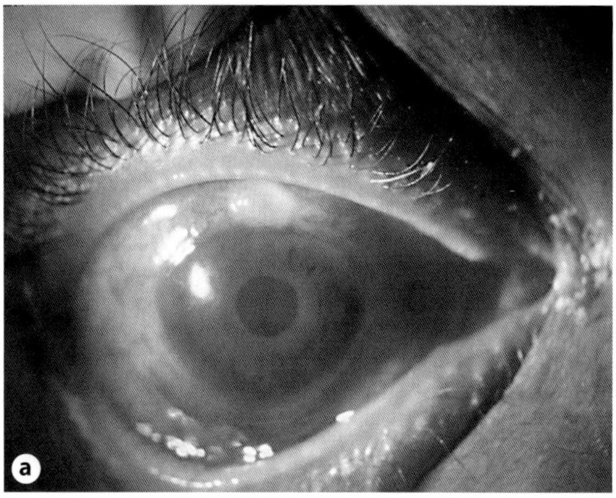

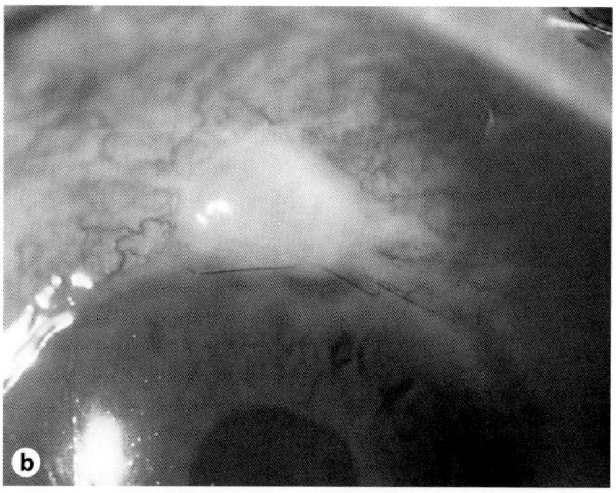

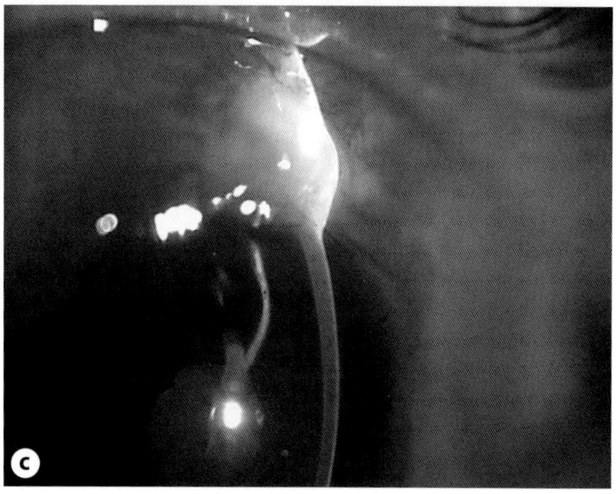

Fig. 2. Post-trabeculectomy blebitis. A 60-year-old woman presented with a 2-day history of pain and red eye. Visual acuity was 20/30 with clear media. **a** Frontal view. Note the cloudiness of the filtering bleb. **b, c** Higher magnification oblique views demonstrating conjunctival injection and cloudiness of fluid within the filtering bleb.

Table 4. Post-trabeculectomy endophthalmitis

Type of infection	Characteristics
Blebitis	Bleb infection without vitreous involvement that usually progresses to endophthalmitis. Clinical features may include: • Conjunctival injection • Purulent material in bleb • Pain (may not be present) • Decreased vision (may not be present)

Bleb-associated endophthalmitis	Usually develops months to years after glaucoma filtering surgery. Clinical features may include:
	• Acute onset: same microbiological spectrum and clinical features as acute postoperative endophthalmitis (e.g. pain, decreased vision, hypopyon, vitreous inflammation). Same mechanism (entrance of organisms intraoperatively)
	• Late onset: microbial penetration of intact conjunctiva is likely mechanism although other causes (e.g. wound leak) occur.
	  • Clinical features include pain, decreased vision, conjunctival injection, cloudy/purulent bleb (view with low intensity light, oblique illumination), bleb leak (uncommon, check Seidel test)
	  • Most common pathogens include *Streptococcus* species (30%), *Staphylococcus* species (30%), Gram-negative organisms (28%), *Enterococcus* species (7.5%), and others [13]

Table 5. Risk factors for post-trabeculectomy endophthalmitis

Risk factor
Conjunctivitis: must treat!
Blebitis: must treat!
Early wound leak (positive Seidel test)
Dacryocystitis
Thin-walled cystic bleb
Presence of seton (usually with conjunctival erosion)
Preceding upper respiratory tract infection
Contact lens wear
Contaminated eye drops
?Adjunctive use of 5-fluorouracil

cancer associated with group G streptococcal infection), as well as blood and urine culture. Eye involvement is bilateral in 25% of cases, so one should be certain to examine the fellow eye carefully when assessing an obviously inflamed eye.

Gram-positive bacteria are the most common cause of endogenous endophthalmitis. The most frequent among these organisms are *Streptococcus* species: *Streptococcus pneumoniae* and *viridans* associated with meningitis, endocarditis; group G *Streptococcus* associated with skin wounds (elderly) and malignancy (also *Clostridium* species); group B *Streptococcus* associated with meningitis (neonates) and immune-compromised adults; *S. aureus*, and *Bacillus cereus* (associated with intravenous drug abuse; classically exhibit ring-shaped corneal ulcer with brownish anterior chamber exudate). In contrast to postoperative endophthalmitis, coagulase-negative *Staphylococci* are uncommon. Enteric Gram-negative bacteria are the most common cause of Gram-negative endogenous endophthalmitis (e.g. *Escherichia coli, Klebsiella pneumoniae, Haemophilus influenzae, Pseudomonas aeruginosa,* and *Serratia* species). *N. asteroides*, an acid-fast bacterium that can

Host risk factor
Immune compromised (e.g. cancer, AIDS,
diabetes mellitus)
Indwelling catheter (e.g. hyperalimentation,
Foley catheter)
Intravenous drug abuse
Abdominal surgery
Long-term antibiotic use
Renal dialysis
Gastrointestinal abscess
Endoscopic procedure

cause endophthalmitis (e.g. subretinal abscess), can arise from a pulmonary focus.

Fungi account for more than half the cases of endogenous endophthalmitis. The most frequently encountered fungal organism is *Candida albicans* (75–80% of endogenous fungal endophthalmitis cases). These cases often begin as focal choroiditis with spread to retina and then vitreous cavity; the presence of white vitreous opacities forming a 'string of pearls' is typical. *Aspergillus* species are the second most frequent cause. *Aspergillus* endogenous endophthalmitis has been reported in immunocompromised patients (e.g. status after heart, lung, or liver transplantation; patients with leukemia), among intravenous drug abusers, in patients with endocarditis, and in patients with chronic pulmonary disease using corticosteroids. *Aspergillus* endogenous endophthalmitis is typically associated with submacular choroidal abscess ± subretinal hypopyon.

Other causes of endogenous endophthalmitis include protozoa (e.g. *Toxoplasma gondii*), parasites *(Toxocara canis), Pneumocystis carinii* (especially AIDS patients), viral infection [e.g. cytomegalovirus, acute retinal necrosis (due to herpes zoster, herpes simplex)], tuberculosis, and syphilis.

The presentation of endogenous endophthalmitis is quite variable, ranging from mild anterior uveitis to panophthalmitis [14], and depends in part on the organism's virulence. The more anterior and localized the inflammatory response, the better the prognosis. *H. influenzae*, *Neisseria meningitidis*, and *S. pneumoniae* can cause endophthalmitis in otherwise healthy individuals. A number of host risk factors, however, have been identified (table 6).

One should consider routine screening eye exams for patients at high risk. Patients undergoing orthotopic liver transplant seem to be unusually susceptible to invasive pulmonary aspergillosis and *Aspergillus* endophthalmitis, with the eye being the second most frequent site of non-pulmonary infection.

Posttraumatic Endophthalmitis
This subject has been reviewed in detail [15]. The frequency of posttraumatic infectious endophthalmitis is ~7%, but is reported as 30% after rural penetrating trauma and 11–26% if there is an intraocular foreign body (IOFB). The condition differs from postoperative and endogenous endophthalmitis in its microbiology and worse clinical course (~30% retain visual acuity ≥20/400). The worse prognosis may also be due to the effects of the injury and delay in diagnosis of infection. Risk factors for posttraumatic endophthalmitis include: lens disruption, IOFB, plant- or soil-related injury, rural environment, delayed primary repair, and penetration with a contaminated missile (e.g. tree branch, farm implement).

S. epidermidis is the most common pathogen causing posttraumatic endophthalmitis. *B. cereus* is among the most aggressive pathogens causing this condition. *B. cereus* is ubiquitous in the environment and causes posttraumatic endophthalmitis particularly in the setting of an IOFB and with vegetable or soil contamination. The presence of a corneal ring infiltrate with panophthalmitis and retinal necrosis is highly suggestive of the diagnosis. Other causes include *Streptococcus* species, *P. aeruginosa* and other Gram-negative organisms, fungi, and mixed flora.

Risk factor
Retained lens fragments (can have true hypopyon or, more commonly, pseudohypopyon)
Retained IOFB (e.g. cotton fibers)
Operative trauma (e.g. iris damage)
Exacerbation of pre-existing uveitis (e.g. sarcoidosis; can be associated with true hypopyon)
Phacolytic glaucoma (can be associated with pseudohypopyon)
Phacoanaphylactic endophthalmitis
Sympathetic ophthalmia
Toxic reaction to drugs
- Hypopyon: thrombin, rifabutin in HIV-positive patients
- Granulomatous uveitis: metipranolol, cidofovir

TASS

Table 8. Some causes of TASS

Cause
Irrigating solution or ophthalmic viscoelastic (e.g. pH, osmolality, additives)
Ophthalmic instrument contaminant (e.g. detergent/endotoxin residue)
Ocular medications (e.g. concentration, pH, osmolality, preservative)
IOL (e.g. polishing/sterilizing compound)

Adapted from Mamalis et al. [16].

Sterile Postoperative Inflammation
A number of factors can cause sterile postoperative endophthalmitis (table 7).

Toxic anterior segment syndrome (TASS) is associated with blurred vision, pain, and red eye with onset typically 24–48 h after anterior segment surgery [16]. Inflammation is most severe in the anterior segment (vs. acute postoperative infectious endophthalmitis, in which vitreous inflammation is most severe). Hypopyon, diffuse corneal edema, and a dilated (irregular)

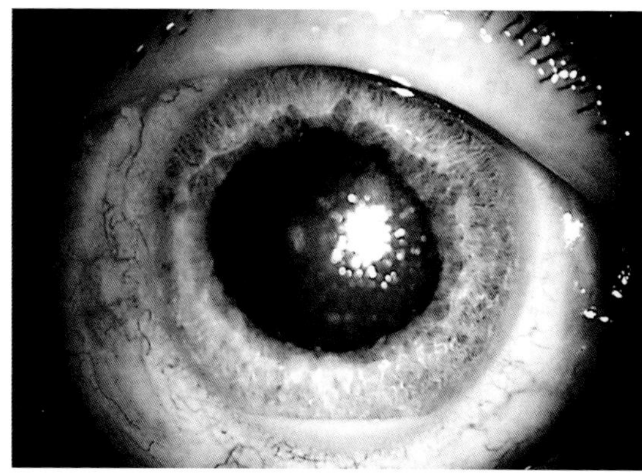

Fig. 3. Sterile hypopyon after intravitreal thrombin use. This 22-year-old insulin-dependent diabetic woman had undergone pars plana vitrectomy 24 h earlier for traction retinal detachment secondary to proliferative diabetic retinopathy. Intravitreal thrombin (100 U/ml) was used to control extensive intraocular bleeding during surgery. The vitreous culture was negative, and the hypopyon resolved with intensive topical corticosteroid use. Reproduced with permission from Kresloff et al. [1].

pupil are present typically. TASS is always Gram stain- and culture-negative, usually improves with corticosteroid treatment, and is more common in diabetic patients. Causes of TASS usually involve environmental and toxic control issues (table 8).

Masquerade Syndromes
Various conditions can mimic infectious endophthalmitis (table 9; fig. 3).

Postoperative Uveitis: When to Culture

It is not simply the clinical findings, but also the setting that influences the decision to obtain tissue for culture, smear, and sensitivity (table 10). For example, the presence of hypopyon 24 hours after intravitreal thrombin for diabetic vitrectomy would not necessarily mandate biopsy and culture of intraocular fluid. On the other hand, 3+ cell

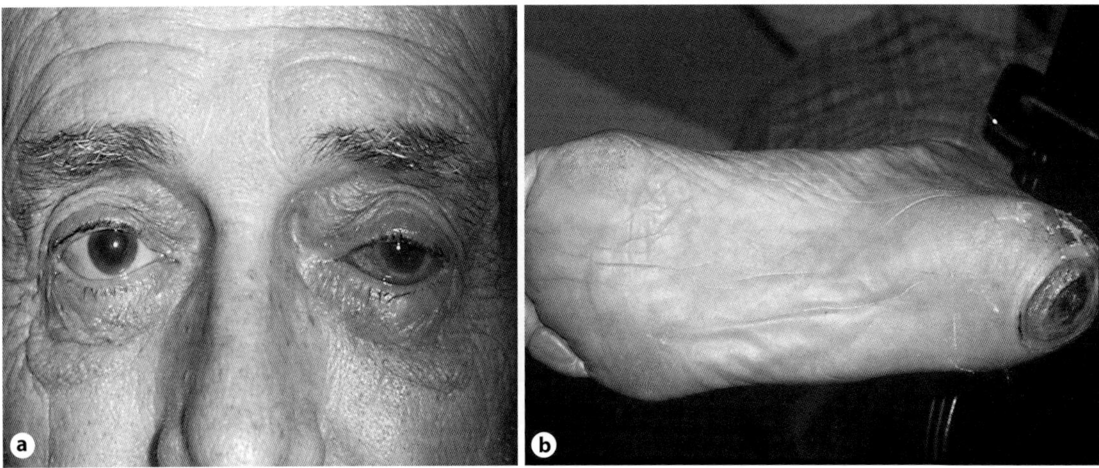

Fig. 4. Skin ulcer associated with endogenous endophthalmitis. A 60-year-old man with insulin-dependent diabetes mellitus presented with metastatic endophthalmitis OS from a foot ulcer. Sometimes culture/smear from a Janeway lesion (erythematous hemorrhagic lesion on the palm or sole seen in endocarditis) is positive. **a** Note small hypopyon in left eye. **b** Painless (due to neuropathy) foot ulcer.

Table 9. Conditions mimicking infectious endophthalmitis

Condition
Sterile hypopyon
• Thrombin
• Behçet disease
• TASS
Hyphema (dehemoglobinized blood)
Corneal ulcer with hypopyon
Retinoblastoma (pseudohypopyon comprising tumor cells)
Leukemia (pseudohypopyon comprising tumor cells)
Intraocular large cell lymphoma (typically mimics granulomatous uveitis)
Metastatic tumor (may create mass-simulating granuloma or abscess)

and flare with fibrinoid anterior chamber reaction 24 h after suture removal probably would mandate such action.

The decision to culture patients with possible endogenous endophthalmitis should be made in consultation with the medical/surgical team caring for the patient and often involves discussion with an infectious disease specialist (table 11).

In some cases of endogenous endophthalmitis, it is not necessary to obtain intraocular material for culture. For example, one can diagnose CMV retinitis in HIV+ patients on the basis of the clinical findings (although one can obtain aqueous for PCR confirmation of the diagnosis). Patients with typical findings of acute retinal necrosis (e.g. confluent peripheral retinitis with retinal hemorrhage and vitritis after a recent episode of herpes zoster dermatitis) usually undergo vitreous biopsy (for PCR) because they are treated with intravitreal antiviral agents. Patients with typical findings of *T. gondii* endophthalmitis need not undergo diagnostic biopsy (e.g. present of bilateral chorioretinal scars with retinitis adjacent to an area of scarring and positive IgG and/or IgM for toxoplasma), although it may be convenient to obtain material for PCR if one is treating the patient with intravitreal dexamethasone and clindamycin [17]. Finally, one usually diagnoses syphilitic endophthalmitis via the presence

Table 10. Postoperative inflammation: when to culture

Setting

Excessive intraocular inflammation associated with an alteration in globe integrity (e.g. suture removal)
Hypopyon (in the absence of known predisposing factor, e.g. intravitreal thrombin use, corneal ulcer in phakic eye without vitritis would not necessarily mandate biopsy)
Vitritis precluding a view of the optic nerve
White plaque and chronic intraocular inflammation unresponsive to corticosteroids
Beaded opacities in the anterior chamber or vitreous unresponsive to corticosteroids
Opacified filtering bleb (intraocular culture may not be useful if there is no anterior chamber or posterior segment inflammation)
Intraocular inflammation unresponsive to corticosteroids
History of exposure to contaminated material (e.g. vegetable matter, soil, or injury in a rural environment)

Table 11. Endogenous endophthalmitis: when to culture

Setting

In the presence of systemic infection with signs of acute or chronic intraocular inflammation but in the absence of positive extraocular cultures
In the presence of culture-positive systemic infection with signs of intraocular inflammation unresponsive to appropriate antibiotic therapy
In the presence of host risk factors with signs of acute or chronic intraocular inflammation and no apparent extraocular source of infection (and no response to anti-inflammatory therapy in chronic cases)
To rule out suspected malignancy after a negative systemic workup

of a positive serum or CSF FTA-ABS or MHA-TP or RPR.

What to Culture and Smear

Acute and Chronic Postoperative Infectious Endophthalmitis

It is most important to culture the vitreous, which is the seat of infection. In one study, 82% of endophthalmitis cases grew identical flora from the vitreous and external surface [7]. In cases of chronic postoperative endophthalmitis, in addition to culturing the aqueous and vitreous humor, one also should culture intraocular plaque if present. (Gram stain and ultrastructural studies may be critical in view of the fastidious nature of these organisms.) In recalcitrant cases, one may consider removing the lens capsule and IOL, especially for *P. acnes* and filamentous fungi. In cases with infected filtering blebs, one may consider culturing a contact lens (if used), the aqueous and vitreous humor, and possibly the bleb contents. (The risk of creating hypotony due to bleb leak must be weighed against the need for tissue diagnosis in management of potentially aggressive organisms.)

Endogenous Endophthalmitis

Generally, one cultures blood, urine, wounds, and, if indicated clinically, the CSF. The history and physical exam may mandate specific studies such as transesophageal echocardiography and culture of skin ulcers, dental caries, and/or indwelling catheters (fig. 4). The yield from the vitreous can be as robust as from blood culture

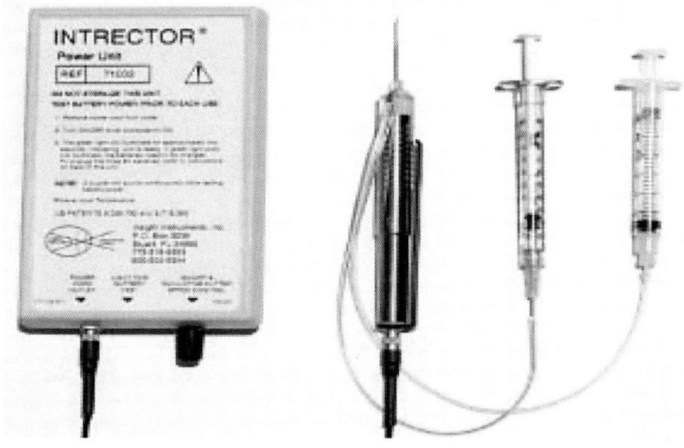

Fig. 5. In-office vitreous biopsy. Under subconjunctival (or retrobulbar) anesthesia, a sterile lid speculum is placed. The ocular surface and lashes are sterilized with topical 5% povidone-iodine. A sharp-tipped 23-gauge automated vitreous cutter is advanced into the eye through the pars plana [3 mm (aphakic/IOL) or 4 mm (phakic eye) posterior to the limbus] with the patient sitting at the slit lamp. One directs the probe just posterior to the IOL or into the mid vitreous cavity (phakic eye) with the cutting port facing the posterior segment. After the biopsy is complete, one injects intravitreal antibiotics via the pars plana using 5/8th inch 30-gauge needles attached to tuberculin syringes.

in properly selected cases. One may perform fine needle aspiration of an intraocular abscess if no definite extraocular source is identified, and if there is no vitritis.

Posttraumatic Endophthalmitis
In addition to culturing the aqueous and vitreous humor, one also should submit any excised tissue or foreign matter for culture, smear, and sensitivity testing. In one study, however, IOFBs were contaminated with bacteria in 5 (26%) of 19 eyes without signs of infection [18].

How to Culture

One may culture the ocular surface with a sterile cotton swab. Aqueous humor can be biopsied using a 5/8th inch 30-gauge needle attached to a tuberculin syringe (0.1–0.2 ml fluid aspirate). An undiluted vitreous sample may be obtained in the office using a sharp-tip 23- or 25-gauge vitrectomy probe (0.5 ml aspirate; fig. 5) or in the operating room using a 20-, 23-, or 25-gauge vitrectomy probe (1.0 ml aspirate). To provide an undiluted sample in the operating room without causing globe collapse, one may infuse air while excising the vitreous. In one study, the vitreous cassette

fluid was positive in 76% of cases, and the vitreous biopsy was positive in 43% of cases [19]. If the view of the fundus is limited, one should consider obtaining preoperative echography to rule out the presence of choroidal detachment, IOFB, and/or retinal detachment and to determine whether a posterior vitreous detachment is present (facilitates safe posterior vitreous cortex removal). If choroidal detachment or media opacity precludes safe placement of an infusion cannula (even 6 mm) through the pars plana, then use an infusing light pipe or begin by infusing into the anterior chamber with a 23-gauge needle while excising vitreous debris with the vitrectomy probe. Rarely, the crystalline lens or IOL must be removed to improve visualization or to remove all micro-organisms completely (3-port approach). Generally, only a core vitrectomy is done (until retina or a bright red reflex is visible) initially. One can return to the operating room in approximately 1–2 weeks when the eye is less inflamed to perform a more meticulous vitrectomy, which may reduce the chance for infection-associated retinal detachment. If a seton is present and definitely infected, it may be necessary to remove it. If the seton is not definitely infected, one may attempt to salvage it by treating the patient with appropriate intraocular and systemic antibiotics and applying a scleral patch graft over the exposed hardware approximately one week later.

Processing the Biopsy Specimen

Intraocular fluids are incubated at 37°C and inoculated on sheep blood agar, US CDC and prevention anaerobic blood agar, chocolate agar, thioglycolate broth, and sabouraud dextrose agar (with gentamicin, without cyclohexamide at 25°C). A much simpler approach is to inoculate aerobic and anaerobic blood culture bottles instead of solid media. One should culture chronic endophthalmitis specimens for 2–3 weeks due to the slower growth of anaerobes and fungi. Routine staining (Gram, Giemsa, KOH) can aid in identification of organisms before culture data are available. Light and transmission electron microscopy can be quite helpful in identifying *P. acnes*, which is fastidious. The smear can also assist one in identifying non-infectious causes of inflammation (e.g. zonal granulomatous inflammation with phacoanaphylactic endophthalmitis; lens-laden macrophages in phacolytic glaucoma). One should interpret smears cautiously. Only ~2/3 smears in culture-positive cases are consistent with the organisms cultured. Both *Aspergillus fumigatus* and *Pseudallescheria boydii* display thin septate hyphae and dichotomous branching, yet these fungi have different antifungal sensitivities (*P. boydii*: miconazole; *A. fumigatus*: ketaconazole, amphotericin B).

Treatment

Acute Postoperative Endophthalmitis
Typically, patients are treated with intravitreal and topical antibiotics and, in selected cases, systemic antibiotics (table 12). The mainstay of treatment is intravitreal antibiotic injection. One reason to avoid using aminoglycosides is the risk of macular infarction (at doses of 400 µg). Ceftazidime, which is more effective against Gram-negative organisms than aminoglycosides and has a better safety profile, is physically incompatible with vancomycin and must be injected in a separate syringe. If the organism is vancomycin resistant (e.g. enterococci), one might use ampicillin + an aminoglycoside + systemic ciprofloxacin. If no improvement or stabilization is apparent within 48–72 h after initial treatment, one should consider pars plana vitrectomy (if not yet done) or repeat vitreous biopsy for culture and smear as well as repeat injection of intravitreal antibiotics. Generally, subconjunctival antibiotics are not used due to relatively poor penetration of the vitreous cavity. If there will be a delay between presentation and availability of intravitreal antibiotics, then one might inject subconjunctival antibiotics as a temporizing measure. Most topical and subconjunctival antibiotics have poor vitreous penetration (even in aphakic eyes).

The EVS explored the use of systemic ceftazidime/ciprofloxacin and amikacin for acute postoperative endophthalmitis. Most EVS isolates, however, were Gram-positive, and this particular combination of antibiotics is not particularly effective against *S. epidermidis*. In contrast, intravenous vancomycin and ceftazidime have significant intravitreal penetration in inflamed eyes and are effective against the majority of organisms cultured in EVS cases. In view of the limitations of the EVS study design, one should base the decision to use systemic antibiotics on the clinical findings and one's estimate of the ability of the host to fight the infection. Systemic and intravitreal corticosteroid use improves outcomes in preclinical models of endophthalmitis and in some clinical studies, but the finding is not consistent [20]. Relative contraindications to systemic steroid use must be borne in mind (e.g. history of diabetes mellitus, systemic fungal infection, tuberculosis).

The EVS, which enrolled patients presenting with endophthalmitis within 6 weeks of cataract or secondary IOL surgery, found that if the

Table 12. Treatment of endophthalmitis

Route of administration	Drug	Dose
Intravitreal	ceftazidime	2.25 mg/0.1 ml
	vancomycin	1.0 mg/0.1 ml
	dexamethasone[3]	400 µg/0.1 ml
Subconjunctival	vancomycin	25 mg/0.5 ml
	ceftazidime	100 mg/0.5 ml
	dexamethasone[3]	6 mg/0.5 ml
Topical	vancomycin	50 mg/1.0 ml
	ceftazidime	100 mg/1.0 ml
	prednisolone acetate 1%[3]	10 mg/1.0 ml
Systemic[1]	vancomycin[2]	1 g i.v. every 12 h
	ceftazidime[2]	1 g i.v. every 8 h
	prednisone[3]	1 mg/kg every morning (5–10 days)

[1] Used only at the discretion of the treating physician (usually in the treatment of late-onset endophthalmitis associated with conjunctival filtering blebs and in posttraumatic endophthalmitis).
[2] Modify dose for abnormal renal function. Do not use ceftazidime in penicillin-allergic patients.
[3] Do not use if in the judgment of the treating physician, corticosteroids are contraindicated (e.g. systemic prednisone in a patient with diabetes mellitus; fungal infection; tuberculosis without isoniazid prophylaxis).

presenting visual acuity was hand motions or better, then vitreous biopsy and intravitreal antibiotic injection was the best treatment approach. If the initial vision was light perception, then immediate pars plana vitrectomy and intravitreal antibiotic injection was best [21]. In the EVS, almost 1/3 of patients required an additional procedure after the initial one. Patients treated with immediate vitrectomy were three times more likely to achieve visual acuity of 20/40 or better (33 vs. 11%), twice as likely to achieve 20/100 or better (56 vs. 30%), and were less likely to incur visual acuity of 5/200 or worse (20 vs. 47%).

Not all patients fit the EVS enrollment criteria (e.g. posttraumatic endophthalmitis patients). In these cases, the following guidelines may be helpful. If vitreous inflammation is severe enough to preclude view of optic nerve and major retinal vessels on indirect ophthalmoscopy, or if progressive inflammation develops despite initial antibiotic therapy, or if the case has not improved despite initial therapy, then one should proceed with pars plana vitrectomy and intravitreal antibiotic injection.

Chronic Postoperative Endophthalmitis
In patients with chronic postoperative endophthalmitis, if the inflammation is not severe, one can delay antibiotic therapy until smear, culture, and sensitivity data are available from biopsy specimens. If inflammation is severe, one should follow the protocol for acute postoperative endophthalmitis (i.e. prompt intravitreal antibiotics, topical/systemic/subconjunctival antibiotics, ±corticosteroids, and vitrectomy as judged necessary). In cases of *P. acnes* or fungal endophthalmitis, one should remove all areas of involved lens capsule and cortex (dilate the pupil widely with flexible iris retractors), and inject antibiotic within the capsular bag. Remove

the IOL and capsular bag if there is no response to previous limited capsulectomy (removal of remaining sequestrum). Treatment of *P. acnes* or fungal endophthalmitis with antibiotic injection alone is likely to fail without vitrectomy if there is significant vitreous involvement. Intravitreal vancomycin (1 mg/0.1 ml) is an effective choice for *P. acnes* cases. For fungal endophthalmitis, voriconazole (100 µg/0.1 ml intravitreal and 200 mg p.o. b.i.d. or 200–400 mg i.v. b.i.d.) is an effective choice against *Aspergillus*, *Fusarium*, and *Candida* species. In one study, it was more effective than amphotericin B (5–10 µg/0.1 ml intravitreal and 0.4–0.6 mg/kg i.v. daily) [22]. Fluconazole (200 mg p.o. b.i.d.) has good intravitreal penetration, but is probably not as effective as amphotericin B in severe cases. *P. boydii* is often resistant to amphotericin B but is sensitive to intravitreal miconazole (25 µg/0.1 ml) or fluconazole (25 µg/0.1 ml).

Conjunctival Filtering Bleb-Associated Endophthalmitis

Patients with blebitis are treated with frequent topical antibiotics. Many surgeons also add oral antibiotics (e.g. ciprofloxacin) and, occasionally, subconjunctival antibiotics. One examines the patient daily to determine whether there is evidence of intraocular inflammation and the need for intravitreal antibiotics and possibly vitrectomy. In cases of frank endophthalmitis, one should proceed immediately to vitrectomy and intravitreal antibiotic injection (e.g. vancomycin and ceftazidime) due to the presumed virulence of the causative organisms. For the same reason, some surgeons routinely supplement treatment with systemic vancomycin and ceftazidime treatment. During vitrectomy, one avoids instrumenting the filtering bleb, which not infrequently can be salvaged.

Endogenous Endophthalmitis

If vitritis is severe enough to obscure a view of optic nerve/macula, management is similar to acute postoperative endophthalmitis with light perception vision. Also, biopsy is indicated if non-ocular cultures are negative or if no improvement is observed after reasonable period of observation while treating the patient with antibiotics. Syphilitic endophthalmitis is an important exception to the rule that severe vitreous inflammation mandates pars plana vitrectomy. Parenteral penicillin alone is highly effective. (One should anticipate the Jaresch-Herxheimer reaction and treat it with aspirin.) If vitreous involvement is minimal and culture/smear shows fungus, one may consider a trial of oral fluconazole or voriconazole without vitrectomy or intravitreal antibiotics due to the fact that the primary site of infection in endogenous endophthalmitis is usually the choroid, and these agents penetrate the vitreous cavity well. Occasionally, patients with endogenous fungal endophthalmitis (e.g. associated with intravenous drug abuse) have no evidence of systemic disease. In such cases, vitrectomy and intravitreal voriconazole or amphotericin B alone may cure the infection.

One should biopsy the area that is primary site of infection, which may not be the vitreous cavity. If available, use non-ocular culture and sensitivity data to guide the choice of antibiotics. In the absence of these data, empiric therapy (intravitreal and systemic vancomycin, ceftazidime) is begun after vitreous/anterior chamber biopsies are obtained.

Posttraumatic Endophthalmitis

As a rule, one should excise all IOFBs. Although intraocular cilia can cause infection, they may be observed if discovered after primary repair and if the eye is quiet. If cultures of excised material are positive for a virulent organism, if there is hypopyon, or if the inflammatory signs and/or pain are in excess of what is expected based on the injury and/or extent of surgery, then one should treat the patient aggressively for infectious endophthalmitis. One should consider early vitrectomy + intravitreal antibiotics strongly in high-risk cases (e.g.

soil contamination, 'dirty' IOFB) regardless of the inflammation severity on initial exam.

Conclusion

Effective treatment of infectious endophthalmitis depends on early recognition of infection, proper biopsy and culture of material, and proper selection of antibiotics. When, what, and how to biopsy and treat endophthalmitis depends on the clinical setting and findings. The prognosis depends heavily on the culture result (better prognosis if culture negative), the time of onset [better prognosis if late onset (unless associated with trabeculectomy)], and the virulence of the pathogen (worst outcomes typically are associated with *Streptococcus* species, Gram-negative species, and *Bacillus* species).

Sterile Uveitis

One can treat phacoanaphylactic endophthalmitis by removing the lens material with surgery and administering corticosteroids. Sympathetic ophthalmia is treated with topical, periocular, systemic, and even intravitreal steroids. Steroid-sparing agents (e.g. cyclosporine, azathioprine) are important adjunctive therapy and permit one to avoid the complications of chronic steroid use. To treat phacolytic glaucoma, one controls the IOP (antiglaucoma medications) and inflammation (corticosteroids) and removes retained lens material (e.g. with vitrectomy).

References

1 Kresloff MS, Castellarin AA, Zarbin MA: Endophthalmitis. Surv Ophthalmol 1998;43:193–224.
2 Aaberg TM Jr, Flynn HW Jr, Schiffman J, Newton J: Nosocomial acute-onset postoperative endophthalmitis survey. A 10-year review of incidence and outcomes. Ophthalmology 1998;105:1004–1010.
3 Olson JC, Flynn HW Jr, Forster RK, Culberson WW: Results in the treatment of postoperative endophthalmitis. Ophthalmology 1983;90:692–699.
4 Han DP, Wisniewski SR, Wilson LA, Barza M, Vine AK, Doft BH, Kelsey SF, et al: Spectrum and susceptibilities of microbiologic isolates in the endophthalmitis vitrectomy study. Am J Ophthalmol 1996;122: 1–17.
5 Johnson MW, Doft BH, Kelsey SF, Barza M, Wilson LA, Barr CC, Wisniewski SR, Endophhalmiis Vitrectomy Study Group: The endophthalmitis vitrectomy study. Relationship between clinical presentation and microbiologic spectrum. Ophthalmology 1997;104:261–272.
6 Group EVS: Microbiologic factors and visual outcome in the endophthalmitis vitrectomy study. Am J Ophthalmol 1996;122:830–846.

7 Speaker MG, Milch FA, Shah MK, Eisner W, Kreiswirth BN: Role of external bacterial flora in the pathogenesis of acute postoperative endophthalmitis. Ophthalmology 1991;98:639–649, discussion 650.
8 Menikoff JA, Speaker MG, Marmor M, Raskin EM: A case-control study of risk factors for postoperative endophthalmitis. Ophthalmology 1991;98:1761–1768.
9 Taban M, Behrens A, Newcomb RL, et al: Acute endophthalmitis following cataract surgery: a systematic review of the literature. Arch Ophthalmol 2005;123: 613–620.
10 Herretes S, Stark WJ, Pirouzmanesh A, Reyes JM, McDonnell PJ, Behrens A: Inflow of ocular surface fluid into the anterior chamber after phacoemulsification through sutureless corneal cataract wounds. Am J Ophthalmol 2005;140: 737–740.
11 Prophylaxis of postoperative endophthalmitis following cataract surgery: results of the ESCRS multicenter study and identification of risk factors. J Cataract Refract Surg 2007;33:978–988.
12 Mandelbaum S, Forster RK, Gelender H, Culbertson W: Late onset endophthalmitis associated with filtering blebs. Ophthalmology 1985;92:964–972.

13 Leng T, Miller D, Flynn HW Jr, Jacobs DJ, Gedde SJ: Delayed-onset bleb-associated endophthalmitis (1996–2008): causative organisms and visual acuity outcomes. Retina 2011;31:344–352.
14 Arroyo JG, Nguyen LT, Zarbin MA: Endogenous endophthalmitis initially misdiagnosed as anterior uveitis. Ann Ophthalmol 2000;32:199–200.
15 Bhagat N, Nagori S, Zarbin M: Post-traumatic infectious endophthalmitis. Surv Ophthalmol 2011;56:214–251.
16 Mamalis N, Edelhauser HF, Dawson DG, Chew J, LeBoyer RM, Werner L: Toxic anterior segment syndrome. J Cataract Refract Surg 2006;32:324–333.
17 Soheilian M, Ramezani A, Azimzadeh A, et al: Randomized trial of intravitreal clindamycin and dexamethasone versus pyrimethamine, sulfadiazine, and prednisolone in treatment of ocular toxoplasmosis. Ophthalmology 2011;118:134–141.
18 Mieller WF, Ellis MK, Williams DF, Han DP: Retained intraocular foreign bodies and endophthalmitis. Ophthalmology 1990;97:1532–1538.
19 Donahue SP, Kowalski RP, Jewart BH, Friberg TR: Vitreous cultures in suspected endophthalmitis. Biopsy or vitrectomy? Ophthalmology 1993;100:452–455.

20 Albrecht E, Richards JC, Pollock T, Cook
C, Myers L: Adjunctive use of intravitreal dexamethasone in presumed bacterial endophthalmitis: a randomised trial.
Br J Ophthalmol 2011;95:1385–1388.

21 Results of the Endophthalmitis Vitrectomy Study. A randomized trial of
immediate vitrectomy and of intravenous antibiotics for the treatment of
postoperative bacterial endophthalmitis.
Endophthalmitis Vitrectomy Study
Group. Arch Ophthalmol 1995;113:
1479–1496.

22 Marangon FB, Miller D, Giaconi JA,
Alfonso EC: In vitro investigation of
voriconazole susceptibility for keratitis
and endophthalmitis fungal pathogens.
Am J Ophthalmol 2004;137:820–825.

Marco A. Zarbin, MD, PhD
Institute of Ophthalmology and Visual Science-New Jersey Medical School
Room 6156, Doctors Office Center
90 Bergen Street
Newark, NJ 07103 (USA)
Tel. +1 973 972 2038, E-Mail zarbin@earthlink.net

Subject Index